ROYAL SOCIETY *of* MEDICINE

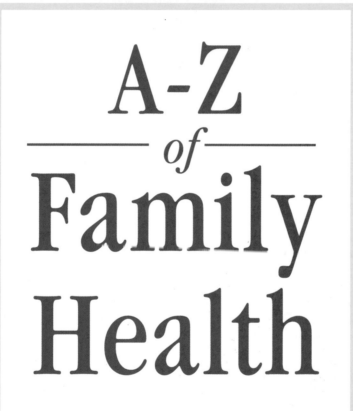

A-Z
of
Family
Health

DR PAUL GIANGRANDE

BSc, MD, MRCP, MRCPath

CONSULTANT HAEMATOLOGIST, CHURCHILL HOSPITAL, OXFORD

HAMLYN

This edition published in 1991 by
The Hamlyn Publishing Group Limited,
part of Reed International Books,
Michelin House, 81 Fulham Road,
London SW3 6RB

ISBN 0 600 57138 6

Conceived and produced by Breslich & Foss,
Golden House, 28—31 Great Pulteney Street
London W1R 3DD

A catalogue record for this book
is available from the British Library

Designer: Ted Kinsey
Design assistant: Sarah Crouch

Illustrators: Stan Johnson, Susan Kinsey,
Sally Launder, Simon Roulstone and
John Woodcock

Project editor: Tessa Rose

Typeset by Setrite, Hong Kong
Film originated by Mandarin Offset in Hong Kong

PREFACE

Our understanding of disease is increasing at such a rapid rate that even practising physicians find it difficult to keep up to date with the latest thinking in specialist areas within medicine. The Editorial Board of the Royal Society of Medicine perceived a need for a book that would enable the general reader to draw on the experience and expertise of the medical specialists to whom patients are often referred. The result is the *RSM A−Z of Family Health*, which contains nearly 1000 entries on individual subjects, each written by an expert within that area.

In choosing the subjects for discussion, we had three principal aims. Firstly, we sought to provide specific information on a wide range of disorders, as well as the related therapy. However, we must emphasise that we would in no way wish to dissuade people from seeking medical advice and help from their family doctor. Secondly, we wished to promote a healthy lifestyle and encourage people in the belief that many diseases are preventable. We have, therefore, included entries on such subjects as smoking and obesity. And thirdly, we sought to provide an invaluable source of background knowledge to specific medical matters that are increasingly discussed in the media, such as AIDS, salmonella and haemophilia.

As we all continue to become more aware of the need for knowledge in order to achieve and maintain good health, I hope that this book will help to bridge the gap between the public and the sometimes obscure and technical world of modern-day medicine.

Dr Paul Giangrande, Oxford 1991

CONTRIBUTORS

Dr J. Ashworth, MD, MRCP
Dr S. Barter, FRCR, MRCP
Major J. D. C. Bennett, BSc, DCH, FRCS
Mr R. Bird, FRCS
Mr A. L. Blower, FRCS
Dr A. K. Burroughs, MRCP
Dr P. L. Callaway, MRCP
Dr A. Forbes, BSc, MD, MRCP
Dr I. P. Hicks, FRCR, MRCP
Dr R. Joshi, MRCPath
Dr G. H. Lear, MRCP
Dr C. A. Lee, MA, MD, FRCP, MRCPath
Dr D. M. Luesley, MD, MRCOG
Dr E. Maher, BSc, MD, MRCP
Dr G. Patton, MD, MRCPsych
Dr R. Pounder, MA, MD, FRCP
Dr C. W. E. Redman, MD, FRCS, MRCOG
Dr T. Roberts, BSc, PhD, MRCP
Dr I. Rowe, MD, MRCP

ABDOMEN

The enclosed space below the chest (thoracic cavity) and above the pelvis. A powerful fan-shaped muscle called the diaphragm forms the roof of the abdomen and separates the organs housed there (pancreas, gall-bladder, liver and kidneys) from the heart and lungs. The front and sides of the abdominal wall are covered by several layers of flexible muscle, which move with respiration and can be safely distended during pregnancy. At the back of the abdomen lies the vertebral column with its large and powerful supporting muscles on either side.

There are several weak spots in the abdomen where the lower abdominal muscles meet the upper muscles of the leg in the groin. Here loops of intestine may force their way through the muscles to lie under the skin and form local bulges or hernias, which enlarge as pressure increases within the abdomen; in coughing, for instance.

The digestive tract or alimentary canal enters the abdomen as the oesophagus (gullet) via a small hole in the diaphragm. The stomach is an expansion of this digestive tube, which receives secretions from various organs, such as the pancreas and gall-bladder, in order to begin the digestion process. The tract continues as the small intestine, where digestion is completed, and the large intestine.

ABORTION

A termination of pregnancy, with expulsion of a fetus from its mother before it achieves viability (ability to live outside its mother's body or to draw breath alone). The definition of viability and the time at which it is reached varies from country to country. In the United Kingdom viability is defined in law as being

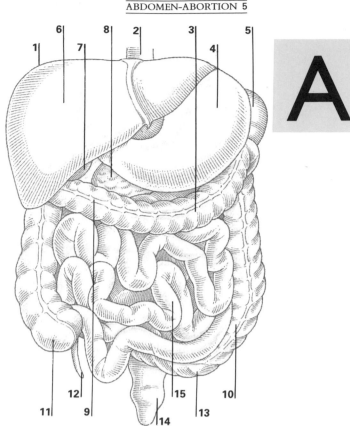

The abdominal organs: **1** diaphragm; **2** oesophagus; **3** transverse colon; **4** stomach; **5** spleen; **6** liver; **7** gall-bladder; **8** pancreas; **9** duodenum; **10** large intestine; **11** caecum; **12** appendix; **13** sigmoid colon; **14** rectum; **15** small intestine.

reached at 24 weeks' gestation. Termination of a pregnancy after this time is illegal. In other EC countries the average upper limit at which a fetus may be expelled legally is 12—14 weeks. The World Health Organization recommends that a fetus weighing 500 g (18 oz) or less be considered as an abortion; this definition would generally correspond to a gestational age of between 20 and 22 weeks.

Abortion can either be spontaneous, often called a miscarriage, or can be induced artificially. There are various stages of spontaneous abortion. A threatened abortion is characterized by bleeding from the vagina and usually occurs in the first 12 to 13 weeks of pregnancy. Often the bleeding will stop by itself without treatment other than rest. In an inevitable abortion the bleeding is heavier, and crampy, period-like pains in the lower abdomen indicate that the cervix is opening. If the ensuing abortion is complete the entire contents of the uterus (womb) are expelled. Often, however, it is incomplete and parts of the placenta (afterbirth) remain inside the uterus. This debris is cleared from the uterus by means of a curette (see *D & C* in order to prevent infection and vaginal bleeding. The patient is given a short anaesthetic while this is accomplished. Most spontaneous abortions are the result of severe abnormalities in the very small fetus. It is estimated that miscarriage may occur in up to 45 per cent of all pregnancies.

An induced abortion can be performed legally, when it is known as a therapeutic termination of pregnancy, or illegally, when it is known as a criminal abortion. The law defining the grounds on which an abortion can be performed legally differs from country to country. In pregnancies of less than 12 weeks the uterus is usually emptied surgically via the cervix by scraping the lining with a curette during a short anaesthetic. At a later stage of pregnancy this becomes difficult and unsafe, so drugs such as prostaglandins are used. These are either injected into the uterus or placed in the vagina.

A more liberal attitude to abortion in many countries has decreased the need for criminal backstreet abortions and as a result there has been a parallel decline in the illness and number of deaths caused by infection.

ABSCESS

A collection of pus formed after infection with bacteria. The microorganisms usually responsible are staphylococci, although a considerable number of other bacteria may be implicated. An abscess may result from direct infection of a wound, local spread from an adjacent site of infection or, less commonly, spread through the bloodstream from a distant site. It is formed from dead white cells called neutrophils which flood the area of the wound in order to digest the invading bacteria and die after successfully destroying them. The abscess enlarges as the dead neutrophils accumulate.

Abscesses can occur in all organs and tissues, including the brain and lungs. The skin is frequently affected, particularly in the areas of the armpits and genitals. The area affected by an acute abscess is very tender and throbs as a result of swelling and inflammation. In some cases whole body systems are disturbed and there are also symptoms of malaise (a general feeling of being unwell) and fever. Occasionally the enlarging abscess will press on neighbouring structures. As the infection progresses, a wall of fibrous scar tissue forms round the abscess, which may then become chronic. This is a natural defence mechanism, but it may prevent penetration by antibiotics; surgical drainage of the abscess may then be necessary. More commonly the abscess will burst, relieving the pain and triggering the healing process. In most cases, early treatment with antibiotics will halt the development of the abscess. Surgical drainage is necessary if the abscess is internal and pus plentiful.

ACHALASIA

A disease of unknown origin which affects the sphincter or valve at the end of the oesophagus (gullet) and the muscles that line the oesophageal wall. Food is moved along the oesophagus by means of a continuous series of muscle contractions called peristalsis. In achalasia a combination of abnormally strong muscle contractions and a defect in the relaxation mechanism of the muscles causes an obstruction during eating as food is retained in the oesophagus instead of being passed along it to the stomach.

Two common symptoms of achalasia are pain in the middle of the chest and regurgitation of undigested food. The most efficient method of diagnosis is a barium meal — gastroscopy (see *Endoscopy*) can miss it. Treatment is usually by stretching the valve with a special balloon or by cutting the overactive muscles.

ACHONDROPLASIA

An inherited condition which causes skeletal disproportion. In one-third of cases achondroplasia arises without a family history. Symptoms appear at birth or in the first year of life as insufficient cartilage or replacing bone is laid down at the ends of the limb bones. As a result of this deficiency the legs and arms are short in relation to the trunk, which is relatively normal, and very broad. Other physical characteristics are fingers of all the same length, an enlarged top half of the skull and a flattened nasal bridge. Curvature of the spine (scoliosis) may also be a feature. Achondroplastics are of normal intelligence. In later life the skeletal disproportion may cause premature osteoarthritis and childbirth complications. There is no treatment for this condition.

ACIDOSIS

Increased acidity of the blood or lowered blood pH. (pH is the measurement used to gauge the alkalinity or acidity of a fluid on a scale of 0 to 14: pH7 is neutral (water), less than 7 acid, and more than 7 alkaline.)

Acidosis occurs as a consequence of an underlying medical condition and may be respiratory or metabolic in origin. Pneumonia, pneumothorax (a respiratory disorder of the newborn) and chronic bronchitis are conditions in which respiratory acidosis commonly arises. Other causes include respiratory depression through drugs, increased pressure within the skull and conditions limiting chest (thoracic) movement. Metabolic causes of acidosis include diabetic ketoacidosis, severe diarrhoea, kidney failure and aspirin (salicylate) poisoning. In both types of acidosis the body will try to correct the abnormality by adjusting its levels of carbon dioxide and bicarbonate in relation to each other. Symptoms, signs and treatment are all dictated by the underlying cause.

ACNE

There are two types of acne: acne vulgaris and acne rosacea. The first type is caused by blockage and inflammation of the fine hair follicles and the natural oil-producing glands (sebaceous) of the face, chest and back. It varies in appearance from mild greasiness of the skin together with some blackheads to severely inflamed cysts in rare cases. Acne vulgaris is commonly seen in adolescence and occasionally during other periods of hormonal turbulence (for example, when starting or stopping the contraceptive pill or during steroid therapy) and almost always improves spontaneously during the late teens or early twenties. It usually responds to a lengthy course of treatment with antibiotics over many weeks. Inappropriate use of corticosteroid (qv) therapy applied to the skin can severely exacerbate the condition. Very severe cases of acne vulgaris can benefit from a Vitamin A derivative that has recently become available. However, this treatment must be supervised by a specialist because of the risk of side-effects.

The cause of acne rosacea is unknown. Typically this type of acne occurs in middle age and presents as redness and inflammation of the facial skin. Like acne vulgaris it responds to treatment with antibiotics. It is made worse by the consumption of alcohol and hot or spicy food.

ACROMEGALY

A condition caused by the over-secretion of growth hormone by a benign tumour (adenoma) of the pituitary gland at the base of the brain. It occurs after normal growth has ceased (compare gigantism). There are both local effects, due to pressure from the tumour, and distant effects, due to the hormone. Among the local effects are headaches and blindness in the outer halves of each visual field (bitemporal hemianopia). Distant effects produce a slow increase in size of the soft tissues and bones; enlargement of the skull, forehead and jaw may cause dental problems. Other skeletal changes include curvature of the spine (scoliosis) and expansion of the hands and feet. The tongue enlarges, as do the internal organs. Paraesthesiae (abnormal sensations) of the hands may occur due to the median nerve being trapped at the wrist, beneath the carpal ligament. Associated disorders include high blood pressure (hypertension) and diabetes mellitus. Other hormones produced by the pituitary (such as ACTH) may also be secreted in excess, producing symptoms of Cushing's syndrome (qv).

Treatment is aimed at reducing the levels of growth hormone by eliminating the pituitary gland by surgery or irradiation. Replacement therapy with some other pituitary hormones, such as cortisone, may then be necessary.

ACTH (ADRENOCORTICO-TROPHIC HORMONE)

A hormone which stimulates the secretion of corticosteroid hormones from the adrenal glands. The production of ACTH is closely regulated by the levels of corticosteroid (qv) in the bloodstream. If these are high, ACTH production is inhibited; if low, the pituitary gland at the base of the brain releases ACTH. ACTH is also produced in response to stress, injury and low levels of glucose in the blood (hypoglycaemia). Benign tumours (adenomas) of the pituitary can release excess ACTH, as can malignant tumours of other organs (such as the lung) on rare occasions. ACTH deficiency arises if the pituitary is destroyed for any reason (hypopituitarism). Over- or under-secretion of ACTH produces Cushing's syndrome (qv) and Addison's disease (qv) respectively.

ACTINOMYCOSIS

A rare infection caused by a bacterium (*Actinomyces israelii*) normally found in the mouth. It produces swellings around the jaw. The infection progresses slowly, but if left untreated it eventually discharges a thick, mucoid pus which has minute yellow flecks in it (known as 'sulphur granules'). The infection can also spread to involve the brain, lungs or the gut, particularly if the patient's immunity is lowered. Treatment is with a prolonged course of penicillin.

ACUTE (ILLNESS)

Medical term for an illness that starts suddenly, or becomes rapidly worse over a 48-hour period. The acute period ends as suddenly as it begins, in either restoration of health, chronic illness, or death. Typically acute illnesses are caused by an infection or thrombosis (blood clot). Some are self-limiting and get better on their own (a common cold, for example). Others require rapid medical attention to prevent disability or death. If the illness lasts longer than 48 hours it is sub-acute, and after six weeks it is known as chronic.

ADDISON'S DISEASE

Chronic failure of the adrenal glands to produce hormones in response to the body's requirements, especially cortisol (hydrocortisone), aldosterone and androgens (sex hormones). In the majority of cases the condition is caused by shrinkage of the glands as a result of autoimmune disease. For reasons that are as yet unknown, the body produces antibodies against its own adrenal cortical cells. Other causes are tuberculosis, metastatic cancer and removal of the glands (adrenalectomy, qv).

Symptoms consist of increasing tiredness, weakness, weight loss, loss of pigmentation, and abdominal discomfort and diarrhoea. Pubic and armpit hair may also be lost. Blood pressure is low. The diagnosis is usually made by giving the patient the pituitary hormone corticotropin (ACTH, qv), which controls the adrenal glands, and showing that the normal response (increased production of cortisol) is absent. Treatment consists of taking oral cortisol twice daily. The dose is increased during times of infection, stress or injury, situations in which the normally functioning adrenals would automatically increase cortisol production. Patients who are also shown to be deficient in aldosterone are given the steroid fludrocortisone as a replacement. SEE ALSO *illustration on page 144*

ADENOIDS

A fleshy mass of lymphoid tissue found in the enclosed space behind the nose and above the palate (post-nasal space). Lymphoid tissue is important

Adenoids **(1)** achieve their maximum size in children aged between 3 and 5 years. They slowly shrink thereafter and usually disappear altogether by puberty.

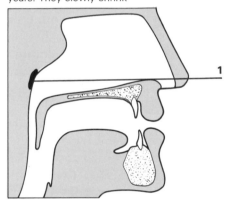

for the production of antibodies, which are essential for immunity. Adenoids enlarge in response to unfamiliar viruses and strains of bacteria.

When enlarged, the adenoids may obstruct nasal breathing, causing the child to breathe through the mouth and to snore. Catarrh accumulates in the nose. As the Eustachian tube (the passageway from the post-nasal space to the ear) becomes blocked, air pressures cannot be equalized, leading to temporary deafness.

ADENOMA

A benign tumour derived from glandular tissue. Adenomas are most commonly found in the intestine, endocrine glands and in the milk ducts of the breasts. Some adenomas secrete hormones and an accumulation of secretions within the tumour may cause cysts to form.

They are usually removed surgically.

ADHESIONS

Fibrous bands of internal scar tissue. The body responds to internal injury, infection or inflammation by exuding from its surfaces fluid containing white cells and chemicals, which limit the damage and begin the repair process. These cells thinly coat the bowel, Fallopian tubes, and other viscera within the abdomen and also line the walls of the abdominal cavity itself. In effect they form a continuous membranous skin which attaches the viscera to the back of the abdominal cavity. In conditions such as peritonitis and salpingitis, this coating (called peritoneum) becomes inflamed, with the result that the surfaces of the affected viscera adhere to each other and adhesions are formed as the repair process tries to combat the inflammation. In many cases adhesions are of no consequence, but sometimes they can cause a blockage in the intestine or in the Fallopian tubes.

Treatment is by surgical division, but sometimes the adhesions reform

Adhesions form when fluids released by the body to combat inflammation of the peritoneum cause the affected viscera to stick together.

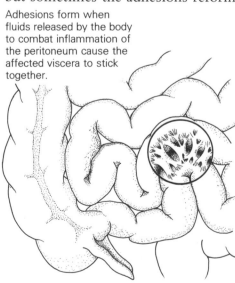

ADRENALECTOMY

Surgical removal of one or both adrenal (suprarenal) glands. Each of these lies above and close to one of the kidneys. The adrenals are responsible for producing a number of hormones, including adrenaline, corticosteroids (such as cortisone), mineralocorticoids (such as aldosterone) and sex hormones (such as androgens). Adrenalectomy of one or both glands is performed in cases of over-secretion of one or more of these hormones being caused by a tumour; for example, in Conn's syndrome, Cushing's syndrome or phaeochromocytoma.

Bilateral adrenalectomy (removal of both adrenal glands) was formerly used to treat metastatic cancer of the breast or prostate with the hope of reducing pain in the affected bones, but this has now been largely superseded by hormone-manipulating drugs and radiotherapy.
SEE ALSO *illustration on page 144*

ADRENOCORTICO-TROPHIC HORMONE

see *ACTH*

ADVERSE REACTION

An unwanted or unexpected effect caused by any substance, usually a drug, that comes into contact with the body; a side-effect. All drugs sanctioned for use in humans may have possible adverse effects; these are indicated in prescribing information, as are indications of potential effectiveness.

Most countries have central organizations responsible for monitoring adverse reactions, especially to newer drugs. Adverse reactions may be prevented by a combination of measures, including using certain drugs only when there are good reasons for doing so, only using drugs that are familiar, ensuring that correct doses are given and taken, knowledge of a patient's previous reactions to similar drugs, avoidance of additional drugs that may increase the risk of adverse reaction and taking into account pre-existing conditions (such as pregnancy, kidney or liver impairment, or age).

AFFECTIVE DISORDER

A disorder in which disturbance of mood (affect) is the central feature. An affective disorder is said to be present in a person whose moods persist or are so intense that they cause him or her or others to suffer. Changes in activity and in patterns of concentration, eating and sleeping will often accompany the disturbance.

The course of affective disorders is variable, some people having a single episode (which can last weeks, months, even years), others having many.

Treatment includes antidepressants, electroconvulsive therapy, tranquillizers, lithium and psychotherapy.

AFTERBIRTH

see *Placenta*

AGENESIS

Complete failure of an organ to develop between the sixth and eighth weeks of fetal life — the period of organogenesis, when the organs of the fetus are formed. The term also refers to failure of part of an organ to develop; for example, agenesis of the corpus callosum, the part of the brain which conveys information from one cerebral hemisphere to the other.

AGORAPHOBIA

The term 'agoraphobia' literally means fear of the market-place or open space. In practice agoraphobia often refers to a constellation of phobias arising from a fear of public scrutiny or falling ill away from home. Sufferers may also report a fear of enclosed spaces (claustrophobia), a fear of crowds or situations from which escape is difficult, such as the theatre or the hairdresser; or anxiety about vomiting, or fainting, or using public toilets. The great majority of sufferers are women. In severe agoraphobia a sufferer may not be able to leave home without being accompanied by a trusted person. Others may have their anxiety about being away from home alleviated by pushing a pram or shopping trolley. The symptoms of agoraphobia will sometimes be a sign of depression or another psychiatric disorder. Commonly used treatments are behaviour therapy, beta-blockers such as propranolol, and antidepressants.
SEE ALSO *Claustrophobia*

AGRANULOCYTOSIS

A reduced number of neutrophils (qv) (a type of white blood cell) in the blood-stream, resulting in severe infection. The condition can occur without evident cause but more often it arises as an abnormal response to a specific drug (see *Idiosyncracy*). The symptoms are fever and death of tissue (necrotic lesions) in the mouth and throat.

In some cases recovery is spontaneous once the drug is no longer taken, but usually treatment is required. This involves blood transfusion (often repeated) until the bone marrow recovers sufficiently to produce active neutrophils again. The process may take weeks or months. In rare cases the bone marrow does not recover and the condition is fatal.

AGRAPHIA

The inability to write due to brain damage caused by injury or disease such as stroke or tumour. It is usually seen in association with alexia (inability to comprehend written language) or acalculia (difficulty in counting) and right/left disorientation.

AIDS (Acquired Immune Deficiency Syndrome)

A disease resulting from infection with the retrovirus known as the Human Immunodeficiency Virus (HIV). The principal groups at risk in the Western world are homosexuals and intravenous drug users. It is clear, however, that the disease may be transmitted by heterosexual intercourse; in Africa, for example, this appears to be the principal mode of transmission. Cases have also been reported in haemophiliacs who have used batches of factor VIII (a protein essential for normal blood clotting) contaminated by the virus, and in recipients of blood transfusions. All donated blood is now tested for the presence of antibody to the virus. In addition, materials for haemophiliacs are now rendered completely free of the risk of infection by heat treatment.

Infection with the virus is established by detection of antibody to the virus in a person's blood: a person with a positive test is referred to as anti–HIV seropositive, or HIV positive in lay terms. This does not mean that he or she has AIDS, although some people will eventually develop it.

Most of the symptoms of AIDS result from an impaired immune system as the virus attacks helper lymphocytes (a type of white blood cell). Symptoms of progressive AIDS include mild fever, weight loss, diarrhoea and skin disorders. As a consequence of impaired immunity, patients are predisposed to a variety of infections, including certain unusual opportunistic ones which are rarely seen in the general population, such as pneumocystis carinii pneumonia, cryptococcal meningitis and tuberculosis. Oral and oesophageal candida (qv) (thrush) is common. Kaposi's sarcoma (qv) is a tumour that may arise in patients with AIDS.

There is no cure for the disease and a vaccine is not yet available. For these reasons much effort has been expended on public education directed at the prevention of transmission. The importance of using condoms, for example, has been stressed as these greatly reduce the risk of transmission by sexual intercourse.

The early diagnosis and prompt treatment of life-threatening opportunistic infections prolong the patient's life. The drug zidovudine has seen shown to increase the lymphocyte count in patients with AIDS, and to reduce the incidence of opportunistic infections. It may increase the patient's chances of survival but it is not a cure.

AKINESIA

An inability to initiate movement. This condition is seen in Parkinsonism (see *Parkinson's disease*) and other diseases in which the basal ganglia (groups or nuclei of nerve cells) in the centre of the brain are affected. Typically, the patient is unable to get out of a chair or to begin walking (the feet 'freeze' to the floor). If such movement is difficult, but not impossible, the term hypokinesia is used.

ALBINISM

An inherited disorder which affects the eyes or skin or both. It is caused by defects in the formation of the skin pigment melanin involving abnormalities in the production of the enzyme tyrosinase. The several varieties of albinism differ in their mode of inheritance, clinical features and underlying biochemical abnormality.

Oculocutaneous albinism is the major variety and affects both the eyes and skin. It is inherited in a recessive manner and is characterized by white hair, pink-white skin that does not tan, and blue or pink irises. Albinism which affects only the eyes (ocular albinism) is inherited in a sex-linked manner. The variety which affects only the skin (cutaneous albinism) is inherited in a dominant manner. In normal individuals melanin provides a natural screen against the sun's harmful rays. Its absence makes both the eyes and skin extraordinarily sensitive to sunlight. Albinos are therefore more prone to skin cancer. Eyesight is also impaired.

There is no treatment, but sun screens, tinted glasses and avoidance of sunlight are helpful measures.

ALCOHOLISM

Continued excessive consumption of alcohol. There is an important distinction between physical forms of alcoholism, in which disease is predominantly of the liver, and psychological forms in which damage is caused by the disruption of home and working life.

Once allowance is made for alcohol content, there is no difference in the risk from different drinks: a $\frac{1}{2}$-pint of beer, a modest glass of wine and a single measure of spirits all have about the same alcohol content, conveniently termed 1 unit. Consumption in excess of 21 units per week for a man, or 14 units for a woman, leads to an increased health risk. The long-term abuser of alcohol who is on the way to liver disease typically drinks heavily and consistently, often holds down a taxing job and does not get drunk; after several years, permanent liver damage occurs in the form of cirrhosis, leading in turn to complications that often prove fatal. Chronic pancreatitis may also develop. Blood tests can warn of impending irreversible liver damage.

The patient with psychological alcoholism is more likely to be a binge drinker with problems at work and at home, and may have convictions associated with drunkenness. Memory lapses and the deliberate alteration of lifestyle to facilitate drinking may be early pointers to cases of this form of alcoholism.

Patients with either form are at an increased risk of death from heart disease. They are also prone to permanent memory loss, psychosis and other neurological ailments, which are related in part to thiamine (vitamin B_1) deficiency.

In order to deal with the withdrawal symptoms that may accompany the cessation of drinking, a minor tranquillizer may be prescribed for 5–10 days. Disulfiram and calcium carbimide, both of which cause unpleasant reactions when alcohol is taken, may be useful in preventing relapse into drinking. For other alcoholics, a self-help organization, group psychotherapy or special inpatient treatment units may be beneficial.

ALKALOSIS

Decreased acidity of the blood or increased blood pH. (pH is the measurement of hydrogen ion concentration in fluid: a low pH is acid, pH7 is neutral (water), and a high pH is alkaline). Alkalosis may be respiratory or metabolic.

In respiratory alkalosis, carbon dioxide levels are reduced, and bicarbonate levels fall to compensate. It is caused by rapid, deep breathing in conditions such as pulmonary oedema (abnormal accumulation of fluid in the lungs), pneumonia, hyperventilation as a result of stress, and excessive artificial ventilation.

In metabolic alkalosis, bicarbonate increases, and carbon dioxide increases to compensate. It occurs when bicarbonate is taken in large amounts for 'indigestion', in potassium depletion and in prolonged vomiting.

Symptoms, signs and treatment depend on the underlying cause.

ALLERGEN

see *Antigen*

ALLERGY

An immune response in a sensitive individual to a normally harmless substance. The substance which causes the reaction is called the allergen. Symptoms are provoked by exposure to natural substances, which cause antibodies to be formed (antigens). The term allergy is usually restricted to atopic reactions (see *Atopy*) which often run in families. The antibody involved in most allergic reactions is immunoglobulin E (IgE). The cells synthesizing this antibody are found chiefly in the respiratory and gastro-intestinal tracts — that is, near the sites where antigens are commonly encountered. The antibody circulates throughout the body and is often found in increased levels in atopic individuals. On encountering its specific antigen (allergen), IgE liberates histamine and similar substances, which are responsible for some of the typical symptoms associated with allergy. Examples include nettle-rash (urticaria), bronchospasm in asthma and inflammation of the lining of the nose (rhinitis) in hay fever. These symptoms may be controlled by anti-histamines, bronchodilators and, if necessary, adrenaline.

Skin prick tests may be used in the diagnosis of allergic conditions, although a person's history will usually suggest the diagnosis. A drop of antigen, dissolved in glycerin, is placed on the skin and the superficial layer is lifted with a needle. Only a tiny amount of allergen is introduced into the skin and the risk of a violent reaction is very low. A positive reaction consists of redness and a weal at the test site which reaches its largest size after 15—20 minutes.
SEE ALSO *Desensitization*

ALLOGRAFT

An abbreviation of 'allogenic homograft', a graft (or transplant) made from a donor who is genetically dissimilar to the recipient. In clinical practice the term covers all grafts from any human donor who is not an identical twin of the recipient.

The donors are usually brain-dead victims of road accidents or cerebral haemorrhages.
SEE ALSO *Rejection*

ALOPECIA

Hair loss. Physiological hair loss, also referred to as male pattern baldness or androgenic (male-hormone dependent) alopecia, may occur to some extent as part of the normal ageing process and involves a gradual reduction in the ability of the hair follicle to produce hair in response to hormones. There is currently no method available for reversing the process. Androgenic baldness of early onset appears to be genetically determined and to be transmitted by unaffected females to some of their male off-spring, though the exact pattern of inheritance is not yet clear. Gradual thinning of the hair in women generally occurs much later in life than in men (usually well after the menopause).

Any serious medical illness can cause generalized hair loss. Occasionally, sudden and very extensive hair loss may occur after minor physical stress (such as pregnancy) before rapidly regrowing again; this is referred to as telogen effluvium.

Alopecia areata refers to inexplicable hair loss, usually affecting the scalp in a patchy fashion and sometimes involving other hairy sites. (The term alopecia totalis is used if all body hair is shed.) Small patches of hair may regrow spontaneously, though more extensive loss may be permanent. The cause of alopecia areata, which occurs most frequently in adolescents and young adults, is not known. Treatment is ineffective.

Scarring skin disorders that only affect the scalp or are part of a more generalized disease process can sometimes cause permanent baldness within the scars. Ringworm, for example, is a fungal infection of the skin which will mimic one of the above-mentioned forms of alopecia when it affects the scalp.

ALPHAFETO-PROTEIN (AFP)

A protein which is normally present in the tissues of a fetus. It can also be detected in adults in conditions such as pregnancy and certain forms of cancer. Its function is unknown but its measurement (either in blood or in the amniotic fluid which surrounds the baby in the womb) can be used to detect some fetal abnormalities or, in the case of adult tumours, to monitor the course of those tumours.

AFP can be detected in maternal blood during pregnancy and can be used as a screening test for certain malformations if measured between the sixteenth and eighteenth weeks of pregnancy. Approximately 1 in 20 mothers who have a raised level at this time will have an abnormal fetus. Abnormalities require confirmation either by ultrasound examination and/or by amniocentesis (qv).

The usual abnormalities causing such a raised level are neural tube defects (spina bifida and anencephaly). Other abnormalities may also cause a raised level: for example, of the kidney and the gastrointestinal tract.

AFP is raised in multiple pregnancies and in a minority of entirely normal pregnancies.

ALZHEIMER'S DISEASE

The commonest form of dementia, affecting around 5 per cent of people over the age of 65. The onset is slow and usually becomes apparent at around the age of 70. Early symptoms, such as difficulty with memory or accentuation of longstanding personality characteristics, are often put down to old age by relatives. The disease progresses inexorably, with the sufferer often coming to believe that he or she is living in some previous place or time. He or she may fail to recognize relatives and friends, or become lost after wandering away from home. Some patients develop delusions. In the late stages a sufferer becomes physically feeble, incontinent and unable to speak. Death usually follows around five years after the disorder first becomes apparent, though in younger patients the course of the illness may be quicker. The disease has become more common, in part due to the greater number of elderly in the general population. The cause is unknown, though there is evidence for a genetic predisposition in some cases. As yet there are no treatments effective in altering the course of the disorder.

AMBLYOPIA

Defective vision for which there is no physical cause. Amblyopia cannot be corrected by spectacles and is usually permanent.

Amblyopia can occur for a number of reasons. In young infants if a non-paralytic squint (so-called concomitant squint because it is constant in all directions of gaze) is left untreated there is progressive psychological suppression of the image from one eye as the child tries to overcome the double-vision (diplopia) produced by the squint. Eventually irreversible amblyopia may result as the affected eye falls into disuse ('lazy eye'). Amblyopia may also be caused by differences of refraction in the lenses of the eyes, even if a squint is not present. The condition may also occur in pipe tobacco smokers (possibly as a result of intoxication with cyanide in the tobacco smoke, but more probably due to associated B vitamin deficiency) and in methanol poisoning (from methylated spirits).

AMENORRHOEA

A temporary or permanent absence of menstrual or monthly periods. Amenorrhoea may be primary or secondary. Primary amenorrhoea is said to occur when periods fail to start at the normal age (12–16 years). In most cases puberty is simply delayed and periods will start naturally in their own good time. In a few, rare, cases of primary amenorrhea, the passage of menstrual blood may be blocked because of failure of the vagina to develop or abnormal development of the hymen (the membrane which partly covers the virginal vagina). In the latter type of case, surgical treatment will be needed.

Secondary amenorrhoea occurs in women who have previously menstruated; the term is usually used to define cases in which there have been no menstruations for over six months. It can be caused by some normal physiological process or by disease. Pregnancy, for example, is the most common event leading to a temporary cessation of periods. Other physiological causes are lactation (see *Infant feeding*) and the menopause.

Hormones disrupted by emotional upsets like examinations or a change of job may cause amenorrhoea. Severe illness and certain drugs can also lead to cessation of periods, and rapid loss of weight (due to dieting or anorexia nervosa) is not an uncommon cause. Weight-related amenorrhoea reverses and periods start again when the ideal weight for an individual is achieved. Women who have just stopped taking the pill may experience temporary cessation of periods. If periods do not start again within six months of stopping the pill then a doctor should be consulted; a few simple tests may be required to establish the cause, although in most cases nothing abnormal is found and periods return spontaneously.

AMNESIA

Loss of memory, presumed to be due to damage to the neural pathways in the brain which control memory. Amnesia may be found in several forms and in a number of conditions.

Post-traumatic amnesia follows head injury and may last for minutes or weeks, depending on the severity of the injury. Loss of memory that extends to the period before the injury is termed retrograde amnesia and usually lasts only a few seconds. Amnesia may also be found in association with organic brain disease such as stroke, brain tumour or dementia. Transient global amnesia, an unusual variety of stroke, is characterized by memory loss for several hours followed by complete recovery; it is thought to be due to transient impairment of the blood supply to areas of the brain serving memory. Amnesia is a well observed early feature of pre-senile dementias.

Hysterical amnesia is thought to be a response to stress but is difficult to distinguish from feigned amnesia, which is often used by criminals as an attempt to escape punishment.

AMNIOCENTESIS

A procedure carried out in pregnant women to determine the genetic make-up of a fetus and so diagnose many inherited or genetic conditions as well as determine the sex of a fetus. Cases of spina bifida, Down's syndrome and, later in pregnancy, fetuses affected by rhesus disease can all be detected by amniocentesis. The procedure is usually carried out at around 16–18 weeks' gestation, as this is the earliest time that reliable tests can be obtained. It carries a small risk of miscarriage; around 1 per cent over the normal risk.

A mother may be offered a termination of pregnancy if a genetic condition is discovered.
SEE ALSO *Chorionic villus biopsy*

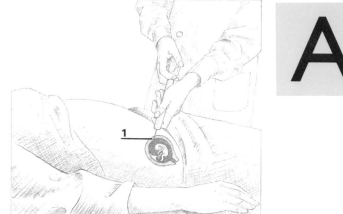

A

Amniocentesis involves obtaining a specimen of the amniotic fluid surrounding the fetus for analysis. A thin needle is inserted through the abdominal wall under ultrasound guidance and takes the sample **(1)**. The fluid contains cells from fetal skin and various biochemical waste products from the fetus.

AMOEBIASIS

An infestation of the colon, common in tropical countries and not rare in the West. The agent which causes it, *Entamoeba histolytica*, may live and multiply in the large bowel without producing symptoms for months or years; however, in some cases the amoebae become invasive, causing ulceration of the bowel and possibly thrombosis of the adjacent veins. Amoebae can travel to the liver through the veins that drain the gut and may create a liver abscess there.

Less commonly, amoebiasis affects the skin, producing deep, painful ulceration, usually around the anus.

Symptoms are variable in severity; they include diarrhoea, possibly bloody, and tenderness around the affected bowel. Diagnosis is by stool examination and artificial production of the bacteria (culture). Treatment with the drug metronidazole is fast (5–8 days) and effective.

AMPHETAMINE

This class of drugs is now almost exclusively used by drug abusers

Amphetamines were formerly used as appetite suppressants in the treatment of obesity; this practice is now discouraged because of the danger of addiction. One of their few contemporary medical applications is to counteract the uncontrollable bouts of sleepiness and muscular weakness characteristic of, respectively, narcolepsy and cataplexy. However, more effective remedies, such as tricyclic antidepressants, are now available, so even this application seems in doubt.

AMPUTATION

Surgical removal of a limb or portion of a limb, or of any other appendage. The most commonly performed limb amputation is that of the leg. This may be below the knee, at knee level or mid–thigh. It may be required in situations such as peripheral vascular disease, diabetes (which may cause gangrene) and injury.
SEE ALSO *Mastectomy*, *Prosthesis*

AMYLOIDOSIS

A rare progressive disease in which a waxy translucent material called amyloid ('starch-like') is deposited between the cells of tissue. Like starch, this material stains violet with iodine when it is biopsied (hence the name). It is known to be composed of a fibrous protein that is generally formed from antibody proteins. Amyloidosis usually occurs in response to chronic inflammation in the body. The organs commonly involved are the liver, spleen, kidneys and heart. In some cases renal or cardiac transplantation is performed, but eventually amyloid may be deposited in the transplanted organs. Death usually occurs from kidney failure or heart failure.

ANABOLIC STEROID

Also known as androgens or male sex hormones, anabolic steroids are substances normally produced by the testes, but small quantities are produced by the ovaries and the adrenal glands. Testosterone is the main testicular androgen but it is also produced, in smaller quantities, in women. Peak secretion occurs in men at puberty and causes the adult appearance of the external genitalia, together with muscular development, increased strength and physical vigour. In women excess androgens produce masculinization (see *Virilism*). Very rarely, some benign tumours secrete androgens in patients of both sexes.

A female fetus exposed to excess androgens before birth can be born with abnormal genitalia, making it difficult to determine its true sex.

Synthetic anabolic steroids (such as stanozolol) are used by some sports competitors. Such abuse can in the long term cause permanent damage to health, such as liver disease and even the development of tumours in the liver and elsewhere.

ANAEMIA

Literally, lack of blood or of red corpuscles in the blood. This is measured by the level of the red pigment haemoglobin. Anaemia causes symptoms of fatigue and lassitude, with palpitations.

Iron deficiency is the commonest cause of anaemia throughout the world. It results in small (microcytic) red cells which are also pale (hypochromic) because of the reduced haemoglobin. The causes of iron deficiency anaemia are blood loss (as in heavy periods), increased demands (as in pregnancy), poor absorption (as in coeliac disease) or poor diet.

Megaloblastic anaemia is a group of anaemias in which the red cell precursors are large with an abnormal nucleus. This is commonly due to a deficiency of vitamin B_{12} or folic acid. These vitamins may be deficient because they are poorly absorbed, because of poor intake (by vegans, for example, who eat no animal produce at all), and because of increased demands (as in pregnancy). Megaloblastic anaemia responds to appropriate treatment: vitamin B_{12} by injection or folic acid tablets.

Haemolytic anaemia results from an increase in the destruction of red cells, so that they have a shorter than normal life span of 120 days. This excessive red cell breakdown often produces jaundice and also causes an increase in young red cells (reticulocytes) as the body attempts to replace the cells being destroyed. Abnormalities within the cell or the membrane, or outside the red cell, may cause this type of anaemia. Haemolytic anaemia can also be inherited (sickle cell disease, for example, or acquired (as a result of an autoimmune process). One other variety of haemolytic anaemia is haemolytic disease of the newborn, which is generally caused by rhesus incompatibility (see *Rhesus factor*).

Many anaemias are associated with other clinical illnesses such as rheumatoid arthritis, chronic kidney failure or cancer. Such anaemias do not respond to treatment of the specific condition but of the underlying medical problem.

ANAESTHESIA

The means by which a person is rendered insensible to pain, either by being made unconscious (general anaesthesia) or by some procedure that blocks the sensation of pain from the affected part (local anaesthesia).

Nothing must be eaten or drunk for six hours before a general anaesthetic to ensure the stomach is empty in case of vomiting. A premedication drug helps the patient to relax. General anaesthesia may be induced with a drug administered via a needle into a vein (usually in the back of the hand) or by gas via a mask. The medical assessment before the procedure and careful monitoring during the operation have made general anaesthesia very safe.

If more limited local pain control is required, anaesthesia can be achieved by a variety of applications such as local injections or sprays, and may be applied by a non-specialist. Anaesthetists themselves also use these techniques in a more sophisticated manner — for example, applying drugs to the epidural space for pain-free childbirth without the loss of general sensation. Remarkable control of pain can also be achieved by techniques such as hypnosis and acupuncture, but these methods are less commonly employed.

ANALGESIC

A drug that is used for the relief of pain. The three most commonly used simple analgesics are aspirin, paracetamol and ibuprofen. Paracetamol is used exclusively for the relief of pain. Aspirin and ibuprofen not only relieve pain but also decrease the inflammation that may cause certain types of pain. Simple analgesics provide relief of pain lasting 4—8 hours, so regular dosing may be required to provide sustained relief from chronic pain. Despite their widespread use, and availability without prescription, simple analgesics are associated with a number of well-recognized side-effects or complications; both aspirin and paracetamol can be extremely dangerous when taken in excess, and aspirin should not be taken by children under 12 years of age because of its suspected involvement in the causation of Reye's syndrome.

More potent analgesics are usually derived from opium, the most common examples being morphine and diamorphine (heroin); pethidine is a synthetic morphine-like drug. These powerful analgesics, which also have a sedative effect, are called narcotics; they can only be prescribed by a doctor and are subject to strict control because of their ability to cause addiction. However, they can be used without fear of addiction for the short-term management of severe pain — for example, after an accident or surgery.

ANAPHYLAXIS

An immediate hypersensitivity reaction to a substance to which an individual has gradually developed an antibody as a result of previous exposure. On previous occasions of exposure to the provoking agent the affected individual had usually experienced some reaction, but a milder one. Reactions to bee and wasp stings or to certain drugs (especially penicillin — see *Antibiotic*) account for most cases of anaphylaxis; it occurs very rarely with some foods, notably nuts and shellfish.

Hypotension, swelling (especially of the face and tongue), nettle rash (urticaria), vomiting, abdominal pain and bronchospasm are the signs of anaphylaxis and are due to specific antibodies causing a rapid release of a substance called histamine from specialist cells (the mast cells) found in tissues throughout the body.

Anaphylaxis may prove fatal and need urgent medical treatment consisting of an injection of the hormone adrenaline. Bee sting hypersensitivity is probably the only allergic condition in which desensitization (qv) gives useful protection.

ANASTOMOSIS

The word derives from the Greek, meaning a 'new mouth', and in medicine is used to describe a surgically fashioned join between two hollow tubes in the body (such as the bowel or a blood vessel). The surgery is typically performed after the removal of a piece of diseased or damaged bowel (a resection); the join between the two ends of bowel is the anastomosis. The join is made by means of stitches (see *Ligation*) or staples, the latter applied with a special metal stapling gun.

ANDROGEN

see *Anabolic steroid*

ANENCEPHALY

Gross malformation of the fetal head and brain. The fetus is usually stillborn or dies soon after birth. The abnormality is probably caused by a number of genetic, environmental and social factors and affects approximately 5 babies per 1,000. There is a 1 in 20 risk of a subsequent pregnancy being affected. Anencephaly can be detected early in pregnancy by ultrasound examination, and at 16 weeks by raised levels of alphafetoprotein (qv) in the mother's blood and amniotic fluid.

ANEURYSM

A localized dilatation of the walls of a blood vessel (usually an artery) due to weakening as a result of a degenerative condition (such as atherosclerosis – see *Atheroma*), an infection or a congenital defect. The most common aneurysm is abdominal aortic aneurysm, which is often found incidentally and appears as a palpable pulsating swelling in the abdomen. It may leak, causing pain in the abdomen or back, or rupture spontaneously, producing profound shock (due to internal haemorrhage) and early death if emergency surgery is not performed. Such aneurysms are treated by replacement of the affected artery with a synthetic graft.

Other types include ventricular aneurysm, which is caused by weakness and dilatation of the wall of the left ventricle (one of the two lower chambers of the heart) after a heart attack; and a congenital berry-shaped aneurysm of the circle of Willis (arterial blood vessels at the base of the brain). Rupture of the latter type leads to subarachnoid haemorrhage (qv). In such cases neurosurgical obliteration of the aneurysm may be possible if the patient survives the initial bleed.

ANGINA PECTORIS

Chest pain due to disease of the coronary arteries, which supply blood to the muscle of the heart. The first attack often occurs unexpectedly during the course of customary effort, such as climbing stairs or walking up an incline, particularly after a meal or in cold weather. An emotional upset may provoke an attack. The pain varies in severity from discomfort to crushing or vice-like; it is felt beneath the breast-bone and lasts a few minutes. If pain is felt in the upper abdomen it is often attributed by the patient to indigestion. It may radiate to the jaw, neck, shoulder and arms. The left arm is affected more fre-

quently than the right, and pain and pins and needles may be felt in the fingers. Similar attacks may recur for years but in some cases may increase in severity and frequency over a period of weeks; this indicates critical cardiac ischaemia which may result in a heart attack.

Routine examination rarely reveals any abnormality and the ECG (see *Electrocardiography*) is often normal but may record changes on exercise.

The hallmarks of angina are its provocation by effort and its relief by rest or by drugs (such as glyceryl trinitrate) which dilate the blood vessels. Avoidance of unnecessary exertion will reduce the likelihood of attacks. Angina is usually managed by drugs. Nitrates are available as skin patches which are stuck on as plasters; the drug is absorbed through the skin and has a long-acting preventative effect. In severe cases coronary artery bypass grafts may be required to provide relief from recurrent attacks. This open-heart surgery requires the bypassing of blocked or narrowed arteries by grafts, usually taken from veins in the leg.

Some patients may be suitable for treatment by angioplasty. This relatively new technique involves dilating the narrowed parts of the coronary arteries under local anaesthetic. A balloon attached to a fine tube or catheter is placed across the narrowed segment at the time of cardiac catheterization and inflated. This widens the narrowed segment, thus restoring blood supply to the heart muscle. The long-term outcome of such treatment is, as yet, unclear, but it does save the patient from open-heart surgery.
SEE ALSO *Coronary heart disease*

ANGIOGRAPHY

see *Arteriography*

ANGIOMA

A benign tumour of blood vessels, some of which are often called haemangiomas (qv). Many adults have one or two small angiomas on the chest or trunk (called Campbell de Morgan spots) and these are of no significance. Sometimes quite large angiomas may be present at birth (called strawberry marks or naevi because of their appearance), but these usually completely disappear during the first one or two years of life.

Port-wine stains are another form of angioma present at birth. They are completely flat and comprise a localized collection of enlarged blood vessels. This form of angioma is permanent, though sometimes laser treatment can improve its appearance. Many angiomas in internal organs are arteriovenous (that is, they contain areas where arteries and veins communicate directly without intervening capillaries). Such angiomas in the brain may cause epilepsy or subarachnoid haemorrhage or may give the symptoms of a brain tumour.

ANGIONEUROTIC OEDEMA

A rare disorder, inherited in an autosomal dominant manner, which is caused by a deficiency in a plasma protein called C1-esterase. (Plasma is the fluid component of blood.) Symptoms include the development of a few deep, large swellings in the tissues which may occur spontaneously or after minor injury. The swellings may be preceded by redness (erythema) and itching (pruritis). They are often tender and last for several hours or even days. There may be recurrent bouts of abdominal pain.

Acute attacks may be controlled with an infusion of fresh plasma in hospital. The drugs testosterone and danazol are effective in the prevention of attacks (prophylaxis).

ANIMAL BITE

Animal bites carry the risk of infection and for this reason may be more serious than other wounds. One of the most serious infections is rabies, a virus which infects dogs and foxes. Other complications are those related to the particular wound inflicted. Bites from large animals may tear out muscle and sever small arteries and veins, making the repair of such injuries difficult. To test an animal bite, a tetanus boost is given to combat the introduction of tetanus spores and sometimes an antibiotic to fight bacterial infection is deemed a wise precaution.

ANKYLOSING SPONDYLITIS

A chronic inflammatory disorder of unknown cause which predominantly affects the spine. It usually begins in early adult life, men being more commonly affected than women. There is a strong genetic predisposition to the disease associated with the inheritance of an antigen known as HLA B27. The classic signs are low back pain and stiffness; these are most marked on getting up in the morning or after periods of immobility. Joints at the base of the spine are usually affected first, and the disease tends to move up the spine. Other joints, such as the hip and knee, may also be involved, and there may be accompanying inflammation in other areas of the body, notably where ligaments and tendons meet the bone. The condition may sometimes also be associated with inflammation in the eye. It is characterized by periods of exacerbation and remission. In time, fusion (ankylosis) of the spinal joints tends to occur and, in some cases, results in permanent spinal deformity.

Treatment may involve physiotherapy and NSAIDs (qv).

ANOREXIA NERVOSA

A disorder whose central features are self-induced weight loss through extreme dieting, amenorrhoea (loss of monthly or menstrual periods), and marked concern about weight and eating. Sufferers, who are predominantly young women, may also use means such as excessive exercising, self-induced vomiting, laxatives and diuretics to lose weight. Onset is usually between the ages of 12 and 22 years. The cause of the disorder is unknown. Factors which may be important are social pressure, a genetic predisposition and a personality characterized by conscientiousness and striving for high achievement.

The initial phase of treatment focuses on restoring weight. In extreme cases, this treatment will often consist of behaviour therapy and will take place in hospital. Psychotherapy and therapy involving discussions with the patient's family may be used as treatments after a normal weight has been regained; medication has little place. The outlook seems poorer for women who fall to a very low weight, have been ill for a long period of time, or develop the illness later in life. Around 5 per cent of all anorexia patients die within eight years, with a further 15 per cent remaining at a very low weight for many years.
SEE ALSO *Bulimia nervosa*

ANOSMIA

Loss of the sense of smell. Anosmia is usually due to nasal obstruction, such as chronic inflammation. Alternatively, damage to the nerve itself (as in skull fracture, for example) prevents stimuli from being transmitted to the brain where they are perceived as smells. Influenza may temporarily damage the mucous membranes of the nose and cause anosmia. The flavour of food depends on the sense of smell and so anosmia sufferers may experience reduced taste sensation.

ANOXIA

Total lack of oxygen. The term is usually employed to describe brain damage after cardiac arrest, when the oxygen supply to the brain is cut off as blood ceases to flow. Three minutes of total cerebral anoxia will cause irreversible brain damage and death. Less prolonged disturbances to blood flow will produce reversible damage, although some residual neurological problem often remains.

ANTACID

A mixture of alkalis, taken by mouth in the form of either a white liquid or tablet, used to neutralize acid within the stomach and relieve mild indigestion. The alkalis are usually salts of aluminium, calcium or magnesium, sometimes mixed with sodium bicarbonate (which is a potent alkali). Traditionally, and to make them more palatable, antacid mixtures have a peppermint or fruit flavouring that may also provide some of the relief for indigestion. Antacids are taken after meals, during the night or during periods of prolonged fasting. Aluminium- and calcium-based antacids tend to cause constipation, while magnesium-based antacids tend to cause diarrhoea. Many proprietary antacid mixtures contain a balance of these different salts.

ANTENATAL DIAGNOSIS

Detection of abnormalities in the embryo or fetus. Techniques used for antenatal diagnosis may be classed as invasive — for example, amniocentesis, chorionic villus biopsy or sampling and fetoscopy; or non-invasive — for example, ultrasound.

Amniocentesis (qv) allows the sex of the fetus to be determined (for pregnancies at risk of sex-linked genetic disorders), the detection of fetal chromosome abnormalities (for example, Down's syndrome), the testing of enzyme levels to detect inborn errors of metabolism, biochemical tests on the amniotic fluid, which surrounds the baby in the womb (for example, alphafetoprotein to detect spina bifida), and fetal DNA diagnosis. The number of single-gene disorders that can be detected by fetal DNA analysis is increasing rapidly.

Chorionic villus sampling (qv) is performed at 8—12 weeks of pregnancy; it allows fetal chromosome analysis and is usually the preferred technique for DNA analysis.

Fetoscopy (qv) can provide samples of fetal blood, skin and liver, and allows inspection for syndromes involving facial or limb defects.

Fetal ultrasound (qv) scanning has no proven hazard and can reveal a wide range of congenital malformations of the nervous system (for example, anencephaly, spina bifida and hydrocephalus), severe congenital heart disease, limb defects, kidney abnormalities (such as absence of one or both kidneys, or hydronephrosis) and some gastro-intestinal defects.

X-rays (qv) can reveal abnormal skeletal development.

Most antenatal diagnosis has been directed to the detection of serious fetal abnormality with a view to termination of pregnancy, but in a small number of conditions it may be possible to give some form of treatment before birth (fetal blood transfusion or surgery for hydrocephalus or hydronephrosis, for example).

ANTEPARTUM

Antepartum, or antenatal, refers to the time between the conception and birth of a baby. If a woman's menstrual periods occur regularly every month the length of the antepartum period is taken to be 40 weeks (280 days) from the first day of the last menstrual period, the time from conception being 14 days less. The opposite of antepartum is postpartum meaning 'after childbirth'.

ANTHRAX

A rare infectious disease caused by a bacterium that can remain potentially active for many years. Anthrax is a disease of animals, such as cattle or sheep, and is only rarely transmitted to man, by direct contact with an infected live animal or with its products (fleece or hide, for example). Anthrax affects exposed areas of skin and causes sores that usually become black and scabby with a surrounding ring of purplish blebs (fluid-filled blisters). There may be generalized symptoms, such as fever and malaise (a general feeling of being unwell), which may prove fatal. More usually the patient responds promptly to treatment with high doses of penicillin; it is also possible to immunize those at high risk.

ANTIBIOTIC

A drug which combats infecting organisms. Antibiotics act on bacteria, viruses, fungi, protozoa and worms.

Penicillin is the archetype and is particularly active against the organisms responsible for many types of pneumonia and meningitis, respectively pneumococci and menigococci; it is 'bacteriocidal', that is, it directly kills the organisms against which it is active. The many newer variants of penicillin have a broader spectrum of activity because they are sometimes effective against microorganisms that have become resistant to the archetype. They include ampicillin and amoxycillin, which are valuable in the treatment of chest and urinary infections; flucloxacillin, active against staphylococci; and expensive intravenous forms, such as ticarcillin and piperacillin, which are useful in septicaemia.

Allergy to penicillin is not rare and usually first shows itself as a skin rash. Allergic people should avoid all penicillins, as subsequent use can cause severe bronchospasm and anaphylaxis. Erythromycin provides a useful alternative to penicillin in allergic patients.

Cephalosporins are drugs derived from penicillins and are particularly useful in the treatment of infections from intestinal organisms and septicaemia, being less toxic to the ear and kidney than the older group of drugs called aminoglycosides.

Sulphonamides are now little used antibiotics, not least because they are 'bacteriostatic': rather than killing bacteria, they only prevent further proliferation. Their use is limited to treating pneumocystis pneumonia and helping to prevent septicaemia in patients undergoing bone marrow transplantation by combining them with trimethoprim (co-trimoxazole).

ANTIBODY

Special protein molecules (immunoglobins) produced in the body as part of the immune response against bacterial and viral infection. Antibodies are produced by white cells called B lymphocytes in order to bring about the destruction and elimination from the body of antigens, which are the agents of the infection. Each antibody is antagonistic to a specific antigen and no other. Once it has been produced it remains in the blood long after the antigen has been destroyed and is capable of recognizing it on a subsequent encounter. Occasionally antibodies are produced which act against normal body tissues (autobodies – see *Autoimmune disease*).

Antibody formation cannot occur until quite late in embryonic development. A child in the womb is therefore protected by antibodies derived from the mother's circulation. Antibodies in the breast milk continue this protection through the first few weeks of life. Rarely maternal antibodies can be harmful to the fetus, as in rhesus incompatibility (see *Rhesus disease*).

Antibodies can also be specifically induced, by vaccination.

ANTICOAGULANT

A drug used to treat clots in the veins and arteries. The major anticoagulants are heparin, streptokinase, urokinase and warfarin (the most commonly used oral type). Heparin inhibits blood clotting; this type is not absorbed if taken orally and so has to be given by injection. It acts rapidly but its effect is not long lasting. Heparin is therefore used to start anticoagulation in a patient who has a deep vein thrombosis while a longer-acting remedy such as warfarin is taking time to work. It is also useful for treating venous thrombosis in pregnancy because it does not cross the placenta from mother to fetus. Other drugs may increase or decrease the action of warfarin and so careful monitoring is required. The main side-effect of warfarin treatment is bleeding and careful control is therefore essential.

Streptokinase and urokinase are enzymes which work by activating plasmin, a protein in blood which dissolves clots. They are rarely, if ever, used in the treatment of deep-vein thrombosis. However, their use in arterial thrombosis is increasing.

ANTICONVULSANT

This term covers several different groups of drugs employed to control epileptic seizures. These include the benzodiazepine group (such as diazepam), which are given intravenously, chlormethiazole and the short-acting barbiturate, thiopentone sodium.

The aim of anticonvulsant therapy is to prevent seizures without incurring side-effects such as drowsiness or difficulties with coordination or speech. Different agents tend to be more effective in different types of epilepsy. For example, ethosuximide is particularly effective in controlling the petit mal absences of childhood; phenytoin is one of the mainstays of treatment of grand mal attacks; and carbamazepine is found to be useful in temporal lobe epilepsy.

High levels of anticonvulsants in the blood are associated with toxic effects, such as ataxia and nystagmus in the cases of phenytoin and carbamazepine respectively.

ANTIDEPRESSANT

A type of medication principally used in the treatment of depression and sometimes in the treatment of neuroses, schizophrenia and bulimia nervosa. There are two main drug types used in the treatment of depression: tricyclic depressants and monoamine oxidase inhibitors (MAOIs).

Tricyclic antidepressants, for example imipramine and amitriptyline, are the most commonly prescribed. They are thought to bring about an improvement in depression by acting on particular neurotransmitters (the chemicals responsible for communication between nerve cells) known as monoamines, the activity of which is disturbed in depression.

Tricyclic antidepressants may produce a number of side-effects including dry mouth, blurring of vision, postural hypotension, sweating and constipation, and sedation. Generally they would not be prescribed for a person with a history of glaucoma, prostate problems or recent heart problems. Care is needed in prescribing them for patients who are already taking certain medications for high blood pressure (hypertension). Tricyclics are taken for an initial period of six weeks and if effective are continued for six months or longer. There may be a delay of up to three weeks before any therapeutic effect is felt.

Monoamine oxidase inhibitors, such as phenelzine, are less commonly used because of their more serious side-effects (such as high blood pressure). They require a special diet which avoids certain foods, including specific cheeses, Chianti (the only red wine on the list of foodstuffs to be avoided), meat and yeast extracts, pickled herrings and chicken liver.

More recent antidepressants (such as mianserin, lofepramine, fluoxetine) have different side-effects and may be used in cases where the more traditional tricyclics or MAOIs cannot.

ANTIGEN

Antigens (sometimes called allergens in allergic diseases) provoke an immune response by reacting with lymphocytes (a type of white blood cell) and with the antibodies produced by lymphocytes. Substances derived from bacteria, viruses, plants (pollen, for example) and animals (such as hair) may all act as antigens.
SEE ALSO *Rejection*

ANTIHISTAMINE

A drug aimed at blocking the action of the chemical histamine, which is released from the mast cells (a type of white blood cell) in response to a variety of stimuli. Many of the obvious symptoms of hay fever and allergic rhinitis, such as watery and itchy eyes and nose and repeated sneezing, are caused by the action of histamine. Antihistamines are useful drugs in the treatment of these conditions, but they may not alleviate the symptoms entirely and have no effect on nasal blockage. The main side-effect of antihistamines is sedation and people taking them should not operate machinery or drive a car. Some newer preparations may avoid this problem.

ANTIPYRETICS

Measures used to reduce the effects of pyrexia, the medical term for a fever exceeding 37.5°C (99.5°F). The term antipyretic refers specifically to a drug whose action is on the temperature-regulating centre, the hypothalamus in the brain. The most commonly used and best known antipyretic is aspirin, though this should be avoided in children — paracetamol is an adequate substitute.

In addition to treatment with drugs, fanning and tepid sponging are also of value in lowering body temperature.

ANTITOXIN

An antibody capable of neutralizing the adverse effects of a bacterial toxin or poison. For example, immunization against tetanus stimulates the production of an antitoxin in the person injected which will neutralize the effects of the tetanus toxin should infection subsequently occur. Diphtheria immunization protects in a similar way. Direct administration of the antitoxin (obtained from people who have been previously immunized) can induce a hypersensitive reaction.

ANURIA

Non-production of urine. Normally the kidneys make urine all the time, and it is passed intermittently from the bladder. If no urine is made then anuria is said to have occurred. (Retention, by contrast, occurs when the urine is made but not passed from the bladder). The usual causes of anuria are dehydration, shock or septicaemia. Rapid treatment of the causative condition (such as intravenous fluid for dehydration, blood transfusion and antibiotics) can sometimes reverse shutdown. Failure of urine production can also occur if both ureters (the tubes leading from the kidneys to the bladder) are blocked by cancer or if the final stages of kidney failure (qv) have been reached; renal dialysis and eventually renal transplantation are the treatment in these cases.
SEE ALSO *Glomerulonephritis, Pyelonephritis*

ANXIETY

Anxiety is a universal emotion which

a person usually experiences when faced with a threatening situation. The physical symptoms of anxiety include a feeling of tightness in the chest, nausea, sweating, light-headedness, palpitations and breathlessness. Mild forms of these symptoms are normal in situations like speaking in public or taking an examination. Some level of anxiety will probably be a spur to performance.

If anxiety is persistent, of such severity as to impair performance or it suddenly appears and interrupts a normal daily routine, it is usually viewed as abnormal. This pathological anxiety is a central symptom in the neuroses, and is often seen in other psychiatric disorders such as depression, schizophrenia and dementia. Anxiety linked to a particular object or situation is known as phobic anxiety. Otherwise it is referred to as generalized or free-floating anxiety.

AORTIC REGURGITATION

A form of valvular heart disease. Under normal circumstances, blood ejected from the left ventricle (one of the lower chambers of the heart) into the aorta (the main artery from the heart) is prevented from leaking back into the heart by the closure of the aortic valve. If the aortic valve is diseased and becomes 'incompetent', then blood can regurgitate back into the left ventricle, increasing the workload of the heart.

The causes of aortic regurgitation include rheumatic fever, ankylosing spondylitis, Reiter's syndrome and syphilis.

The principal symptom is breathlessness on exertion, but chest pain on exercise (angina pectoris qv) may also occur. Murmurs are characteristics of valvular heart disease and can be detected by stethoscope. Techniques used in the treatment of aortic regurgitation include echocardiography (to assess heart size and performance) and cardiac catheterization.

AORTIC SCLEROSIS

Hardening of the aortic valve. This condition is frequently encountered in the elderly and is responsible for a murmur similar to that produced by aortic stenosis (qv). It is not serious and treatment is rarely required.

AORTIC STENOSIS

Narrowing (stenosis) of the aortic valve of the heart. Narrowing of the valve may be congenital or the result of disease, and is often associated with disturbances in rhythm (arrhythmias) and/or ischaemic heart disease (see *Ischaemia*). The patient may faint on exertion, as cardiac output cannot increase to cope, and a murmur is often audible over the front of the chest. The narrowing of the valve means that the left ventricle has to work harder to maintain the circula-

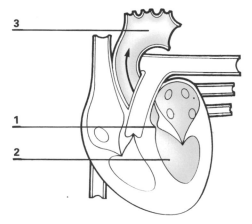

The aortic valve **(1)** lies between the left ventricle **(2)**, the principal heart muscle, and the aorta **(3)**, the main artery. All oxygenated blood leaving the heart must pass through the valve. Narrowing of the valve results in the left ventricle having to work harder in order to maintain the circulation.

tion; the left ventricle therefore thickens (hypertrophies) and this causes changes which are easily picked up on an ECG.

Treatment is by surgically replacing the affected valve.

APGAR SCORE

A means of evaluating and recording the condition of a baby at birth. This assessment is made during the vital first few minutes of life (usually one and five minutes after birth).

A score of 0, 1 or 2 is given to each of five observations of the baby. These are the baby's heart rate, breathing, floppiness (muscle tone), movements and colour. The scores are added together to give an overall assessment of the baby's condition, with a maximum possible score of 10.

APHAKIA

An eye without its crystalline lens; this occurs in cataract (qv). As a result the lens becomes cloudy and reduces the amount of light reaching the retina (the light-sensitive membrane at the back of the eye), so rendering the image perceived misty and indistinct. Cataract develops as a result of old age, diabetes, injury and, rarely now, rubella infection during pregnancy. When vision is seriously impaired the lens is removed surgically and the patient given a thick, convex spectacle lens to restore sight. However, this type of replacement may take a little while to get used to as it enlarges the image by a third and slightly distorts it. The most recent advance in this area is the use of plastic lens implants to replace the diseased lens.

APHASIA

see *Dysphasia*

APNOEA

The absence of breathing or any respiratory effort.

APPENDICITIS

Inflammation of the appendix, a small, worm-like, blind-ended pouch situated off the first part of the large intestine (the caecum). When the mouth of the appendix gets blocked, or the walls become infected, the appendix swells up and becomes inflamed. While this occasionally clears up without treatment, perforation usually follows, causing a local abscess or generalized peritonitis. The usual course of action is to remove the appendix surgically (appendicectomy). Typically, a patient with appendicitis feels unwell, and has central abdominal pain which moves to the right side; this is accompanied by vomiting and occasionally diarrhoea. The symptoms vary with the position of the appendix, and in the young and the elderly, which can make the diagnosis difficult.

'Grumbling' appendicitis describes intermittent attacks of acute appendicitis which partially resolve but which nevertheless usually require appendicectomy in the end. Gangrenous appendicitis is a particularly severe form of appendicitis, with early perforation and peritonitis. It occurs after obstruction of the blood supply to the appendix and is treated by appendicectomy.

ARNOLD-CHIARI MALFORMATION

A common cause of obstructive congenital hydrocephalus (qv). In this condition the roof of the fourth ventricle (cavity) of the brain lies below the level of the foramen magnum (where the brain-stem passes through to the spinal cord); the exit is blocked and, at a higher level, there is congenital narrowing (stenosis) of the aqueduct of Sylvius, the canal between the third and fourth ventricles. This obstructs the flow of cerebrospinal fluid, which bathes the brain and spinal cord, and can lead to increased pressure in the ventricular system, which dilates enormously, causing the head to enlarge. Intelligence may be impaired, as the cerebral cortex is reduced to a mere shell. The condition may also cause dilatation of the central canal of the spinal cord and produce syringomyelia (qv).

Treatment is by insertion of a valved shunt between the ventricle of the brain and the right atrium of the heart to relieve the excess pressure.

ARRHYTHMIA

Any variation from the normal rhythm of the heart beat. The term covers bradycardia, heart block, ectopic beats, extrasystole, atrial flutter and fibrillation, tachycardia and ventricular fibrillation; see individual entries for details of these.

Normal regular contraction of the heart depends on its natural pacemaker, known as the sinuatrial node (SA node). This is a collection of cardiac muscle fibres which initiate contraction by spontaneously sending out impulses over the atria (upper chambers of the heart) and to another similar node called the atrio-ventricular node (AV node). These impulses then travel down a band of specialized muscle fibres called the Bundle of His which in turn transmits the inherent atrial rhythm to the ventricles, causing them to contract.

The AV node and the Bundle of His also possess pacemaker properties which are usually suppressed by the SA node. The SA node is stimulated by the hormone adrenaline, causing the heart rate to speed up, and is depressed by the vagus nerve, causing it to slow down. If the function of the SA node is depressed for any reason, then pacemaker activity can emerge from the AV node and Bundle of His and establish an abnormal rhythm.

One common cause of an arrhythmia is ischaemic heart disease (see *Ischaemia*), which damages the conduction mechanism, but arrhythmias may be provoked in healthy individuals by excessive intake of caffeine, heavy smoking and anxiety. Clinical examination and an ECG (qv) will usually reveal the type of arrhythmia.

ARTERIOGRAPHY/ ANGIOGRAPHY

The demonstration on X-rays of the circulatory system by means of a contrast medium injected into an artery is called arteriography, while a similar demonstration of arteries and veins is called angiography. (Contrast medium is an organic iodine-containing liquid which is opaque to X-rays and will therefore highlight the internal structure of any cavity or tube into which it is placed. It is excreted via the kidneys.)

The injection may be made directly by needle into the required artery, or more usually by catheterization from a distant blood vessel. Catheterization involves puncturing the femoral artery in the groin with a hollow needle under local anaesthetic. A guide wire is then passed through the needle into the artery. The needle is removed and a long, thin tube (the catheter) is threaded over the guide wire. The wire is then removed and the catheter manipulated in the arterial system using X-ray screening. The X-rays produce an image on a TV monitor, and so the catheter can be precisely guided to its required position. An injection of contrast medium is given through the catheter and a rapid series of X-ray films taken to follow the passage of the medium in the artery and other vessels under study.

Arteriography is performed to investigate vascular diseases of blood vessels, particularly aneurysms, stenosis, thrombosis and embolism, as well as to investigate the heart and coronary arteries. It may also be used to form a clearer picture of some tumours.

Recently the technique has started to be used as a means of treatment. For example, catheters can be used to dilate an area of narrowing (stenosis); by injecting blood-clotting substances down branches of arteries that are bleeding, haemorrhage can be controlled; and the blood supply to tumours may be reduced using this method, resulting in a reduction of their size. In cases of cancer, drugs may be instilled directly into the artery which supplies a tumour, thus avoiding some of the side-effects caused by administering such toxic compounds throughout the body.

ARTERIOSCLEROSIS

see *Atheroma*

ARTERITIS

A group of conditions characterized by inflammation in the walls of arteries (vasculitis, qv); these include polyarteritis nodosa (qv) and vasculitis associated with diseases such as rheumatoid arthritis (qv) and systemic lupus erythematosus (qv).

Giant cell (temporal) arteritis is a not uncommon form of arteritis which involves the arteries in the head. It occurs after the age 55 years and in women more frequently than men. Onset is often insidious, starting with a headache which may be severe and concentrated in the region of the inflamed artery. The area over the temporal arteries may be tender. The most serious complication involves the eyes, and may lead to sudden blindness. Anaemia, fever, malaise (a general feeling of being unwell) and weight loss may accompany the condition. Features of polymyalgia rheumatica (qv) appear in about 50 per cent of cases. Blood tests and biopsy of the temporal artery (on the side of the head) are used to help make the diagnosis. The condition usually responds well to treatment with steroids.

ARTERY

Arteries are the high-pressure vessels which transmit blood to the capillaries or tiny blood vessels, where gases are exchanged with the body tissues.

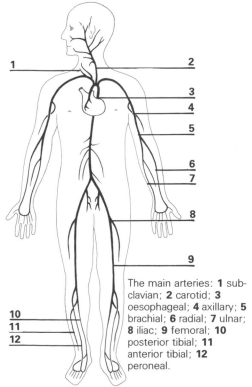

The main arteries: **1** subclavian; **2** carotid; **3** oesophageal; **4** axillary; **5** brachial; **6** radial; **7** ulnar; **8** iliac; **9** femoral; **10** posterior tibial; **11** anterior tibial; **12** peroneal.

In case of obstruction, in many organs an extensive network of 'collateral' arteries can sometimes take over the supply and prevent tissue death (infarction). However, if blockage (occlusion) occurs where such collateral circulation is inadequate or the artery affected is a so-called 'end-artery' and the exclusive means of supply to a tissue (for example in parts of the brain), infarction will result.

ARTHRITIS

Inflammation of the joints, although the term is often used loosely to indicate any disease process affecting the joints. The symptoms are pain and stiffness in the joints. Acute arthritis may develop for many reasons; for example, as a result of both infection within the joint (septic arthritis) and infection distant from the joint (Reiter's syndrome, rheumatic fever), or because of the development of crystals within the joint (as in gout and pseudogout). Arthritis may also be chronic, as in rheumatoid arthritis, ankylosing spondylitis or osteoarthritis.

ARTHRODESIS

A bone operation in which a diseased joint (usually the knee) is removed and the bones are united with each other and fixed in one position. This procedure reduces deformity, eliminates instability and relieves pain in the area concerned, but at the cost of total loss of movement. Arthrodesis has largely been replaced with the improved techniques of arthroplasty (qv).

ARTHROGRAPHY

A technique used to visualize the structure of joints. A solution of special contrast medium, which highlights the areas of interest, is injected directly into the joint cavity before X-ray pictures are taken. The examination is usually performed under local anaesthesia. Almost any joint cavity can be visualized in this way, although the knee is the one most frequently investigated. Using this technique damage to the menisci of the knee (commonly but incorrectly referred to as 'cartilages') may be observed; similarly, damage to ligaments of the joint or rupture of the back of the capsule (cavity) of the joint can be diagnosed.

ARTHROPLASTY

An operation which aims to reconstruct a joint so that pain, stiffness and deformity are relieved. At its simplest this may be achieved by removing one or both of the surfaces that form the joint or articulation without subsequently attempting to get the bones to fuse. The reconstructed joint may allow movement but the range is never full, and the joint is not always painless. Pieces of material with low-friction surfaces may be placed between the bone ends in an attempt to reduce stiffness and improve stability and movement.

The most effective arthroplasty is the replacement of both components of the joint with artificial ones (prosthesis). Excellent prostheses are available for the hip and are now routinely used. Prostheses are now available for many other joints, including the knee and elbow.

ARTHROSCOPY

Internal examination of a joint (usually the knee). Arthroscopy is performed under a general anaesthetic and involves introducing into the joint a very narrow fibre-optic telescope

(endoscope) via a tiny incision. It is possible to remove any foreign bodies and to perform a meniscectomy (removal of some cartilage) endoscopically. This has considerable advantages over an 'open' operation; in particular, there is no scarring, recovery is more rapid and the stay in hospital is considerably reduced.
SEE ALSO *Endoscopy*

ARTIFICIAL INSEMINATION

The placing of sperm in the lower female genital tract by means other than sexual intercourse. It is usually accomplished by collecting a sperm sample and placing it in the upper vagina or lower part of the cervix (the neck of the womb), but in some cases it can be injected directly into the uterus (womb) or Fallopian tube. Both procedures can be performed on outpatients and are usually painless.

There are two forms of artificial insemination: artificial insemination by the husband (AIH), and artificial insemination by a donor (AID). AIH is used if, for reasons of illness or disability, the male partner is unable to complete normal intercourse. It is also used in cases of chemical abnormality of the mucus plug in the cervix preventing the passage of sperm. In this situation the partner's specially prepared sperm can be injected directly into the uterus or Fallopian tube; this technique is called GIFT (gamete intra-Fallopian transfer).

Donor sperms (AID) are used in situations where the male partner has a low or absent sperm count or is known to carry a dangerous hereditary disease. Donors remain anonymous and are carefully selected. Donor sperm can be stored in sperm banks for long periods without loss of subsequent fertility. Couples who

undergo AID are carefully counselled to ensure that they understand the genetic and social implications of having a child that is the mother's but not the male partner's.

ARTIFICIAL LIMB

see *Prosthesis*

ARTIFICIAL RESPIRATION

The use of mechanical breathing aids in patients who cannot maintain sufficient respiratory effort; also known as assisted ventilation.

Artificial respiration is achieved by connecting a cyclical air pump (ventilator) to a tube inserted into the trachea (windpipe). This endotracheal tube has an inflatable cuff, ensuring an airtight fit. If an obstruction of the upper airway prevents the introduction of an endotracheal tube or longer-term ventilation is envisaged, it is sometimes necessary to make an opening in the windpipe (tracheostomy).

Ventilators may be set to be triggered by the patient's own respiratory effort. If the patient 'fights' the ventilator, then sedatives and a paralyzing agent are given and the machine is set to automatic mode.
SEE ALSO *Ventilator*

ASBESTOSIS

A lung disease (pneumoconiosis) caused by the inhalation of asbestos dust and fibres. Asbestos is a naturally occurring mineral and has a number of industrial applications. It is used in the manufacture of paper and cardboard, for example, and as an insulating material. There are three types of asbestos: white, blue (crocidolite) and brown. White is the most widely utilized. Blue is the most dangerous.

The commonest feature of asbestos exposure is the development of fibrous deposits (plaques) in the pleura (the membrane between the lung and chest wall). In time these may calcify (harden); otherwise they are harmless. Up to a quarter of people with pleural plaques will later develop fibrosis of the lung. The symptoms of this condition are breathlessness and a deterioration in lung function. The condition is difficult to treat.

Asbestosis is also associated with an increased risk of malignancy; the incidence of lung cancer in asbestosis patients is increased, especially if the person smokes. There is also a dramatic rise in the incidence of an otherwise rare tumour of the pleura, called mesothelioma.

ASCITES

An abnormal accumulation of fluid in the abdominal (peritoneal) cavity.

Ascites is seen in heart failure, including some types of pericarditis, and is a feature of kidney disease (for example chronic kidney failure, and the nephrotic syndrome). Diseases of the liver, such as cirrhosis, are frequently associated with ascites. The condition is also caused by blockage (occlusion) of the veins draining the gut into the liver or of the veins draining the liver into the general circulation, and abdominal malignancies, especially those of the ovary. Ascites may also be a response to infection — for instance, abdominal tuberculosis, and other inflammatory diseases such as acute pancreatitis.

ASPHYXIA

Asphyxia, or suffocation, is the condition produced by a blockage of the airway. Carbon dioxide levels increase and oxygen levels decrease as gases cease to be exchanged; this stimulates respiration, causing violent respiratory efforts, the blood pressure and heart rate to rise sharply and the blood to become acidic. Eventually the respiratory efforts cease, the blood pressure falls and the heart rate slows. If artificial respiration is not started the heart will stop beating within 4–5 minutes.

ASPIRATION

This term literally means 'sucking out'. It is used to describe two different phenomena. First, the removal of collections of fluid or pus which is performed with guidance from ultrasound or X-rays. Secondly, the act of breathing vomit into the lungs which results in a severe type of pneumonia requiring vigorous treatment with antibiotics and physiotherapy. The patient may also need mechanical assistance with breathing. The risk of this type of aspiration increases when a person is drunk or unconscious. In either of these circumstances the danger can be reduced by placing the affected individual on his or her side so that any fluids run out of the mouth. In unconsciousness due to a general anaesthetic the risks are reduced by starving the patient beforehand and using endotracheal tubes while the anaesthetic is effective.

ASTHMA

A common condition characterized by reversible obstruction of the airways (bronchi) caused by contraction of the smooth muscle surrounding them (bronchospasm). The symptoms, wheezing and breathlessness, may be triggered by exposure to a wide range of allergens (see *Allergy*). Asthma can start at any time before middle age. In

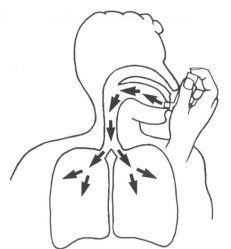

Of the many types of inhaler available to asthmatics, two are most commonly used. The first contains steroids and is taken regularly to prevent an attack. The second is used only during bronchospasm and contains an agent which relaxes the smooth muscle of the airways.

childhood asthma is often associated with other allergic conditions, most commonly hay fever and allergic dermatitis. Frequently other family members are similarly affected; this is extrinsic or atopic asthma. In asthma starting in later life there may be no evidence of an individual or familial atopy; this is intrinsic or non–atopic asthma.

Some people experience symptoms only on exercise, whereas others can pinpoint animal hair, house dust or grass pollen as the trigger. Many asthmatics are made worse by smoky or dusty conditions. Rarely certain foods, notably dairy products, may produce asthmatic symptoms. Emotional stress can precipitate an attack but does not cause asthma. Other factors which may induce an attack are respiratory infections and aspirin. Skin tests can help asthmatics recognize and avoid the factors likely to cause an attack; however, many people with extrinsic asthma react to several allergens and skin tests may not necessarily reflect the cause.

Bronchospasm in the asthmatic is assessed by measuring the peak expiratory flow rate on a hand–held meter: the force of expiration is measured by blowing hard into a tube which measures air flow in litres of air forced out per minute. Variability in readings throughout the day, in particular a morning 'dip', is characteristic. More sophisticated tests of lung function may be performed in hospital respiratory laboratories.

Symptoms are usually well controlled by regular medication given either by inhaler or tablets. Medication in tablet form is given to those unable to use inhalers efficiently. The long–term use of inhaled steroids does not produce the complications of oral treatment, as only a fraction of the dose is required.

Although generally a mild condition, asthma may take the form of an acute attack; if this fails to respond promptly to the usual therapy, medical help should be sought immediately.

ASTIGMATISM

The condition found when the eyeball is not symmetrical. In astigmatism light rays entering the eye are not focused clearly on the retina (the light-sensitive membrane at the back of the eye) and this causes blurring.

A cylindrical lens that has a different power of refraction along the vertical axis from the horizontal is used to correct the condition. A large degree of astigmatism makes the fitting of contact lenses difficult.

ASYSTOLE

The complete absence of electrical and consequently mechanical activity of the heart, usually as a result of a heart attack. Asystole is also known as cardiac arrest. Once asystole occurs the circulation of blood stops and loss of consciousness is rapid. Death will follow unless immediate measures are taken. Occasionally a sharp blow to the front of the chest can cause normal heart activity to resume. Drugs to stimulate the heart, such as adrenaline, are usually required and are sometimes given directly into it. Long-term treatment of asystole involves fitting a pacemaker (qv).

ATAXIA

Unsteadiness or lack of coordination. It results from a person's inability to control accurately the range and precision of his or her movements. Ataxia caused by a defect in the sensory pathways that convey information from the extremities is called sensory ataxia. A patient with this form of ataxia often has a high-stepping gait and walking is much worse in the dark. He or she may fall if the eyes are closed.

Disease of the cerebellum may also result in ataxia since this part of the brain is concerned with the fine coordination of movement and judgment of distance. The patient is unsteady and walks in a drunken manner. He or she has difficulty in stopping suddenly or turning. Many inherited forms of cerebellar ataxia are known, including Friedreich's ataxia, a progressive form usually beginning in childhood.

In the majority of cases there is no effective treatment.

ATELECTASIS

Collapse of part of the lung, due to blockage of the small airways leading to that area. The most common cause of blockage is through secretions from the cells lining the airways after general anaesthesia and surgery. Treatment is by physiotherapy to dislodge the blockage. If the condition is not treated, infection can follow, leading to pneumonia.

ATHEROMA

Deposits of abnormal material within the arteries. Atheroma is responsible for the condition called atherosclerosis (also known as arteriosclerosis). The atheromatous deposits are predominantly of fatty (lipid) origin and form when there is excessive fat circulating in the blood. In Western populations they form to a variable extent with increasing age. Hereditary factors, smoking, diabetes mellitus and a high-fat diet (particularly the saturated fats found in red meat and milk products) predispose to atheroma. Limiting total fat intake and, especially, reducing the proportion of animal fat in the diet, and reducing or, better, giving up smoking are wise precautions for everyone. Some people with very high levels of fat in their blood (mostly cholesterol and triglycerides) may require drug treatment in addition to dietary change.

ATHEROSCLEROSIS

see *Atheroma*

ATHETOSIS

A form of involuntary movement. The person affected makes slow writhing movements, particularly of the limbs and sometimes of the face, grimacing too. Most cases are congenital and due to either birth injury or a dysfunction of formation of certain nerve cells in one part of the brain (the putamen).

ATOPY

An atopic individual commonly suffers from asthma, allergic rhinitis or atopic dermatitis (eczema). The tendency is inherited and 80 per cent of sufferers have a close relative who is also atopic. Atopic status can usually be determined by skin testing to a battery of common allergens (antigens). The tests are performed by introducing a minute amount of allergen just beneath the skin. A reaction is positive if a weal and redness develop around the skin prick. Once developed, positivity reactions to the allergen may be seen long after symptoms have ceased. As many as 25–30 per cent of the population are found to have positive skin tests. Some of these individuals remain symptom-free, and others have only a few symptoms, but 10–15 per cent of the population will develop an atopic allergic condition.

SEE ALSO *Allergy*

ATRESIA

Failure of normal development of an isolated part of the body while the unborn child is still in the uterus (womb). The affected organ is withered or blocked, producing symptoms immediately after birth. Biliary atresia results in the development of severe jaundice, as the bile ducts are not formed properly. Oesophageal atresia means that the oesophagus (gullet) is blocked, and the baby cannot feed. Other parts of the bowel can also be affected by atresia, resulting in blockage of the intestine. Atresia produces a medical emergency in the days immediately after birth and usually demands some form of urgent surgical correction to save the life of the newborn baby.

ATRIAL FLUTTER

A disturbance in heart rhythm (cardiac arrhythmia) caused by a rapid electrical discharge from an area within the atria (upper chambers) of the heart. Heart rates are between 80 and 150 beats per minute, and may be regular or irregular in rhythm. Atrial flutter is often found in association with atrial fibrillation (see *Fibrillation*), and is invariably a short-term by-product of heart disease. Palpitations, dyspnoea (breathlessness) and syncope (temporary loss of consciousness) may all be associated.

Electrocardiography (qv) is essential for diagnosis of atrial flutter. Termination of the flutter is achieved by means of drugs or a form of electric shock treatment.

ATROPHY

The reduction in size of a previously normal organ or tissue. This is usually due to a decrease in the number of individual cells, but may also be caused by a reduction in the size of the cells or a combination of both. Atrophy which occurs as a result of normal physiological processes is sometimes called involution – for example, a reduction in the size of the ovaries at menopause. In some cases of atrophy (Alzheimer's disease of the brain, for instance) the cause is still not clear.

AUDIOMETRY

The measurement of hearing function. The threshold of sound perception is the quietest sound the average normal hearing person can hear. It is given the value of zero decibels (dB). Of the many types of audiometry available, two are most commonly used to test hearing function. In the first an audiogram is plotted like a graph, with the minimum sound intensity (threshold) plotted for different sound frequencies. In speech audiometry spoken words are given at different loudness levels. The number of words correctly heard is expressed as a percentage for each intensity and the results plotted as a graph. This is a useful measure of the degree of disability in deafness but takes a long time to perform. It can also help identify the site of the cause of deafness.

The results obtained may give a useful guide to treatment with hearing aids or by other means.

AURA

A particular sensation commonly experienced by epileptics before a seizure and directly related to the location in the brain of the sources of the electrical impulses that provoke epilepsy (qv). Frequently experienced auras include a sense of fear, a welling up in the throat, an unpleasant smell, diverse visual and auditory hallucinations, and abnormal tactile sensations in the limbs. Such auras give a clue as to the site of the epileptogenic focus. Auras are usually short-lived and are followed by the general epileptic seizure, comprising loss of consciousness, rigidity or rhythmic movement, tongue-biting and incontinence.

AUSCULTATION

The clinical art of listening to the body, usually through a stethoscope. It is used especially in order to identify heart, lung or abdominal sounds or abnormal sounds over blood vessels.

Auscultation of the heart is useful in suspected valvular disease, as the turbulent flow of blood through a stenosed (narrowed) valve produces 'white noise' (like the noise you hear when a radio is not tuned in properly). Similarly, the sound of blood regurgitating through a leaking valve can also be heard through a stethoscope. Severe ischaemic heart disease produces other heart sounds.

Examination of the lungs is also highly dependent on auscultation. In pneumonia the normally quiet breath sounds become harsh and the timbre of the voice changes when they are heard through the stethoscope. Breath sounds are quietened if the pleura (the membrane around the lungs) or pleural fluid becomes thickened. Heart failure produces wet lungs, and additional sounds are produced as the opening of the small airways becomes noisy.

Abdominal auscultation determines whether the bowel is functioning; food is propelled by contraction, and this may be heard as a series of 'squelches'. If the bowel is obstructed, these sounds become less frequent and adopt a much higher pitch.

As in the heart, fast blood flow through a narrowed artery produces a noise or bruit. Excessive blood flow through the veins is sometimes audible as a hum and may sometimes indicate an arteriovenous fistula.

Antenatal examination of an unborn child by means of auscultation confirms that the fetus is alive; it is also a way of checking that the fetal heart rate is within the normal range. SEE ALSO *Murmur*

AUTISM

A severe mental disorder of infancy and childhood in which symptoms appear before 3 years of age. Autism is uncommon and affects about 1 in 5,000 children. The cause is unknown, though there is some evidence for a genetic predisposition. Abnormal behaviour may be noted from birth, when the baby may not respond to the mother's usual displays of affection. In other cases the child may appear to develop normally for a year or two before starting to show the characteristic features of autism; the most obvious of these is lack of emotional contact with other people, often first noticed as a refusal to look others in the eye. Other common features are poor language development, loss of previously acquired language and abnormal speech.

No treatment has been shown to affect the long-term outcome, including the recently popularized 'holding' method (physical contact). Fifteen per cent of autistic children are well adjusted by adolescence, but most others remain severely handicapped.

AUTOANTIBODY

An antibody which fails to recognize an individual's own cells and tissues as 'self' and acts against them. This failure may lead to autoimmune disease. The precise stimulus which triggers the production of autoantibodies is unknown. In some cases a self-antigen may become altered by a virus or a drug in such a way that the immune system regards it as foreign. In others, a self-antigen may already have a structure very similar to that of a foreign antigen which the body would normally react to and eliminate.

AUTOIMMUNE DISEASE

A disease state resulting from an abnormal response of the body's defence system to its own tissues. The trigger which initiates the production of autoantibodies (qv) and autoreactive lymphocytes (types of white blood cell important to the immune system) is unknown. 'Self'-antigens on normal cells may be altered by a virus or a drug, or they may already closely resemble foreign antigens in structure. In some autoimmune disorders, antibodies to a particular organ are produced (organ-specific), whereas in others non-organic-specific autoantibodies are found. The latter react with antigens found on many widely differing organs and tissues and may produce many diverse symptoms.

Many endocrinological disorders are the result of organ-specific autoimmune disease (for example, Addison's disease) and some forms of abnormal thyroid function (such as thyrotoxicosis). An individual may have several autoantibodies reacting to different endocrine glands and thus have symptoms of more than one autoimmune endocrine disease. Pernicious anaemia is an autoimmune disorder. Rheumatoid arthritis and systemic lupus erythematosus are also thought to have an autoimmune origin, although the mechanism is poorly understood.

Relatives of people with autoimmune disorders run a higher than normal risk of developing an autoimmune condition.

AUTOSOME

see *Chromosome*

BACILLE CALMETTE-GUÉRIN

see *BCG*

BACKACHE

Establishing the precise cause of backache in the majority of individuals is not possible. Many attacks are acute and tend to be self-limiting, getting better of their own accord. In others pain may become chronic, often involving periods of mild discomfort interspersed with severe exacerbations.

Acute back pain may be due to a slipped disc (see *Sciatica*), especially if the pain spreads down the leg. Chronic spinal pain may be due to degenerative changes (see *Spondylosis*) or fractures (breaks or cracks in bone), or more uncommonly may be due to inflammation of the joints of the spine (see *Spondylitis*). Rarely, pain may be caused by infections such as tuberculosis or malignant tumours. Sometimes disorders of internal organs such as the kidneys, pancreas or stomach may give rise to back pain.

Acute back pain may require treatment with bed rest in the initial stages. Fortunately, however, most cases resolve spontaneously. Depending on the clinical picture, the doctor may perform tests to look for an underlying cause. In a few patients with structural back conditions surgery may be necessary. A wide variety of forms of treatment is available for chronic 'non-specific' back pain, including physiotherapy, manipulation, local injections and drug therapy. Some patients benefit from osteopathy or chiropractic.

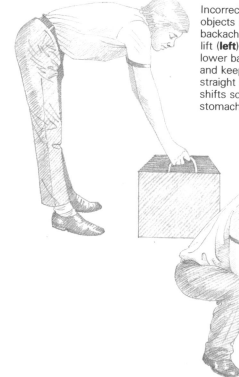

Incorrect lifting of heavy objects is a common cause of backache. Bending forwards to lift (**left**) puts great strain on the lower back. Bending the knees and keeping the spine relatively straight when lifting (**bottom**) shifts some of the strain to the stomach and leg muscles.

BACTERIUM

A single-cell micro-organism capable of asexual reproduction. Not all germs, as bacteria are commonly called, cause disease in humans: the production of yoghurt and blue cheeses also depends on bacteria, for example. There are many classifications, the simplest being based on shape — round (coccus), straight rod (bacillus) or spiral rod (spirochaete) — and on whether the cell wall takes up a particular stain, a testing procedure called Gram's method. Some bacteria have one or more flagellae (small 'whips') which enable them to move; the spiral rod bacteria are mobile without this modification.

Different bacteria require different conditions for multiplication. Some, such as the bacillus responsible for tuberculosis, are very fussy. Others, such as *Escherichia coli* (*E. coli*), are more tolerant and can easily survive on the skin. Only a small group of bacteria are strictly anaerobic (that is, they require the absence of oxygen); these include the microbe responsible for gas gangrene.

The *Rickettsiae* (this group includes typhus) and *Psittacosis* groups are special cases and cannot survive outside parasitized host cells, a feature they share with viruses.

Bacteria are responsible for a wide variety of illnesses, ranging from the trivial (staphylococci cause boils) to the potentially rapidly fatal (such as meningococcal meningitis).

Unlike most viruses bacteria are susceptible to antibiotics, unless they have developed a resistance; this is often due to the drugs being used indiscriminately.

BALDNESS

see *Alopecia*

BARBITURATES

see *Drug dependence*

BARIUM ENEMA

Radiological examination of the large bowel (colon). There are two basic techniques: single-contrast and double-contrast. A double-contrast technique is usually employed, although in children and the elderly a less potent single-contrast study may suffice.

In double-contrast barium enema, dense viscous barium sulphate (a substance opaque to X-rays) is introduced into the rectum through a tube; if the patient is tilted, the barium can be persuaded to flow to the caecum (the first and lower part of the colon on the left). Air is then blown into the colon to distend it and enable a thin layer of barium to coat the wall. X-ray films are taken from different angles so that all parts can be seen. The double-contrast technique allows detailed scrutiny of the mucous membrane lining the bowel for irregular features, such as fine ulceration in early ulcerative colitis.

In the single-contrast study only dilute barium is introduced and this does not provide fine detail.

BARIUM MEAL

Radiological examination of the oesophagus (gullet), stomach and first few centimetres of the small bowel. This technique can detect structural diseases such as peptic ulceration or tumours. It can also provide information on movement of the walls of the oesophagus and stomach and show, for example, whether muscular spasm of the oesophagus impairs swallowing.

In a single-contrast barium meal, only barium sulphate, a substance opaque to X-rays, is swallowed; ulcer-craters are easily filled and a tumour can be seen by X-ray as a 'filling defect' in the barium. In double-contrast studies, carbon dioxide-producing granules or tablets cause the stomach to distend with gas; a small volume of dense, viscous barium is then swallowed to coat the lining of the stomach thinly. This reveals fine detail of the lining as well as ulcers and tumours.

BARRIER NURSING

The nursing care of patients who have an infection and who potentially can transmit their infection to others. Some hepatitis B patients and tuberculosis cases require this type of nursing. The infected patients are nursed in single rooms, away from others. Nursing and other staff or relatives wear gloves, masks and gowns when attending or visiting the patient. Goggles are worn if there is an added risk of the patient's bodily secretions or blood getting into the eyes. After each contact, hands are washed and the protective materials discarded inside the room.

Reverse barrier nursing is required when the patient is at risk of infection from health personnel, other patients or friends and relatives who come to visit. These patients are generally immunosuppressed as a result of bone marrow transplantation or intensive chemotherapy for cancer, or AIDS, for example. Hands are washed, and gloves, gowns and masks are worn and discarded outside the room. These patients require specially purified air and sterilized food.

BCG (BACILLE CALMETTE-GUÉRIN)

A vaccine originally developed by the French scientists Calmette and Guérin,

B

B

consisting of live but inactivated bacteria derived from bovine tuberculosis. When injected into the skin of humans it confers immunity against subsequent infection with tuberculosis. Protection probably starts about six weeks after vaccination and lasts for approximately fifteen years. Occasionally a small ulcer appears at the injection site. This usually heals after a couple of month, leaving a small scar. Rarely an abscess can develop. BCG is recommended for contacts of tuberculosis, health service staff, travellers to areas where tuberculosis is endemic, those living in communities where the incidence is high, student teachers, and school-children between the ages of 10 and 13 years. Immunization of infants in high-risk groups may be carried out soon after birth.

BEDSORE

Bedsores are either acute or chronic. The acute variety are associated with disease or injury of the spinal cord (paraplegia, for example) and often progress with alarming rapidity despite excellent care.

Chronic bedsores are usually found over bony prominences, classically the sacrum (the central bone of the pelvis) and the heel, in patients confined to bed for long periods during severe illness.

The first sign of an imminent bedsore is redness (erythema), followed by breakdown of the skin, and later death or necrosis of the skin and deeper tissues.

Preventative treatment is paramount: measures include a change of posture every two hours, the use of a ripple bed (an air bed) or sheepskin to lie on, and keeping the pressure areas dry and free from sweat and urine. The treatment of established bedsores

centres around meticulous nursing care, together with the desloughing of necrotic tissue and, in severe cases, skin grafting.

BED WETTING

Enuresis is the medical term for bed wetting.

Most children are dry by day at 2 years of age, and dry by night at 3 years. Bed wetting is not considered a problem until after the age of 4, and even then is very common. Twenty per cent of 4-year-olds, 10 per cent of 5-year-olds and 2 per cent of 14-year-olds wet the bed. Sometimes wetting starts again after a period of dryness, and at this point it is important to make sure that there is no underlying disease, such as urine infection. A bout of bed wetting can be brought on by an emotional upset, such as bereavement or the arrival of a new baby.

Treatment rests largely on providing positive encouragement; negative influences, such as physical punishment or humiliation, merely serve to reduce an already low self-esteem and should be avoided. Reinforcement with star charts or other reward systems is sometimes effective in younger children. A buzzer alarm which is triggered automatically when the child wets the bed may help in children over the age of 8. Some older children respond to drug treatment.

BEHAVIOUR THERAPY

A form of psychological treatment in which a person's observable behaviour is the principal target. Behaviour therapy techniques have been successfully applied to a wide range of psychiatric conditions. For example, phobias may be treated either by helping a patient to confront a feared situation slowly (desensitization) or by exposing him or her to it suddenly (flooding). Another technique, exposure with response prevention, is used in obsessional neuroses: a sufferer is exposed to a situation which causes anxiety and is then prevented from making his or her usual ritualistic response. Behaviour therapy strategies have been effective in the treatment of sexual problems such as impotence, premature ejaculation and vaginismus (an extreme tightening of the vaginal muscles, preventing intercourse). They have been used with success too in the problem behaviours found in mental handicap, in the rehabilitation of patients with chronic schizophrenia, and in the treatment of bed wetting.

BELL'S PALSY

Paralysis of one side of the face due to a lesion of the seventh cranial (facial) nerve. The cause is unknown. The condition occurs equally in both sexes and at any age, but especially between the ages of 20 and 50. Paralysis sets in rapidly over two days, leading to difficulty in speaking, eating and blinking. Paralysis may be partial or more severe, and the sense of taste may be lost. High-pitched or loud sounds may cause distress due to paralysis of the inner ear muscles.

Most people recover spontaneously over a period of several weeks, although more severe cases may take three months. Corticosteroids may be of benefit in the early stages.

BENDS

Also called decompression sickness or Caisson disease, bends occurs when a diver who has been breathing air ascends too rapidly to the surface.

Nitrogen gas is a normal constituent of air and during respiration some becomes dissolved in the circulating blood. A rapid ascent through water, however, may cause some nitrogen not to dissolve but to form bubbles in the tissues and blood. These bubbles cause severe pain, particularly around joints, and an obstruction of the arteries. Paralysis or heart attack may result.

Treatment of the condition is by prompt recompression in a pressure chamber, followed by slow decompression. Recovery is often complete, but there may be neurological complications due to irreversible damage to the nervous system.

BENIGN

Of mild or gentle character. The word is commonly used to distinguish between types of tumour. When examined microscopically, benign tumours closely resemble the tissue from which they arise. They generally grow slowly, pressing against the surrounding tissues but not invading them. Benign tumours have little tendency to ulcerate and bleed, and usually do not recur after surgical removal.

Benign hypertension is the common and mild type of raised blood pressure.
SEE ALSO *Malignant*

BERIBERI

An illness caused by deficiency of thiamine (vitamin B_1). There are two forms: wet beriberi and dry beriberi. The other components of the diet determine which form the beriberi takes. In wet beriberi the body is markedly swollen due to water retention caused by heart failure. Sudden death may occur. Dry beriberi leads

B

to severe muscle weakness and numbness in the limbs. The person may become bedridden. In the past beriberi was common in the Far East where polished rice, which lacks thiamine, formed the staple diet. (Vitamin B_1 deficiency can also occur in chronic alcoholism and is the commonest cause of alcoholic neuritis.) Treatment consists of thiamine administration.

BETA-BLOCKERS

A class of drugs which block the receptors in the heart and peripheral blood vessels, known as beta-adreno-receptors. These drugs are particularly effective in the treatment of angina pectoris, because they reduce the work done by the heart, and in the treatment of high blood pressure (hypertension), although the way they help this condition is poorly understood. They are sometimes prescribed to reduce the rate of recurrence following heart attack, or to help in the treatment of certain rhythm disorders of the heart (especially those associated with fast heart rates, such as thyrotoxicosis) or migraine. Performers such as instrumentalists and snooker players sometimes take them to reduce tremor due to anxiety and so improve performance.

In some individuals beta-blockers may precipitate heart failure, and it is important that they are not taken by those who are already suffering from a heart condition involving the conducting system, which controls heart rate and contraction. Beta-blockers may also bring on an attack of asthma; cardioselective types of beta-blocker have less effect on the lungs and so minimize this possibility.

Many different beta-blockers are now available and in general they are all as effective as each other. Some have different properties and some

last longer than others; this may be of advantage in particular situations.

BILHARZIASIS

see *Schistosomiasis, Worms*

BIOAVAILABILITY

This term refers to the proportion of a drug which reaches the circulation unaltered; also known as biological availability. When a drug is injected into a vein it gains access to the whole body via the circulation and its availability is 100 per cent. If the same quantity of the drug is swallowed, however, the entire amount will not necessarily enter the bloodstream, and its availability may be less than 100 per cent.

Reduced bioavailability occurs for both biological and pharmaceutical reasons. Biological causes include destruction of the drug by gastric acid or alteration of it in the gut wall or by the liver before it reaches the circulation. Pharmaceutical formulation of a drug may vary between different manufacturers, and the time it takes for a tablet or capsule of the same drug to dissolve may differ. A doctor has to take such factors into account when prescribing.

BIOPSY

The removal and examination of tissue from the living body for diagnosis. This procedure is generally carried out under local anaesthetic and may be done using a needle or a special instrument (endoscope), or surgically.

Biopsy from the bone marrow, liver, pleura (the membranes surrounding the lungs) and increasingly from breast lumps is obtained using special needles. Specialized instruments are also available which may be inserted through the body orifices, such as the nose, anus and urethra (the tube which drains the bladder), and into the lungs, stomach, intestine and bladder to obtain a sample of tissue from any area which appears suspicious. Lymph nodes, skin and breast lumps are usually biopsied surgically through a small cut in the skin. The tissue obtained by any of these procedures is then sent to a pathologist for microscopic examination.

Biopsy is commonly undertaken to find out if a growth is benign or malignant and, if malignant, to ascertain the type of malignancy. It is sometimes also used to determine how far malignant disease has spread (staging). The use of biopsy is not restricted to tumours, however, and the procedure can also help diagnose blood disorders, cirrhosis, coeliac disease, inflammatory bowel diseases, diseases of muscle and nerve and rare infections.

BIRTH

see *Labour*

BIRTH CONTROL

see *Contraception*

BIRTH MARK

Most so-called birth marks are not present at birth but develop during the early months of life. They result from the abnormal development of skin structures, such as blood vessels (haemangiomas) or the pigment-producing cells (brown or black naevi). Only in rare cases are other structures, such as fibrous tissue or sebaceous glands, involved.

The commonest marks present at birth are 'stork marks', composed of small blood vessels (capillaries). Small and pink in colour, they are found on the eyelids, bridge of the nose and nape of the neck. 'Stork marks' eventually fade away. Extensive capillary haemangiomas (port-wine stains) are uncommon. Other haemangiomas are raised and red (strawberry marks), or bluish. A Mongolian blue spot is found over the lower back and buttocks of 90 per cent of non-Caucasian babies. Its greyish-blue colour (produced by increased numbers of pigment cells) fades with age and is of no significance, but may be confused with bruising. Other pigmented birth marks are uncommon, and may occur anywhere on the skin. Some are large, and occupy the bathing trunk area. The appearance of these giant pigmented naevi can be improved by plastic surgery, but malignancy may occasionally arise later on. Most pigmented naevi (moles) appear in later childhood. Some of the more unusual birth marks are associated with abnormalities of the nervous and skeletal systems.

BLACKOUT

A non-medical description of sudden loss of consciousness, usually due to an inadequate supply of blood to the brain. A blackout due to fainting (syncope) can be caused by a relatively simple problem, such as standing up suddenly, or standing immobile for a long period. However, it may have more serious causes — for example, epilepsy, a change in the rhythm of the heart causing inadequate pumping of blood to the brain, or a temporary blockage via one or more of the arteries supplying the brain.

Repeated episodes of fainting or blackout may require investigation of the blood supply to the heart or brain, together with a test of brain function (an EEG, see *Electroencephalography*).

B

B

BLEEDING

see *Haemorrhage*

BLEPHARITIS

Inflammation of the eyelids. By far the commonest cause of blepharitis is infection with the bacterium *Staphylococcus aureus*. The infection may produce pus with some stickiness of the eyelids.

Treatment involves regular gentle bathing of the eyelids with a mild antiseptic solution and the frequent application of an antibiotic ointment.

A very much more unusual cause of blepharitis is infection with the virus *Herpes simplex* (qv). In this case the infection usually affects the skin surrounding the face. Infection with this virus is potentially very serious and requires treatment with a systemic anti-viral agent to prevent permanent damage to the eye.

BLINDNESS

A visual handicap. In many under-developed countries blindness is found in over 1 per cent of the population, and occurs as a direct consequence of poor living conditions (see *Trachoma*). By contrast, the prevalence of blindness in Europe and the United States is approximately 0.2 per cent of the population. In these areas, cataracts, glaucoma and senile macular degeneration (in which the centre of the retina wastes away) are common causes of blindness, mainly in the elderly. Diabetic retinopathy (qv) is the most frequent cause of blindness in the working population.

BLISTER

A collection of fluid beneath or within the outermost layers of the skin (the epidermis); also known as a bulla. This is usually caused by some form of physical injury, such as a thermal burn or sunburn, from caustic chemicals, bites, and so on. Because of the superficial nature of the injury, recovery is usually complete and does not leave a scar, provided that serious infection is prevented. Treatment usually consists of applying antiseptic poultices or creams.

Other common causes of blisters are viral infections of the skin such as herpes simplex (cold sores) or herpes zoster (shingles). Again, treatment is mainly directed at the prevention of serious secondary infection; new anti-viral medication may help.

A group of rare skin conditions (pemphigoid, pemphigus and dermatitis herpetiformis) is characterized by the appearance of blisters, for which there is no clear explanation. In these conditions it appears that the host immune system attacks certain components of the skin as if they were foreign tissue (an autoimmune attack). Treatment is with drugs, such as corticosteroids, and aims to suppress this attack.

BLOOD

Fluid that circulates the body via the arteries, capillaries and veins, exchanging substances with the bodily tissues. Blood absorbs oxygen from the lungs and food from the digestive system. The food and oxygen are taken to individual cells of the body which give up waste products to the blood. These waste products are then carried to the organs that excrete them: carbon dioxide is carried to the lungs where it is breathed out; and urea and other impurities pass to the kidneys.

The blood moves around the body in blood vessels and is kept in motion

B

by the heart, which acts as a pump. The total volume in an adult is about 5 litres (9 pints). It is made up of liquid plasma with red cells, white cells and platelets floating in it. The red cells are disc-shaped and contain haemoglobin, which carries oxygen and gives blood its red colour. The white corpuscles fight infection; they are capable of independent movement and can enter body tissues through tissue spaces. The platelets and clotting factors in the blood are able to form a 'plug' or clot whenever there is a surface break-age, either inside the body or as a result of a skin wound. In some people, for example haemophiliacs, important clotting factors are missing and special measures have to be taken to protect them.

BLOOD GROUP

Group of people who share a common antigen on their red blood cells. The major blood groups are A, B and O. The presence of the A and/or B antigen defines these classic blood-group systems. Neither antigen is present in the commonest blood group, O (meaning 'zero'). The coexistence of both antigens (in blood group AB) is rare; in the UK, for example, it is found in only 3 per cent of the popula-tion. In these systems an individual possesses antibodies against the antigen he or she has not got; for example, a person with group A blood will have antibodies against group B red blood cells, and vice versa. A transfusion of group B blood into an individual with the group A antigen would therefore be very dangerous and would result in the red corpuscles of the mismatched blood sticking together (agglutinating).

There are many other antigen systems apart from the major groups. In these minor systems (for example, Duffy, Kell and MNS) antibodies are not formed spontaneously against the antigens the individual does not possess and will only develop if trans-fused blood carrying those antigens is received.

Blood groups vary between ethnic groups. Blood group B, for example, is more common in Indians and Africans than Caucasians.
SEE ALSO *Rhesus factor*

BLOOD PRESSURE

The pressure caused by the action of the pumping heart against the resis-tance of the wall of the artery. It is measured using a sphygmomano-meter (qv).

Blood pressure values rise with age. In a normal person it is 120 systolic and 80 diastolic. A raised blood press-ure, if confirmed after a few repeated measurements, requires investigation, except in the very elderly. An adequate systolic blood pressure of at least 90mmHg is required to maintain normal kidney and other organ func-tion. Low blood pressure must there-fore be treated quickly to prevent damage to the body's organs.
SEE ALSO *Hypertension*, *Hypotension*

BLUE BABY

see *Fallot's tetralogy*, *Premature baby*, *Ventricular septal defect*

BOIL

A collection of fluid beneath the outer layers of the skin which (unlike a simple blister) has become infected. Isolated boils are common and usually improve either spontaneously or after treatment with a short course of antibiotics aided by poultices or antiseptic cream. Sometimes, when an abscess has formed and the boil has become completely walled off from

B

surrounding tissue, it is necessary to drain the pus surgically to assist healing. Any area of the body may be affected, although hairy sites such as the genital region and armpits are usually involved. People who recurrently suffer from boils should be checked for diabetes mellitus.

BONE MARROW TRANSPLANTATION

Bone marrow transplantation is performed most commonly for leukaemia, but it can also be used for serious inherited disorders of the blood, such as thalassaemia (qv). Cells from the bone marrow of a donor, obtained by sucking marrow from the pelvic bones, are transfused into a patient to provide a new blood system. Before the transplantation, the patient is treated with drugs or radiotherapy to destroy his or her own bone marrow. For about three weeks before the graft 'takes', the patient has pancytopenia (no blood cells). This means that treatment with antibiotics to stop infection, and transfusions of blood and platelets to stop bleeding, is necessary.

Sometimes the graft may react against the patient: this is called graft-versus-host disease (qv).

BONE SCANNING

The term 'bone scan' is generally taken to refer to an isotope scan of the skeleton. The most common isotope used is technetium combined with a phosphate complex to form a radioactive compound that is then taken up in the skeleton. The compound is injected intravenously and the patient is scanned by a gamma camera about three hours later. Areas where greater amounts of the isotope have been taken up are abnormal and show up on the scan; in many pathological or disease processes increased activity may be seen on a bone scan long before there is any change visible on a plain X-ray.

Many benign lesions take up radioactivity, particularly Paget's disease of bone, osteoarthritis, fractures and osteomyelitis. Malignant tumours of bone, both primary cancers and metastases, also produce high activity.

Detection of metastases is the widest application for skeletal scanning. In up to 30 per cent of patients with cancer of the breast, occult (or hidden) metastases will occur; these metastases produce no symptoms or signs but are unexpectedly found on the scan. Occult metastases are also very common in patients with cancer of the prostate. It is common clinical practice to give any patient who has either of these cancers bone scans every year or so in order to detect bone metastases as soon as they develop.

BOTULISM

A rare but serious and often fatal disease caused by the toxin secreted by the bacterium *Clostridium botulinum*. The toxin is readily destroyed by heating, and so botulism is associated with the consumption of uncooked foods, including some commercially prepared and canned foods.

It is found more frequently in non-acidic foods, such as meat and vegetables, than with fruits. The toxin causes non-specific gastrointestinal symptoms 12—24 hours after consumption and in severe cases muscle paralysis. Difficulty in swallowing is followed by weakness of the limbs and ultimately, as the muscles of respiration are affected, breathlessness. Treatment involves intensive nursing and artificial ventilation in combination with an antitoxic serum.

BOW LEGS

see *Knock knees/Bow legs*

BRADYCARDIA

A slow heart rate, generally implying less than 60 beats per minute (normal is around 80 beats per minute). In some individuals, however, this is not abnormal: for example, athletes often have a constitutional bradycardia; the reason for this is not known. Bradycardia may be found in disease states: for example, after infections, and in patients with thyroid disease or jaundice. Excessive dosage of some drugs, such as digoxin, may result in bradycardia, as may heart abnormalities — after a heart attack, for example. Bradycardia may also occur in conditions affecting the conducting system of the heart (the system of electrical pulses which controls heart rate and contractions); an electrocardiogram (ECG) will help to distinguish this cause. Patients may temporarily lose consciousness (syncope) if bradycardia results in insufficient blood supply to the brain.

BRAIN

The brain is situated within and protected by the skull. It is composed of a mass of interconnecting wells. There are two types of cell: neurones (which transmit electrical messages) and glial cells (support cells). These are organized into special regions and pathways which have specific functions, such as speech, eyesight, hearing, maintenance of vital reflexes such as respiration drive and blood pressure, control over muscles, movement and balance.

The main structures are the cerebral hemispheres, the pons, cerebellum and medulla oblongata. The outer covering is called the meninges.

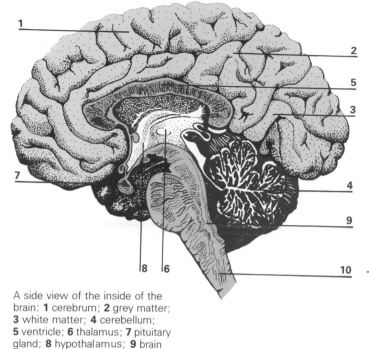

A side view of the inside of the brain: **1** cerebrum; **2** grey matter; **3** white matter; **4** cerebellum; **5** ventricle; **6** thalamus; **7** pituitary gland; **8** hypothalamus; **9** brain stem; **10** spinal cord.

BRAIN ABSCESS

A localized infection within the brain, closely related to and sometimes coexistent with abscesses involving the meninges. The abscess is usually due to bacterial infection but may be caused by fungal agents or certain parasitic infestations such as amoebiasis (qv). The symptoms are those normally associated with brain tumour (severe headache and vomiting, for example) together with those of infection (such as fever).

Approximately one-third of cases arise from the direct spread of pus in the middle ear, mastoid process (the knob of bone behind the ear), paranasal sinus, or skull (after injury or surgery). Another third of infections are carried in the blood, from a lung abscess or infection of the heart valves. Patients with lo vered immunity are at increased risk of developing an abscess, frequently due to rather unusual organisms such as fungi and unicellar organisms called toxoplasma.

B

The condition may require surgery to drain the pus if antibiotic therapy at an early stage is unsuccessful.

BRAIN DEATH

Patients with severe brain damage may have their other vital functions maintained in intensive care units. Criteria have therefore been defined to establish when the brain is dead, even when a heartbeat continues. These criteria include: a positive diagnosis of structural brain damage, irreversibility of the condition causing damage, and loss of function of the brain-stem which controls vital functions such as respiration.

When these criteria have been satisfied and confirmed by two independent medical specialists, brain death can be diagnosed and as a result life-support systems can be discontinued and organs such as the kidneys, heart, lungs, liver and cornea may be removed for transplantation.

BRAIN SCAN

Any method of imaging the brain; the term may be used to mean a CT scan, an isotope scan or a scan by ultrasound or magnetic resonance imaging (MRI) — see individual entries.

BRAIN TUMOUR

Brain tumours usually arise from the brain tissue itself or from its surrounding membranes (meninges), or may occur as a result of the spread of tumours, from the lung or breast for example. Most brain tumours, apart from those arising from the meninges, are malignant, the degree of malignancy varying from low to high-grade. These tumours rarely spread outside the brain. They occur in all age groups and are one of the commonest forms of cancer in childhood.

As the tumours arise within the confined space of the skull and there is considerable swelling of the surrounding brain tissue, symptoms tend to occur while the tumour is still quite small. Early morning headaches and vomiting, personality changes, drowsiness, fits (see *Convulsions*), loss of co-ordination and weakness of the limbs are some of the symptoms that may be found. A CT scan of the brain is usually needed for making a diagnosis. Sometimes this is followed by a biopsy to confirm the type of brain tumour.

The treatment varies, depending on the site and nature of the tumour. If the tumour is surgically accessible, it is removed to whatever extent possible. Sometimes this may result in a cure. Most meningiomas, which are benign, can be removed completely. However, most malignant brain tumours cannot be cured surgically and radiotherapy or chemotherapy may be needed to improve both the chances of survival and quality of life.

BREAST CANCER

The commonest malignant disease of women in England and Wales, responsible for 15,000 deaths annually. It is estimated that 1 in 12 of all women will develop breast cancer during her lifetime. There is no known cause and its natural history is obscure; it occurs most frequently in Western women between 45 and 55 years old, and is rare in the East. It is more common where there is a family history of breast cancer and in women who have never borne children. Any part of the breast may be affected, though it is commoner in the upper outer area. The most common sign is a lump in the breast. With screening programmes and mammography

BREAST EXAMINATION

1 Stand in front of a mirror and feel each breast in turn for any difference in texture; **2** Look for any changes, expecially in the nipples; **3** With both arms raised, look for any swelling or dimpling in the skin of the breasts; **4** Place a pillow under the right shoulder and put your right arm behind your head; **5** Feel the right breast gently, working from the outside towards the centre; **6** Squeeze the nipple to see if there is any discharge.

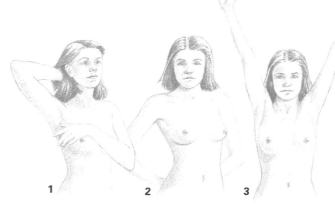

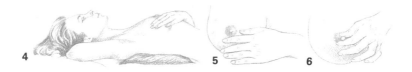

more early tumours are being detected.

Breast tumours spread locally, grow in size and invade increasing amounts of the breast if left untreated. They may invade the skin and pectoral muscles and even the chest wall. They spread via the lymphatic channels to the lymph nodes in the armpits (see Lymphatic system). Spread via the bloodstream produces metastases anywhere in the body. Skeletal (bone) metastases are found most commonly in the ribs, vertebrae and skull. The lungs, adrenal glands and ovaries are also common sites.

Treatment depends on what stage the tumour has reached at the time it is discovered. This involves assessing the size of the lump in the breast, together with the presence of metastases. Treatment may take the form of mastectomy with or without clearance of the nodes in the armpit, or of lumpectomy or local excision (local removal of the tumour preserving the bulk of the breast is usually followed by radiotherapy). Radiotherapy and/or chemotherapy, as well as hormone-manipulating therapy (antioestrogenic drugs), are often used as an adjunct to surgical treatment.

BREAST ENLARGEMENT (in Males)

see *Gynaecomastia*

BREECH

Breech presentation means that the buttocks of the fetus will enter, or already have entered, the birth canal before the fetal head. At 30 weeks' gestation approximately one-third of

Normal presentation   Breech presentation (full)

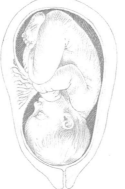
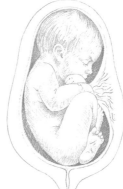

There are three types of breech presentation. In a full breech the legs are bent at the knees and enter the pelvis at the same time as the buttocks. In a footling breech the legs enter

the pelvis before the buttocks. In an extended breech the legs are flexed at the hip and bent upwards alongside the baby's body.

B

fetuses adopt a breech position; the majority will change spontaneously to a head presentation (cephalic) by term (40 weeks) so that only 4 per cent of babies will enter labour as a breech presentation.

Various conditions may cause a breech presentation, such as multiple pregnancies, an abnormally situated placenta, abnormality of uterine (womb) shape or an abnormality of the fetus, but in most cases there is no obvious cause. Most breech presentations are delivered by Caesarean section.

BRITTLE BONE DISEASE

see *Osteogenesis imperfecta*

BRONCHIECTASIS

A chronic chest condition in which the lower airways are largely destroyed and therefore ineffective in transferring oxygen into the bloodstream. Bronchiectasis results from previous severe chest infection but is now rarely a major problem in developed countries other than in patients with cystic fibrosis. Sufferers usually have a continual cough productive of large quantities of yellow-green phlegm (sputum) and have difficulty in breathing (dyspnoea), which may be severe. The fingertips often have a clubbed appearance (see *Clubbing*).

Diagnosis depends on X-ray findings and CT scanning, but bronchography (qv) may be needed to confirm the presence of dilated small bronchi containing pus. Treatment is with antibiotics and postural drainage, a form of physiotherapy (often self-administered) designed to maximize drainage of the secretions from the affected parts of the lung.

BRONCHIOLITIS

A common disease of infancy usually caused by the respiratory syncytial virus (RSV). Inflammation occurs in the small airways within the lungs (bronchioles). The disease is passed on by droplet infection from coughs and sneezes, often from older children or adults in whom RSV causes only a common cold. Susceptible infants develop a more severe illness with breathing difficulty and often with wheezing, which may interfere with feeding. Smaller babies (under 6 months) are worst affected and may need observation in hospital, where tube-feeding (via a tube inserted through the nose) or intravenous fluids can be given if necessary. Oxygen and, in extreme cases, ventilation may be required.

BRONCHITIS

An inflammatory condition of the main airways (windpipe and bronchi) caused by bacteria. Bronchitis may be acute or chronic. Acute bronchitis often follows a common cold, influenza or other viral illness. It is prone to occur in smokers. The condition is signalled by an irritating, unproductive cough and often upper chest discomfort. Most people gradually recover over a few days; a course of antibiotic treatment may be necessary. Cough mixtures may also help.

Chronic bronchitis is a condition characterized by a persistent cough and production of phlegm after continuous exposure to an irritant such as tobacco smoke. Exposure to dampness or infection may exacerbate the condition, which affects more men than women and occurs most commonly in middle and late adult life. Wheezing and retention of phlegm may also be noticed. As the condition

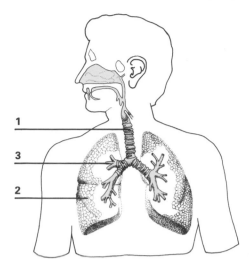

Bronchitis affects the windpipe
(1) and the bronchial tubes in the
lungs **(2)**. In chronic cases the
small airways, or bronchioles **(3)**,
are gradually destroyed.

B

progresses, the small airways are destroyed, leading to emphysema (qv). In periods when the condition becomes much worse, treatment with antibiotics and physiotherapy may be required, as may bronchodilator drugs to relieve constriction of the airways. Chronic bronchitis may eventually lead to heart failure.

BRONCHODILATOR

Drugs which increase the diameter of airways narrowed as a consequence of disease such as asthma and chronic bronchitis. In asthma, for example, these drugs reduce spasm of the muscle in the airways (bronchospasm); salbutamol and terbutaline are commonly used for this purpose. Several types of bronchodilator are available, including pressurized inhalers. Bronchodilators are best inhaled, but may also be administered orally. In some circumstances, inhaled steroids or a course of oral steroids may also be necessary to promote bronchodilation.

BRONCHOGRAPHY

A method of examining the respiratory passages in the lung using a special material called contrast medium which shows up on X-rays.

This examination has largely been superseded by direct imaging of the bronchial tree using a fibreoptic instrument (bronchoscopy, qv) and computerized tomography (CT scan, qv) but may still occasionally be performed in the investigation of bronchiectasis.

BRONCHO-PNEUMONIA

see *Pneumonia*

BRONCHOSCOPY

An examination of the interior of the larger bronchial tubes. Bronchoscopy involves passing a flexible fibreoptic instrument (bronchoscope), usually through the nose, into the tubes that lead into the lungs (the bronchi). The procedure is usually performed under mild sedation, together with local anaesthesia to the nose, throat and larynx (voice-box). The bronchoscope carries a fibreoptic light so that the operator (bronchoscopist) can see into the different bronchi of the lungs. Any disease observed in the lungs can be biopsied and the samples sent to the laboratory for microscopic examination. Secretions can be sucked out of the lungs to diagnose infectious diseases, and in rare instances the bronchoscopist can retrieve a foreign body inhaled by the patient.

BRONCHOSPASM

Narrowing of the bronchial airways, caused by contraction of the smooth muscle that surrounds the bronchi in the lungs.

Episodic bronchospasm is a common, and treatable, symptom of asthma (qv). Constant irreversible

B

bronchospasm is the main feature of chronic obstructive bronchial disease, such as emphysema.

The condition is treated by bronchodilator drugs (qv), which work by relaxing the smooth muscle.

BRUCELLOSIS

An infection commonly caused by the organism *Brucella abortus*. It is spread from cattle to man by the drinking of raw milk; the boiling or pasteurization of milk prevents the condition. The incubation period is about three weeks. Symptoms are usually variable and gradual in onset. They include weakness, loss of appetite and pain in the limbs, back and head, together with constipation, cough, sore throat and pain in the joints. The patient's temperature fluctuates, a characteristic which gave rise to the condition's alternative name, 'undulant fever'. The disease can usually be confirmed by a blood test. Treatment is with antibiotics.

BRUIT

An abnormal sound or murmur (qv) heard through the stethoscope, and usually produced by abnormal or turbulent blood flow. Narrowing (stenosis) of an artery due to disease is commonly signalled by a bruit. For example, a blowing sound heard over the abdomen may indicate an aneurysm or dilatation of the abdominal aorta (the main artery). Both tumour circulation and the normal placenta in a pregnant woman produce turbulent blood flow which gives rise to a bruit sounding like a continuous hum.

BULIMIA NERVOSA

An eating disorder found mainly in young women. Some of the symptoms are similar to those found in anorexia nervosa (qv). Symptoms include bingeing (that is, the consumption of a large amount of food in a short period of time), attempting to get rid of the effects of eating by self-induced vomiting or the use of laxatives, and great anxiety about gaining weight. Sufferers often alternate between periods of rigorous dieting and over-eating. Some use methods such as excessive exercise, diuretics and slimming tablets to control weight. Psychological approaches, such as cognitive psychotherapy, have been shown to be effective treatments.

BUNION

Thickening of the skin and joint at the base of the big toe. This development is related to a common deformity of the toe called hallux valgus, which is commoner in women than men and is seen with increasing frequency with advancing years. The wearing of tight shoes that taper towards the front causes hallux valgus and consequently bunions. Gradually the big toe is pushed over its neighbour digit by the pressure of the shoe, the base of the big toe becomes increasingly prominent, and a protective pad develops, which may become chronically inflamed; the lesion is termed a bunion.

A soft pad to cover the bunion will often relieve pain and discomfort. Comfortable shoes must be worn. In severe cases the hallux valgus may be corrected surgically and the bunion removed at the same time.

BURNS

The term usually refers to tissue damage caused by heat. However, a variety of caustic chemicals and ultraviolet light (such as sunlight) may also induce a burn. Simple superficial burns require immediate treatment with cold water: the affected part is held under cold running water until the pain is relieved. The burn should be regularly and gently cleansed with an appropriate antiseptic fluid and covered with non-stick dressings until healing occurs; painkillers should be taken if required. Sometimes even non-stick dressings may adhere to burn sites, so it is often helpful to apply an antiseptic cream directly to the dressings. Where a burn has resulted in damage to the full thickness of the skin, preventing natural tissue regeneration, then surgical treatment such as skin grafting (qv) may be required. Extensive burns result in the body rapidly losing life-sustaining fluid and electrolytes (salts such as sodium and potassium) through the skin. Such cases must be managed in a specialized unit equipped to provide the high level of care required.

BURSITIS

Inflammation of the bursa, a small sac with a smooth lining (synovial membrane) which produces a thick lubricating fluid (synovial fluid). Bursae are present around joints and bony prominences where they protect the tendons and muscles from rubbing against the bones and joints which they travel across.

The most common cause of bursitis is inflammation due to rheumatoid arthritis. The inflammation causes drying out of the bursa with loss of the synovial fluid, and swelling of the synovium to produce the characteristic nodules of rheumatoid arthritis. The bursa can also dry out as a result of over-use or from inflammation in the synovial membrane to produce pain in the affected muscle when it is moved in a particular way.

Bursitis may be treated by sucking out the fluid that accumulates as a result of the inflammation (aspiration), injection of steroids, or surgical removal of the bursa (bursectomy).

BYPASS

The term 'bypass' has two meanings in medicine. First, it may describe a method of providing artificial circulation and oxygenation, bypassing the heart and lungs, employed in thoracic (chest) and cardiac surgery. This is known medically as a cardiopulmonary bypass.

Secondly, bypass may mean an operation to carry arterial blood from a large artery to a smaller one, thereby circumventing a blockage (often caused by atherosclerosis — see *Atheroma*) in the artery. Coronary artery bypass is the most commonly performed. The patient is put on a heart-lung machine and a piece of reversed saphenous vein taken from the patient's lower leg is joined at one end to the aorta (the main artery) and at the other to one of the coronary arteries beyond the blockage; in this way the blood supply is resumed to a previously bloodless or ischaemic area and anginal pains are reduced.

Artificial materials may be used if the patient has no suitable veins. The results of bypass surgery are good but frequently marred by progression of the atherosclerosis.

CACHEXIA

The marked loss of muscle and fat. Cachexia is found in some chronic and disabling illnesses such as tuberculosis or cancer, despite a normal or increased intake of food. The reason for this is poorly understood, but may be due to a hormone released by the growth.

CAESAREAN SECTION

The removal of a baby from the uterus (womb) through its mother's abdomen. Caesarean section accounts for between 10 and 20 per cent of all births.

There are two types of Caesarean section: elective and emergency. An elective Caesarean is performed on a planned basis to overcome known problems. For example, in cases of the mother's pelvis being small in relation to the size of the baby (disproportion); the presentation or position of the baby making normal delivery impossible or unsafe; or the afterbirth or placenta blocking the birth canal (placenta praevia). An emergency Caesarean is performed when problems develop during labour; for example, a baby with the umbilical cord tightly round its neck may need immediate delivery by this method, as may cases involving maternal illness or bleeding.

The operation may be carried out under epidural anaesthesia rather than general anaesthesia.

CAISSON DISEASE

see *Bends*

CALCINOSIS

A rare condition in which abnormal deposits of calcium salts are laid down just beneath the skin (subcutaneous tissue) in muscle, tendons and certain organs. Calcinosis may occur in flat plaques or in large swellings, or lumps, near larger joints; the latter is called tumoural calcinosis. The cause of the condition is unknown and no treatment is required. Often the signs of calcinosis only show up on X-ray and there are no symptoms.

CALCIUM ANTAGONIST

A class of drug commonly used in the treatment of angina pectoris and high blood pressure; an example is nifedipine. Calcium antagonists work by blocking the entry of calcium ions into certain tissues, notably the smooth muscle that surrounds blood vessels and the electrical conducting tissue of the heart. They prevent blood vessel spasm and produce dilatation instead; called vasodilatation, this allows greater blood flow to the heart muscle and also lowers blood pressure by decreasing resistance to blood flow. Side-effects of flushing, swelling of the ankles and postural hypotension are sometimes experienced when these drugs are used. Calcium antagonists also block the transmission of electrical impulses in the heart and may be used in the treatment of tachycardia (rapid heart rate).

CALCULUS

A 'stone'; a calculus may form in any part of the body, especially in reservoir organs (where fluid is stored) and their passages.

Biliary calculi form within the gallbladder or biliary tree (see *Gallstone*) and may cause inflammation (cholecystitis) and biliary colic.

Salivary calculi are most commonly found in the submandibular salivary gland (below the jaw) or within the duct that drains saliva from the gland to the mouth. They are usually visible on a plain X-ray. Stones within the duct are easily removed through the ear; those within the gland require surgical removal of the gland itself. Salivary calculi are signalled by swelling (often painful) of the affected gland in response to food. Parotid calculi (the parotids are salivary glands behind the jaw) are far less common.

Urinary calculi form within the pelvis of the kidney and cause severe colicky loin pain (uteric or renal colic) with haematuria (blood in the urine) when they pass along the ureter (the tube leading to the bladder). The pain ceases once the stones reach the bladder (vesical calculi); see *Urolithiasis*.

Calculi may also occur in the pancreas and prostate gland.

CALLUS

The term has two meanings in medicine. First, it may describe the hard thick skin that occurs when an area is subject to prolonged friction. The most common site is on the sole of the foot over the 'ball' area.

Callus is also the bone-like reparative substance that forms around the edges and fragments of a broken bone. It is built up in the swelling that surrounds a fracture which slowly ossifies and gives the site increasing rigidity and strength. Callus is slowly reabsorbed during the healing process and eventually disappears completely.

CANCER

The general term for all forms of tumour which are malignant in nature. From the time of Hippocrates until recently, the diagnosis of cancer meant fear and despair for patients but thanks to research, early diagnosis and better treatment almost 50 per cent of people who are newly diagnosed may be alive five years later and some of these may be cured.

Cancer mainly affects the elderly. In most developed countries it is the second most common cause of death after heart disease, accounting for 20 per cent of all deaths. Current estimates suggest that about one-quarter to one-third of people now born in the developed world will develop a cancer in their lifetime. While some cancers are distributed fairly uniformly throughout the world, others have a very high incidence in certain areas — for example, stomach cancer in Japan, or liver cancer in East and South Africa.

Cancer is, in most cases, thought to be derived from a single abnormal cell that has gone wrong and escaped from the normal control mechanism. This theory is supported by the finding that a single cancer cell injected into an experimental animal under the right conditions can cause cancer formation. Cancer cells do not necessarily grow faster than the normal cells of the body. The basic difference between them is that in normal adults the number of new cells produced exactly balances the number lost, while in cancer the number of tumour cells produced exceeds the number that die. Once established, the cancer proliferates relentlessly by invading local tissue and by metastasis and, unless successfully treated, leads to death. Tumours derived from lining or epithelial cells are called carcinomas. Tumours of connective tissue are called sarcomas (qv).

Although a number of factors are known to be associated with cancer in humans, the exact cause of the majority of human cancers is not yet known. It is thought that most cancers are caused by 'multiple hit'. Some people have an inherent genetic predisposition to cancer and this is triggered by exposure to secondary factors. These include cigarette smoke, certain types of food, radiation, chemicals, viruses and excessive exposure to the ultraviolet rays of the sun. It has been suggested that if people stopped smoking cigarettes, reduced their

C

alcohol and fat intake, increased dietary fibre and avoided exposure to strong sunlight, the incidence of cancer might be reduced.

SEE ALSO *Breast cancer, Leukemia, Lung cancer, Melanoma, Myeloma*

CANDIDA

A type of yeast-like fungus which is commonly found on the skin in the mouth, gut and vagina; also known as thrush. It does not normally cause any harm but under certain conditions, such as debilitating illness and prematurity, it can produce disease.

When candida occurs in the mouth and throat it causes soreness and difficulty in swallowing and forms white, cheesy patches called oral thrush. In the vagina it causes itching and discharge; this occurs mainly in women who are pregnant, diabetic or on the contraceptive pill. Candidal infection of the skin tends to occur in moist areas, such as beneath the breast and in the groin.

Candida can be treated easily in most cases by topical antifungal antibiotics. In conditions giving rise to decreased immunity, such as steroid treatment or leukaemia, the infection can spread to the oesophagus (gullet) and lungs and through the blood to other organs, such as the kidneys. In these life-threatening situations, treatment with more powerful antifungal antibiotics is necessary.

SEE ALSO *Fungal disease*

CANNABIS

An illegal psychoactive drug derived from the flower of Indian hemp (*Cannabis sativa*) and which is more commonly known as marijuana. A derivative of the drug is used therapeutically as an antiemetic to prevent vomiting.

CARBOHYDRATE

Compounds composed of sugars and/ or sugar polymers (made up of many relatively simple repeated units) which provide energy. In pure form carbohydrate contains carbon, oxygen and hydrogen. Naturally occurring carbohydrate-rich foods — wheat, rice and potatoes — are composed of starches which are polymers of the simple sugars glucose (dextrose), fructose, maltose and their compounds (sucrose, for example).

Mammals utilize carbohydrate in two forms: in the simple form, as an immediate energy source which can be used by all cells in the body; and as an energy reserve, in the form of glycogen, which is a polymer similar to starch in plants.

Lactose, a sugar made up of glucose and galactose, is the principal carbohydrate in breast milk.

CARCINOID SYNDROME

A condition due to a rare, slow-growing malignant tumour, usually of the small intestine. Symptoms usually only develop once the cancer spreads to the liver, producing metastases. The classic features include episodic facial flushing, fever, acute breathlessness and wheezing, abdominal pain and diarrhoea. These are due to the secretion of a hormone called serotonin by the tumour. The diagnosis is made by detecting the breakdown products of serotonin in the urine.

Treatment of the syndrome proceeds on two fronts and is aimed not only at the tumour, using cytotoxic drugs to kill the cancer cells, but at reducing the effects of the hormonal symptoms by using agents which block them.

CARDIAC ARREST

The sudden cessation of circulation as a result of an electrical disturbance of the heart (ventricular fibrillation or asystole). Consciousness is lost within seconds as the ventricle (one of the two lower chambers of the heart) expels no blood; if circulation is not restored rapidly, brain damage or death may occur from lack of oxygen (anoxia). The condition is recognized by the absence of a pulse; respiration ceases and the pupils dilate shortly after the pulse stops. Heart attack (myocardial infarction) is the commonest cause, although many other conditions and drugs may precipitate cardiac arrest.

Treatment involves restoring both circulation and respiration through first aid. If a single blow to the chest is not successful, then external cardiac compression is required. The patient is placed on a firm surface and the lower sternum or breastbone compressed by 3 cm ($1\frac{1}{4}$ inches) by the 'heels' of both hands at the rate of 60 beats per minute. Ventilation is as important as circulation and mouth-to-mouth resuscitation must be started at the same time. The lungs must be expanded at a rate of 15 times per minute (once every fourth compression). First aid measures can be very effective if the heart is healthy before cardiac arrest, and half of the people with underlying heart disease may be resuscitated. If first aid is successful, further measures may be necessary if anoxia has damaged the brain and kidneys.

CARDIAC CATHETERIZATION

A special study of the anatomy and function of the heart and large blood vessels using X-ray techniques, pressure recordings and blood measurements. It is used in the investigation of congenital heart disease, disease of the heart valves and to study the coronary arteries prior to bypass graft operations.

CARDIOMYOPATHY

Disorder of the heart muscles. The term is usually used to describe two clinical syndromes: hypertrophic obstructive cardiomyopathy (HOCM) and congestive cardiomyopathy (COCM).

In hypertrophic cardiomyopathy, which sometimes runs in families, an abnormality of the heart muscle cell results in a loss of distensibility of the left ventricle (the chamber that pumps blood to the body). Failure of this ventricle to distend properly causes symptoms of breathlessness, fluid in the lungs and fainting. Some patients may develop angina. The heart-muscle, particularly the left ventricle, also overgrows (hypertrophies) and this may cause the valve in the base of the aorta (the main artery) to narrow, obstructing the outflow of blood from the left ventricle. The mitral valve between the left atrium and left ventricle fails to close properly and this combination of valvular stenosis and incompetence leads rapidly to heart failure. Beta-blocking drugs may be effective in reducing the symptoms caused by outflow obstruction.

Congestive cardiomyopathy is not as a rule familial. The term covers a large group of unrelated disorders that tend to present as heart failure. (By convention, heart failure due to ischaemia, high blood pressure, or rheumatic heart disease is excluded from the group.) Principal symptoms are breathlessness, cough, fluid on the lungs and swelling of the legs and ankles. Angina and arrhythmias may

C

be features. Commonly, no cause can be found but other conditions such as alcoholism, thiamine deficiency (beriberi), viral infections, systemic lupus erythematosus, polyarteritis nodosa, muscular dystrophy and thyroid disease may damage heart muscles and cause congestive cardio-myopathy. The treatment is the same as that for heart failure (qv).

CARIES

Dental decay, due to the destruction of the enamel cover of teeth by bacteria in the mouth. It is the most prevalent disease affecting the human race and virtually no areas of the world are spared. Caries affects both sexes of all races and every socio-economic group and once it occurs persists through-out life even though the initial prob-lem is treated. It usually begins shortly after the first teeth erupt.

Tooth decay is thought to be caused by the interaction of food particles (especially sugar) and dental plaque to form an acidic solution which destroys the tooth structure. Dental plaque is a soft, non-calcified bacterial deposit which accumulates naturally on the surface of teeth and is known to con-tain acid-producing bacteria.

Dental caries may be controlled by

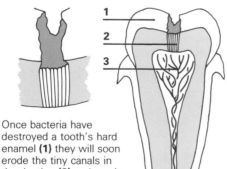

Once bacteria have destroyed a tooth's hard enamel **(1)** they will soon erode the tiny canals in the dentine **(2)** and reach the pulp chamber **(3)** containing nerves and blood vessels. If the decay is left untreated, the tooth will eventually die.

cutting down on sugar-containing foods, fluoridation, brushing the teeth and using dental floss to remove debris from tooth surfaces.

CARPAL TUNNEL SYNDROME

This condition is the result of com-pression of the median nerve as it passes into the wrist through the carpal tunnel. It causes pain and tingling in the area supplied by the nerve, namely the thumb, index and middle finger as well as half of the ring finger and half of the palm. The pain can be severe enough to cause the patient to wake during the night. While the condition usually affects one hand only, both hands may be involved. Some hand muscles may be weak, often inter-preted as 'clumsiness' by the patient, and there may be wasting of muscles associated with the thumb.

Often there is no obvious cause for the compression of the nerve, but it is generally due to swelling of tendon sheaths. The condition is particularly common in middle-aged women, and may also occur in pregnancy, hypo-thyroidism, rheumatoid arthritis and acromegaly. The disease is confirmed by nerve conduction studies.

Although splinting the wrist may help, the best form of treatment is to divide the ligament under which the nerve passes (the flexor retinaculum) surgically at the wrist. This minor operation immediately relieves the pressure on the nerve.

CARRIER

There are two ways in which this term is used in medicine. First, a person may be a carrier of an infec-tious agent. All of us carry many bacteria on the surface of and within our bodies; some of them are harmless but others are potentially harmful and can cause disease, given the right conditions to multiply. An example of carrier status is the 2—15 per cent of the population who carry the *Neisseria meningitidis* bacterium in their nasal passages. This agent is responsible for the outbreaks of meningitis which occur in 8—12 year cycles, especially in groups living in close proximity. Similarly, there are carriers of the organisms responsible for other epidemic infections such as typhoid, cholera and diphtheria. Carrier status is also found with viral agents, notably the millions of carriers of the hepatitis B virus.

Secondly, a person may be a carrier of a hereditary disorder.

SEE ALSO *Dominant, Recessive* and *Sex-linked (Pattern of Inheritance)*

CATARACT

A painless condition in which the lens of the eye becomes cloudy and ultimately opaque, causing blindness of the affected eye. It is found in a number of rare inherited conditions but is seen in developed countries mostly in the elderly (and after some forms of eye injury). Treatment is by removing the affected lens surgically. This, however, causes a major blurring of vision (refractory error), which can only be corrected by thick, pebble-like spectacles. These make binocular vision in which both eyes work together difficult, as the views seen by the normal eye and the lensless eye are of different sizes. This problem is largely overcome by the use of contact lenses, but many old people find these difficult to use. In recent years surgeons have become more skilled in the safe use of artificial lenses implanted within the eye in the position of the natural lens.

CATATONIA

Usually refers to a form of schizophrenia in which a sufferer has a limited ability to communicate his or her thoughts and behaviour is patently abnormal. The abnormalities of behaviour may include maintaining an awkward and unusual posture for a long period of time or making unusual movements that appear to have a special meaning. In severe catatonia a patient may be mute.

Treatment is described under *Schizophrenia.*

CATHETER

A tube, often flexible, which can be inserted into an organ or body cavity to sample, drain or collect fluid. A typical example is a urinary catheter. These catheters are made from materials such as polythene, rubber and silicone rubber. If the catheter is required to remain in the bladder for some time, a special type, called the Foley catheter, is used. It incorporates a balloon at the tip which can be inflated to keep the catheter in place.

Cardiac catheters can be used to enter large blood vessels in the groin,

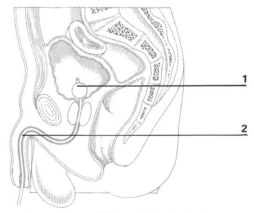

A urinary catheter **(1)** is used if urination is not possible voluntarily; for example, in unconscious patients after surgery or in patients with an enlarged prostate gland. It is passed through the urethra **(2)** to drain the bladder.

and via these the aorta (the main artery) and the heart. Once in position, they can be used to measure pressures and take samples of blood for analysis.

Other varieties of catheter are used to drain fluid from the chest and abdomen in certain conditions, and also to add fluid to the abdomen in the case of patients undergoing peritoneal dialysis for kidney failure.

CAT SCAN

see *CT scan*

CELL

see *Cytology*

CELLULITIS

Diffuse inflammation of the soft tissues producing redness, tenderness, heat and swelling. The term is generally used with reference to inflammation of the skin but essentially the same processes occur in internal organs such as the alimentary tract, lungs and upper airway.

Cellulitis is due to bacterial infection, often occurring after a laceration. Other predisposing factors include obstruction of the sweat glands or vessels in the lymphatic system, exposure to chemical irritants, and in the legs swelling of the tissues under the skin due to obstruction of the veins or heart failure. Once cellulitis has become established it spreads along the path of least resistance, along the planes where the tissue may have split, and also into the lymphatic vessels, producing inflammation. The lymphatics drain towards the lymph nodes, which become enlarged. If the walls of veins are affected, thrombosis (thrombophlebitis) may follow. Abscesses may form. Treatment is with an appropriate antibiotic and drainage of any abscess.

CEREBRAL PALSY

Abnormality of posture and movement resulting from injury to the brain, which may have occurred in the fetus during pregnancy (for example, if the mother had rubella — German measles), during birth (as in brain haemorrhage) or in infancy (for example, meningitis). The area of the brain that is injured determines the type of movement disorder and the part of the body affected. Cerebral palsy affects about 2 in 1,000 5-year-olds.

Diagnosis may be difficult in early infancy. Although brain damage does not get any worse, the signs of the abnormality may change as the baby grows and develops. The commonest form of cerebral palsy is characterized by increased stiffness or spasticity of certain muscle groups on both sides of the body (diplegia); it may affect one or more limbs, or sometimes half of the body (hemiplegia). Other types are athetoid (frequent writhing movements), ataxic (with tremor) and dyskinetic (with variable stiffness). The child's muscles may be weak, or he or she may have difficulty controlling movement; this may be mild, moderate or severe. Common associated features, such as impaired intellect, epilepsy, poor vision and deafness, are important in determining the degree of handicap.

Treatment depends on the cooperation of many disciplines. Special schooling may be necessary in some cases.

CEREBROSPINAL FLUID (CSF)

A colourless fluid present within the ventricular system of cavities in the brain and surrounding the brain and spinal cord. It is formed by filtration

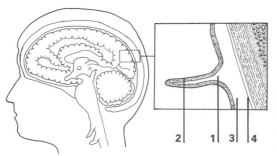

In the brain, cerebrospinal fluid **(1)** lies between three sheets of tissue called the meninges: pia mater **(2)**, arachnoid mater **(3)** and dura mater **(4)**. (See also illustration of Lumbar Puncture on page 181.)

of the plasma that circulates within blood vessels, and contains glucose and small amounts of protein. CSF is produced by special organs lying within all four ventricles. Fluid in the fourth ventricle communicates with a small central canal running the length of the spinal cord. It also passes through three small openings in the roof of the ventricle to communicate with CSF bathing the brain and spinal cord. The average volume of CSF in the human body is 100–150 ml, (4–5 fl oz), of which one-fifth lies in the ventricles. CSF flowing over the surface of the brain is reabsorbed into the cerebral veins.

CERVICAL EROSION

A condition in which the squamous or scaly type of epithelium lining the vaginal cervix is absent from part of it and replaced by columnar epithelium (a single layer of long, narrow cells) and patchy areas of granulation tissue (small masses of formative cells). Cervical erosion is common in women taking oral contraceptives. It may also be congenital. Symptoms such as vaginal discharge and irritation may be present, although there may be none at all. In all cases the area of apparent erosion is biopsied to exclude

malignancy. The most satisfactory treatment is cauterization, either with electrical cautery or by low temperature freezing (cryosurgery).

CERVICAL SMEAR

A screening test whose objective it is to detect pre-cancerous changes in the skin (epithelium) of the cervix (neck of the womb). These changes are thought to occur well in advance of cancer developing.

It is known that many women with abnormal smears will never develop cervical cancer. Nevertheless they do represent a section of the population who are at high risk and need careful follow-up. Minor changes often return to normal without any intervention, but changes that worsen or persist require further investigation, by colposcopy (qv).

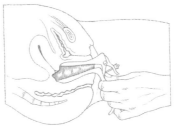

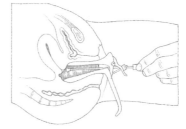

A cervical smear is a painless procedure and takes only a few minutes. The vagina is held open with a speculum **(top)** to allow a sample of cells to be collected from the surface of the cervix **(bottom)** for microscopic examination.

Smears should be performed on all women who have been heterosexually active. They should be repeated every three to five years; more frequently if there has been a history of abnormal smears.

CERVICAL SPONDYLOSIS

see *Spondylosis*

CHAGAS' DISEASE

see *Trypanosomiasis*

CHANCRE

This is usually the first sign of syphilis, a sexually transmitted disease caused by the spirochaete bacterium *Treponema pallicum*; it appears after an incubation period of 9–90 days after intercourse with an infected person. It starts as a small painless lump at the site of infection, which is usually, though not invariably, the genital region. Soon this breaks down to form an ulcerated area with a raised hard border. Lymph nodes adjacent to the chancre also enlarge. Healing takes place after some weeks, leaving a small scar. This constitutes primary syphilis (qv).
SEE ALSO *Spirochaete*

CHANCROID

A sexually transmitted disease. Chancroid is endemic in tropical and subtropical areas and is caused by a bacterium called *Haemophilus ducreyi*, which gains entrance to the body through breaks in the skin. The incubation period is 3–5 days, after which a painful pimple (papule) forms, typically on the genitalia. The pimple eventually ruptures, forming an ulcer. Further ulcers develop in the surrounding skin; these are tender to the touch and bleed easily. The disease may progress rapidly, resulting in massive destruction of tissue.

Treatment is with antibiotics and general measures such as improving hygiene. Further tests are usually carried out to check whether the patient has other venereal diseases.

CHEMOTHERAPHY

Treatment with chemicals or drugs. The term is mostly associated with the use of drugs in the treatment of cancers and leukaemias, but may also be applied to antibiotic treatment. One of two approaches may be adopted: aggressive (radical) chemotherapy, which is designed to effect a cure; and palliative chemotherapy, which aims to relieve symptoms and/or prolong life in cases where there is no expectation or hope of a cure.

Radical chemotherapy is used in the treatment of some patients with lymphoma, leukaemia, testicular teratoma and seminoma, and in a relatively small but steadily increasing proportion of patients with cancer of other organs. The best chance of cure in any of these conditions (assuming that the extent is too great for surgery or curative radiotherapy) is with the first sequence of courses of cytotoxic drugs. Rarely is a single drug sufficient, so regimes of 'combination' chemotherapy have been established. These use three or more drugs, acting in different but complementary ways, to maximize tumour cell death with minimal damage to the patient. Nevertheless, the side-effects that patients experience may be severe, including hair loss (alopecia) marked nausea and vomiting. The effects of the drugs on the bone marrow are also serious, since this becomes profoundly suppressed; as cells in the bone marrow make blood cells, chemotherapy will cause a drastic reduction in the white blood cells necessary to combat infection (thrombocytopaenia). Damage to the nerves, the kidney and the heart may also occur and occasionally patients may die as a result of their treatment rather than directly from their disease. The problems can be anticipated and minimized by antiemetic drugs to reduce vomiting, scalp-cooling to reduce hair loss and a variety of other manoeuvres to 'rescue' the patient from an otherwise dangerously high dose of cytotoxic medication. It is usual for a patient to need upwards of four courses of chemotherapy, spaced at intervals of 3—6 weeks. Hospital admission is generally necessary. The discomfort and risks of radical chemotherapy are justified only by the aim of complete cure.

Palliative chemotherapy aims to improve the patient's quality (and length) of life when a cure is not possible and the hazards of radical chemotherapy cannot be justified. Many women with advanced breast cancer are prescribed tablets of tamoxifen which are free of side-effects; these slow the progression of the tumour, improve the quality of life and postpone death — an example of palliative chemotherapy at its best. Hospital admission should not normally be required.

CHEYNE-STOKES RESPIRATION

An abnormal form of periodic breathing characterized by alternating bouts of non-respiration (apnoea) and deep respiration. The person often lies motionless for 15—20 seconds and then begins to breathe, shallowly at first and then progressively deepening to a maximum, and finally shallowly again, decreasing to another period of apnoea. When breathing is taking place, respirations are regular.

The cause of this type of disturbance lies in the control centre for respiration in the brain (the respiratory centre), which is normally regulated by carbon dioxide levels in the blood. In certain circumstances the respiratory centre becomes abnormally sensitive to these levels. During the periods of apnoea, the carbon dioxide level in the blood rises, and then stimulates the respiratory centre. As breathing becomes deeper, carbon dioxide is eliminated from the lungs, the blood level falls and the stimulus to the respiratory centre decreases; hence breathing becomes more shallow before the next period of apnoea. A cyclical chain of events is, therefore, created.

Conditions in which Cheyne-Stokes respiration is seen include congestive cardiac failure, brain damage due to injury or stroke, or chronic hypoxia (inadequate oxygen in the blood). Treatment is directed at the underlying cause.

CHICKENPOX

A usually mild illness of early childhood caused by the *Varicella zoster* virus (one of the herpes group); also known as varicella. Chickenpox may be life-threatening if it occurs in the newborn or those with immune deficiency (leukaemia patients, for example). The highly contagious infection is spread by droplets from coughs and sneezes and by contact with the rash that is characteristic of the illness. After an incubation period of 2—3 weeks the illness may begin with a day or so of fever and malaise (a general feeling of being unwell) before the rash appears. Initially, this consists of a few flat red spots which rapidly develop into blisters (vesicles). Successive crops of spots appear over about five days, and take a further three to four days to crust over. The infectious period lasts until all the spots have formed crusts.

No specific treatment is necessary for chickenpox, although an antiviral agent (acyclovir) is available for unusually severe cases. Chickenpox does not recur but the causal virus may remain dormant in the sensory nerves after the initial infection and re-emerge in later life to cause shingles (see *Herpes zoster*). There is no generally available vaccine.

CHILBLAIN

An area of painful discoloration of the skin resulting from cold-induced injury to the underlying blood vessels. The most effective treatment for chilblains is gentle rewarming of the affected part at room temperature.

CHLAMYDIA

A group of specialized bacteria. *Chlamydia trachomatis* is an organism that commonly causes infection of the genital tract, leading to non-specific urethritis (NSU) in the male. It can also cause conjunctivitis in the newborn. In the Third World, chlamydia eye infections are the commonest cause of blindness.

Chlamydia is thought to be responsible for 50 per cent of cases of NSU. With this infection men develop pain on passing urine and a discharge from the urethra (the tube which carries urine away from the bladder) 2–3 weeks after sexual contact. Symptoms are uncommon in women, although occasionally severe pelvic inflammatory disease (with pain, fever, and so on) may develop. Treatment is with antibiotics for 2–3 weeks; both partners should be treated and intercourse should be avoided during treatment.

CHLOASMA

A patchy brown discoloration of the skin which usually appears on the forehead and cheeks. It commonly occurs in normal pregnancy and is thought to be due to changes in the levels of oestrogen hormones in the body. In pregnant women chloasma usually, but not invariably, disappears soon after the birth of the baby. A similar pigmentation is seen in some women who use contraceptive pills containing oestrogens. Chloasma is rare in men, but it can occur in both sexes in some epileptic patients taking the drug phenytoin. Chloasma has little clinical significance but can be unsightly.

CHOLANGITIS

A condition caused by blockage of the common bile duct. The bile passages in the liver form the bile ducts, and these join to form a common bile duct which drains bile from the liver into the bowel. Infection commonly occurs if the bile duct is blocked by a gallstone or any disease resulting in narrowing of the duct (such as a growth in the pancreas). The infection and narrowing result in jaundice, fever and rigors. The infection spreads rapidly into the bloodstream, causing septicaemia, with a fall in blood pressure. This combination is called cholangitis.

The treatment of cholangitis involves antibiotics to combat the infection, fluid replacement to improve the blood pressure, and drainage of the bile duct to relieve the jaundice. The modern treatment is to bypass the blockage with a fine tube (called a stent) placed by ERCP (Endoscopic Retrograde Cholangio-Pancreatography), or passed through the skin into the liver with guidance from X-rays. An operation on the common bile duct may be necessary in some cases.

CHOLECYSTECTOMY

Surgical removal of the gall-bladder, performed for gallstones or inflammation of the gall-bladder (cholecystitis).

Cholecystectomy is performed under general anaesthesia through an incision beneath and parallel to the ribs; some surgeons prefer a vertical incision. It is usual for a procedure called an operative cholangiogram to be performed during the operation to ensure that no gallstones remain in the bile ducts. If stones are present in the duct system an exploration of the common bile duct is then performed. Hospital stay is from 5−12 days and convalescence takes 6−12 weeks.

CHOLECYSTITIS

Inflammation of the gall-bladder when it is irritated by a gallstone. Usually the stone causes infection in the gall-bladder or a blockage at its mouth. These both result in inflammation and swelling in the walls of the gall-bladder. The patient suffers a severe pain in the upper abdomen, which is also felt in the right side of the back and may last for several hours. There is sometimes a single stone composed of cholesterol (fat which is made in the liver and excreted in the bile), or many smaller stones made of bile pigments, but a mixture of constituents is the most common. These can be diagnosed with an ultrasound scan or special X-ray called a cholecystogram (see *Cholecystography*).

The acute infection usually settles with antibiotics. However, the diseased gall-bladder needs to be removed by an operation called a

cholecystectomy to prevent further attacks of pain and to prevent the stones passing into the bile ducts and causing obstructive jaundice or cholangitis (qv). Techniques are now being developed for treating gallstones without surgery, either by giving drugs in an attempt to dissolve them or by crushing them with a lithotripter.
SEE ALSO *Jaundice, Stricture*

CHOLECYSTO-GRAPHY

A radiological examination of the gall-bladder which is undertaken to detect the presence of gallstones (calculi) or disease of the wall of the gall-bladder, and to give an indication of whether the gall-bladder is working properly.

The gall-bladder is not normally visible on plain X-rays of the abdomen unless it is hardened (calcified) or contains hardened gallstones (calcified calculi). In order to see it, a special chemical compound is administered; this contrast agent is excreted by the liver and concentrated in the gall-bladder and biliary ducts. Typically two doses of the contrast agent are given orally (oral cholecystogram or OCG), the first on the eve of the examination and the second on the morning of the examination. After X-ray films have been taken, a fatty meal or drink can then be given in order to test for loss of function; a gall-bladder that is working properly will contract as a result of this intake. In many centres cholecystography has now been replaced by ultrasound examination.

CHOLERA

A severe, acute illness caused by the ingestion of water, milk or food con-

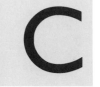

taminated with the *Vibrio cholerae* bacterium. It occurs in hot climates and is associated with poor hygiene. A short incubation period of 1—4 days is followed by vomiting and profuse, watery diarrhoea. These symptoms lead to a marked loss of salt and water from the body and subsequent physical weakness and collapse.

Treatment involves the rapid replacement of water and salts by intravenous fluid infusion ('drip'). Antibiotics may sometimes be given. Vaccination does not provide complete protection but is nevertheless recommended for visitors to countries where the disease is endemic.

CHOREA

A type of involuntary muscular activity, characterized by irregular, non-repetitive and jerking movements. There are two types of chorea: Sydenham's chorea (also known as St Vitus's dance) and Huntington's chorea.

Sydenham's chorea is closely associated with rheumatic fever, of which it is a symptom. The characteristic abnormal movements of both sides of the face and the arms are the result of unknown factors affecting the central nervous system. Speech, chewing, swallowing and respiration may all be affected. See *Rheumatic fever* for treatment.

Huntington's chorea is an autosomal dominant genetic disease in which choreic movements are accompanied by progressively worsening dementia. The condition usually appears between the ages 35 and 45, by which time most patients have had children. However, in a small but significant number of cases the disease becomes apparent before the age of 20. The cause of the disease is not known and there is no treatment.

CHORIOCARCINOMA

A rare tumour of placental tissue; it is the malignant equivalent of a hydatidiform mole (qv). After pregnancy, abortion or hydatidiform mole, any remaining placental tissue not expelled as the afterbirth is usually shed or absorbed by the body. This does not occur after 1 in 10 cases of hydatidiform mole, 1 in 5,000 abortions and 1 in 50,000 normal pregnancies, and the tissue continues to grow and proliferate, forming a choriocarcinoma. As the tissue proliferates it produces large quantities of the hormone human chorionic gonadotrophin (HCG), abnormal bleeding from the uterus (womb) occurs, and the tissue spreads rapidly to the brain, lungs and so on.

All women who have had a hydatidiform mole are followed up closely and their HCG levels monitored. Although uniformly fatal in the past, the outlook for women with this condition has changed dramatically with the advent of increasingly powerful drugs to which this tumour is very sensitive.

CHORIONIC VILLUS BIOPSY

The procedure (otherwise referred to as trophoblast biopsy) whereby a small sample of specialized placental tissue (trophoblast) is removed for examination at an early stage of pregnancy (before 12 weeks). Trophoblast develops at the same time as the embryo and is normally attached to the wall of the uterus (womb). Genetically it is identical to the tissues of the developing fetus and examination of it provides information regarding the genetic structure of the fetal cells. Down's syndrome and Duchenne type muscular dystrophy are two

A sample of chorionic villi is obtained by passing a fine needle on a syringe through the cervix or directly through the abdominal wall so that the tip rests in the placental bed **(1)**. Gentle suction is then applied to collect the sample. The procedure is aided by a speculum **(2)** and ultrasound. The ultrasound probe **(3)** allows the obstetrician an interior view of the mother's womb.

conditions that can be diagnosed at an early stage by using this technique. However, there are certain risks associated with chorionic villus biopsy, the most important being miscarriage, and at present only mothers known to be at risk of carrying an infant with an abnormality are offered the test.

CHOROIDITIS

Inflammation of the choroid, the delicate network of blood vessels just behind the retina (the light-sensitive membrane at the back of the eye). It is usually caused by an invasion of micro-organisms or parasites, especially toxoplasma and toxocara. Historically, tuberculosis, syphilis and leprosy were frequent causes, and still are in certain areas of the world. Choroiditis may be seen in people with AIDS.

The signs of acute infection can easily be seen with an instrument called an opthalmoscope. The main symptom experienced by the patient is blurred vision. Later, white areas with pigmented edges are seen; these may be symptomless. Treatment is with antibiotics and corticosteroids to retard or stop the progress of the disease. Little improvement in vision can be achieved because the damage to the retina is irreparable.

CHRISTMAS DISEASE

A type of haemophilia (qv) in which an inherited deficiency of the blood clotting factor IX results in spontaneous bleeding into the muscles and joints; also known as haemophilia B. It is clinically indistinguishable from the more common type of haemophilia, haemophilia A, in which factor VIII is deficient.

Patients treat themselves regularly at home with injections of factor IX concentrate. Those patients in whom the deficiency is less than severe may only require treatment if bleeding occurs.

CHROMOSOME

A thread-like structure present in the nucleus of a cell; chromosomes contain DNA and its hereditary information. Each chromosome is divided into many individual segments, each known as a gene (qv), which carry the genetic information necessary for the production of a single specific protein. Human cells with a nucleus contain 46 chromosomes arranged as 23 matching pairs: 22 pairs of autosomes and one pair of sex chromosomes. For each pair of autosomes one chromosome is derived from the mother and one from the father. The sex chromosomes are two X chromosomes in a normal female (46XX) and one X and one Y chromosome in a normal male (46XY).

Chromosome abnormalities may be numerical or structural and may occur in both autosomes and sex chromosomes. They are responsible for several disorders. For example, an extra autosome (trisomy) is responsible for most cases of Down's syndrome; an extra X chromosome causes Klinefelter's syndrome (qv), while partial or complete lack of the second X chromosome results in Turner's syndrome (qv). The loss of an autosome is lethal but part of it may be missing, or in the wrong place. The clinical effects of such an occurrence will vary depending on which genes are affected.

SEE ALSO *Dominant* (pattern of inheritance) *Recessive* (pattern of inheritance), *Sex linkage*

CIRRHOSIS OF THE LIVER

A hardening or scarring of the liver, due to one of many different forms of damage to the liver. Common problems causing cirrhosis include excessive alcohol intake, inflammation of the liver due to chronic viral infection (particularly hepatitis B virus), or allergic damage to the liver (chronic active hepatitis or primary biliary cirrhosis). The liver plays an important central role in the general metabolism of the whole human body and if its normal activity is reduced, as in cirrhosis, ill-health will result. The symptoms of cirrhosis include jaundice (retention of the pigment bilirubin, causing a yellow discoloration of the eyes and skin), retention of fluid in the abdomen (ascites) and in the legs

(oedema), a tendency to bleeding (particularly from oesophageal varicose veins) and, ultimately, disturbed mental function.

Established cirrhosis of the liver cannot be reversed, so treatment is aimed at eliminating the cause (for example, alcohol) and dealing with the complications mentioned above. Liver transplantation may be a life-saving treatment for severe cirrhosis.

CLAUDICATION

A severe cramp of the calf muscles, caused by a blockage in the blood vessels supplying the legs. The poor blood flow allows insufficient oxygen to reach the legs and so they are unable to work properly. Both legs are usually affected, but sometimes in varying degree. The disease is almost always due to smoking and has certain characteristic symptoms. A cramp-like pain comes on during exercise (for example, while walking) and prevents further movement. After a short rest the pain disappears only to recur with further exercise when the same distance has been walked. The distance walked, known as the claudication distance, gives an indication of the severity of the blockage in the blood vessels. Without treatment the disease will progress to causing rest pain (the same type of pain experienced with movement now also felt at rest), which is particularly bad at night, and then to gangrene in the foot. If the patient stops smoking, progression of the disease will halt and his or her condition may improve. The narrowed sections of the artery can sometimes be replaced by surgery, easing the pain or preventing gangrene and its treatment by amputation of the affected limb.

SEE ALSO *Angiography*, *atheroma*, *thrombosis*

CLAUSTROPHOBIA

A phobia in which a sufferer reports severe anxiety when in an enclosed space from which escape is difficult, such as a lift, a crowd or an underground train. Although historically a distinction has been made between claustrophobia and agoraphobia (fear of open spaces), there is in reality a great overlap, with sufferers often reporting symptoms of each.

Treatment is described under *Phobia*.

CLEFT LIP

see *Hare lip*

CLEFT PALATE

A condition which arises in the fetus when components of the upper jaw and nose fail to fuse, leaving a Y-shaped gap running from the back of the palate forward to a point just short of the teeth. Often the baby also has a cleft or hare lip (qv).

Cleft palate may interfere with feeding, as the baby may have difficulty making an airtight seal around the teat for sucking, and may regurgitate milk through the nose. An orthodontic plate is used to separate the mouth from the nasal cavity, and also to align the components of the jaw as the baby grows. Cup and spoon feeding may be necessary if sucking proves difficult.

Surgery is usually performed when the baby is about 1 year old, but recently has begun to be possible before birth, in some cases diagnosed *in utero* by ultrasound. Both cleft lip and cleft palate tend to run in families, and there is a 10 per cent chance of malformation being present in other organs. Later problems may include ear infections and abnormalities of dentition.

CLUBBING OF THE FINGERS

A deformity of the ends of the fingers and nails which is associated with a number of illnesses. At first the nail becomes more convex; this progresses to an enlargement of the end of the finger, where the normal 15° angle between the nail bed and the surface of the end of the finger is lost.

Clubbing is routinely looked for by the doctor on physical examination. Five to ten per cent of cases are associated with tumours within the chest, particularly lung cancer. Other underlying conditions include chronic infections in the lung, pneumoconiosis, congenital heart disease with cynanosis and advanced pulmonary heart disease (cor pulmonale). Cirrhosis of the liver, other liver diseases, diarrhoeal states (Crohn's disease, ulcerative colitis and dysentery) and bowel cancer can also cause clubbing.

The fingers will return to normal if the underlying condition is treated. Rarely, clubbing may be hereditary, when it is also known as pachydermoperiostosis. This form is not associated with underlying illness and so does not require treatment.

CLUB FOOT

A deformity of the foot; known medically as talipes. Some cases of club foot have a genetic basis, others result from environmental factors, especially abnormal positions of the fetus in the womb or drugs such as thalidomide.

Some cases respond easily to treatment with strapping. Others are resistant to correction and need surgery to lengthen the tendons and occasionally to reshape the bones. This group of patients often ends up with a short foot, but the treatment is

C

In the commonest type of club foot, equinovarus, the foot points downwards and inwards. The abnormality causes changes in the tendons around the ankle and in the bones of the foot, resulting in permanent deformity by infancy.

effective in correcting the direction of the foot.

COARCTATION OF THE AORTA

A narrowing of the aorta, the major artery arising from the heart. This congenital defect may occur at a number of sites along the part of the aorta which lies in the chest. It results in the pulse and blood pressure rates being different between the two arms or between the legs and the arms. If not detected by clinical examination and X-ray in early life it can lead to high blood pressure (hypertension) and heart failure. Coarctation of the aorta is relatively straightforward to repair surgically.

COCAINE

An alkaloid derived from the leaves of two South American plants (*Erythroxylum coca* and *Erythroxylum truxillense*). Cocaine's medical use is confined to that of a surface local anaesthetic which reduces local blood flow in the eye and the mucous membranes lining the nose.
SEE ALSO *Drug dependence*

COELIAC DISEASE

A congenital condition which results in destruction of the lining of the gut and so interferes with the normal absorption of food. Coeliac disease tends to run in families and arises from an immunological reaction to gliadin, which is a major component of gluten. (Gluten is found in all cereals except rice and corn.) The condition is most often diagnosed in children and is a major cause of failure to thrive and of diarrhoea. It can, however, occur at any age and in varying degrees of severity.

The mainstay of treatment is a gluten-free diet which must be adhered to for life.

COIL

see *Contraception*

COLD, COMMON

A viral infection of the upper respiratory tract, also called coryza. The common cold affects the nasal passages and may involve the pharynx (throat), larynx (voice-box) and trachea (windpipe). Nasal discharge, sneezing and nasal congestion are the usual symptoms, often accompanied by a cough, headache and sore throat. Many viruses can cause the common cold, no single agent being more important. The group known as the rhinoviruses is most frequently implicated. It includes more than ninety different strains; hence the difficulty in developing an effective vaccine. The body's natural defence against a virus, the production of antibodies, only confers protection against re-infection for a year or two. The viruses are transmitted from person to person by droplet infection (carried in the air by coughing and sneezing). Isolation and quarantine are ineffective in preventing the spread of infection: many people will carry the virus without developing symptoms, and the virus is usually excreted 1–2 days before symptoms appear. There is no specific treatment, although aspirin and nasal decongestants are sometimes effective in controlling some of the symptoms.

COLIC

This term may be used in two ways.

First, to describe a type of pain which varies in intensity and is described as 'coming and going'. The pain is usually caused by muscular contraction of one of the body's tubes (bowel, bile ducts or ureter – the tube which leads from the kidney to the bladder), which may be obstructed. Constipation and gastro-enteritis are common underlying causes of abdominal colic at any age. Both biliary colic and ureteral colic are symptoms of obstruction by stones: gallstones are responsible for the first type of colic, and kidney stones for the second.

Secondly, to describe infantile colic, which is a common problem in babies less than 3 months old. It is thought to be related to air swallowing during feeds in the young baby whose sucking and swallowing mechanism is relatively inefficient. In addition there is probably a psychological component related to the interaction between baby and parents. Typically, after the evening feed the baby refuses to settle down to sleep and cries persistently, drawing the knees up as if suffering with abdominal pain. The crying often stops if the child is rocked or picked up by a parent. By 3 months the problem usually clears up. Drug treatment and gripe water are of doubtful benefit.

COLITIS

Inflammation of the large bowel (colon). Colitis is commonly caused either by an infection (dysentery due to salmonella, shigella or amoebiasis), inflammatory bowel disease (ulcerative colitis or Crohn's disease), or more rarely by interruption of the blood supply to the colon in the elderly (ischaemic colitis).

The symptoms of colitis include lower abdominal pain, diarrhoea, and the passing of blood, pus and mucus through the anus. Appropriate investigation may include an examination of the stools to exclude an infection, examination of the rectum and colon using either a rigid tube (sigmoidoscopy) or a flexible fibre-optic tube (colonoscopy – see *Endoscopy*), or a barium enema.

The infectious causes of colitis usually settle spontaneously, but amoebic dysentery always requires treatment with an antibiotic (metronidazole). The condition is usually managed in its acute phase by a form of the drug prednisolone, which is given by injection, by mouth, or by enema or suppositories. A special form of aspirin is used as long-term treatment. Some patients with severe colitis may require a colectomy (removal of the colon), but most patients do not require surgery.

COLLES' FRACTURE

A fracture of the lower end of one of the two bones in the forearm (the radius) which also affects the other bone (the ulna). In effect, both wrist and hand are broken. The fracture is confirmed by an X-ray.

If the deformity is severe it is corrected under an anaesthetic. The fracture is then supported in its correct position by means of plaster of Paris

Colles' fracture typically occurs when a person tries to break an imminent fall by putting the hand out. The wrist breaks across the radius (1) and the tip of the ulna is pulled off (2).

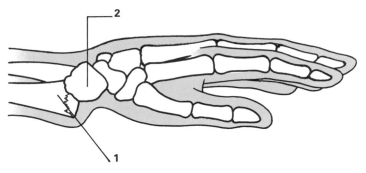

until it is healed. Post-menopausal women are particularly prone to this type of fracture, because of loss of bone substance (see *Osteoporosis*).

COLOSTOMY

Surgery to the large bowel (colon), diverting the normal flow of faeces away from the rectum, and bringing the colon to the surface on the front of the abdomen (the stoma). A colostomy may either be temporary, to allow rest and healing of the bowel beyond the stoma, or it may be permanent. It is usually performed because of disease in the lower colon or rectum — either severe diverticular disease of the colon, or cancer of the colon or

rectum — or as a result of injury. The stoma is covered by a colostomy bag, into which the faeces pass.

COLOUR BLINDNESS

The inability to distinguish certain colours. Colour deficiency is a more accurate term as most of those people affected have normal sharpness of vision but limited colour vision. The cause of colour blindness is not precisely known but is thought to be due to the absence of one of the colouring agents (photopigments) normally found in the cones of the retina (the light sensitive membrane at the back of the eye). There are three types of cone, one of which is receptive to red light, one to green, and one to blue. Colour blindness is classified according to which of these types is affected and how. The prefixes prot-, deuter- and trit- are used to refer to defects of the red, green and blue cones respectively. The suffixes -anomaly and -anopia are used respectively to differentiate colour weakness from a complete inability to distinguish certain colours. Protanopia, for example, describes the inability to distinguish red from green, the commonest form of colour blindness. The various forms of colour blindness can be distinguished by using a test system called Ishihara's charts (qv).

Colour blindness is usually congenital in origin, inherited in a sex-linked manner through the female, who is rarely affected. The condition affects about 8 per cent of males and is permanent.

COLPORRHAPHY

A vaginal repair operation in which the ligaments that support the womb (uterus) are tightened. The operation is usually performed to cure vaginal prolapse but may form part of the treatment to cure stress incontinence of urine. Colporrhaphy is usually performed under general anaesthesia and takes about an hour. All of the surgery is done within the vagina, so there is no abdominal incision; this allows quicker recovery after surgery compared to abdominal operations. The surgeon may insert a catheter (tube) into the bladder during the operation which will be left in place for a few days to avoid any discomfort when the patient passes urine after surgery. Most patients stay in hospital for about a week after the operation.

COLPOSCOPY

A method of examining the neck of the womb (cervix) under magnification. It is used in conjunction with cervical cytology (qv) and enables samples of tissue to be taken accurately from suspicious areas. A binocular instrument called a colposcope is positioned outside the cervix where it obtains a view of the area with the help of a vaginal speculum.

COMA

A state of unconsciousness in which an individual shows a complete lack of response to external stimuli; if the coma is light, painful stimuli may elicit an appropriate response from the patient, such as withdrawal of a limb.

There are many causes of coma including stroke, hypoglycaemia (in diabetes mellitus), ingestion of drugs and poisons and epileptic seizure.

Management of the comatose patient involves maintaining vital functions (breathing, blood pressure and kidney function) while the underlying cause is sought and, if possible, treated.

COMPUTERED/ COMPUTERIZED TOMOGRAPHY

see *CT scan*

CONCEPTION

see *Contraception, Infertility*

CONCUSSION

A short-lived disturbance of those centres in the brain stem which control consciousness. Concussion occurs as a result of a violent blow to the head. People with head injuries who have suffered a loss of consciousness are admitted to hospital for observation, in case of haemorrhaging within the skull (see *Extradural haemorrhage, Subdural haemorrhage*).

CONDOM

see *Contraception*

CONFABULATION

A strategy used by patients with a memory deficit to fill in gaps with plausible coherent statements. It differs from lying in that the confabulator does not realize that his or her replies are incorrect. Furthermore, he or she will rarely question the truth when it is presented. Confabulation occurs in amnesias resulting from brain damage and is most common in the early stages of a type of psychosis called Korsakoff's psychosis. This is a chronic syndrome caused by the thiamine deficiency that may follow long-term alcohol abuse.

CONFINEMENT

see *Labour*

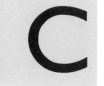

CONFUSION

At a general level, an inability to think with customary clarity and coherence. The term may be used more specifically to refer to an abnormal mental state in which a person's level of consciousness is diminished; this is also known as an 'acute confusional state' or 'delirium'. It refers to a condition, usually of sudden onset, in which a person becomes disorientated, not recognizing familiar people or situations, and restless, failing to pay attention to his or her surroundings. He or she may seem afraid or perplexed and becomes preoccupied with an inner world distorted by illusions, delusions and hallucinations. An acute confusional state may be a sign of a wide range of illnesses, particularly in the elderly. Causes include head injury, chest infection, intoxication with alcohol or drugs, drug or alcohol withdrawal and dementia. Treatment is directed at the underlying cause.

CONGENITAL ABNORMALITIES

Defects of structure or function which originate before birth. Some defects are obvious at birth: Down's syndrome, for example. Others, such as polycystic kidney disease, may only be noticed in later life.

In nearly half of cases no reason can be given. Of those with an identifiable cause, the commonest are genetically determined. Most, such as heart defects, are caused by several factors, but some are due to specific chromosome or gene abnormalities. Nowadays, few abnormalities are the result of the mother taking medicines and drugs during pregnancy; the thalidomide disaster has ensured that all new drugs are thoroughly tested for effects on the fetus (see *Teratogenesis*). Drugs known to be harmful or teratogenic are warfarin (an anticoagulant used in the treatment of blood clots) and alcohol. There is a high risk that some infections acquired during early pregnancy, such as rubella (German measles) and cytomegalovirus, will lead to multiple abnormalities (including heart and brain). The risk of malformation is increased too if the mother has diabetes mellitus.

Some abnormalities, such as anencephaly (absence of the brain), are rapidly lethal, while others can be treated successfully (many forms of congenital heart disease, for example). In the case of genetically determined disorders, genetic counselling is used to establish the risk of future pregnancies being affected. Treatment of the baby is coordinated by the paediatrician, and other specialists are involved according to the abnormalities present.

Routine antenatal screening detects only a minority of congenital abnormalities. However, specialized tests for individual illnesses (such as haemophilia and muscular dystrophy) may be carried out if parents are thought to be in a high risk group.

CONGENITAL DISLOCATION OF THE HIP (CDH)

The upper end or head of the femur (thigh-bone) is shaped like a ball and fits into the socket of the pelvic bone to form the hip joint. In about 1 in 1,000 births it lies outside the socket (the acetabulum), and is therefore dislocated. It is commoner in the first-born child, and with breech deliveries, but also runs in some families.

Dislocation is usually detected when the baby's hips are examined

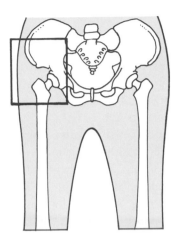 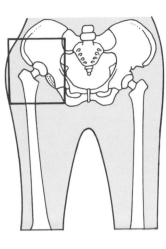

In a normal hip joint (**far left**) the head of the femur fits snugly into the socket. If the hip joint is dislocated (**left**) the head of the femur slips in and out of the socket. This limits movement so that the baby is unable to separate his or her legs when the leg is bent halfway to the tummy. The problem is especially noticeable at nappy changes.

during the newborn period and is confirmed by an ultrasound scan or an X-ray. Treatment involves holding the femoral head in the socket to permit normal growth of the hip joint. This is achieved by placing the baby in a special harness for six weeks. If, as occurs in about one-third of cases, the diagnosis is not made until a while after birth, an operation may be required to position the head of the femur in the acetabulum.

CONGENITAL HEART DISEASE

Malformation of the heart or major blood vessels, present at birth. The abnormalities usually occur early in pregnancy, and may be detected by antenatal ultrasound scan. Some result from maternal infection, such as rubella (German measles), and some are associated with other abnormalities, such as Down's syndrome. Most occur in an otherwise normal baby. Less than 1 per cent of newborn babies are affected.

There are two types of congenital heart disease. Ninety per cent of cases are acyanotic (pink), because the blood is well oxygenated, and consist mainly of obstruction to blood flow, such as a narrowed valve or major artery, or of abnormal communications between the right and left sides of the heart (hole in the heart). Ten per cent are cyanotic (blue), because of mixing of arterial and venous blood which, as a result, is poorly oxygenated, and are mostly either Fallot's tetralogy or transposition of the great arteries (crossing over of the principal artery and veins). A few are more complex. Many different abnormalities may co-exist, making diagnosis and treatment difficult. Acyanotic heart disease may be noticed in the newborn period if a murmur (the noise made by abnormal blood flow) is heard, or if the baby develops heart failure. Sometimes the diagnosis is not evident until later childhood. Cyanotic babies may be blue soon after birth, though some are not blue until later in the first year of life (see *Fallot's tetralogy*). The diagnosis is confirmed by echocardiography (qv) and cardiac catheterization.

Surgery is required for cyanotic and some acyanotic disorders. The chance of a good outcome depends on the complexity of the malformation, and is excellent in the straightforward acyanotic types. Some ventricular septal defects (one form of hole in the heart) close spontaneously and thus do not require surgery.
SEE ALSO *Cyanosis*

CONJUNCTIVITIS

An acute inflammation of the conjunctiva, the delicate membrane covering the exposed part of the eyeball. Conjunctivitis can be caused by viruses, bacteria or allergy. Conjunctival irritation from wind, dust, smoke and other types of air pollution may cause non-infective inflammation of the conjunctiva. Conjunctivitis may also accompany the common cold, illnesses such as measles, and irritation of the cornea due to intense light.

In acute conjunctivitis the eye becomes red and discharges, and may be itchy; the eyelid may be swollen. Antibiotic drops are the main treatment, and in cases of allergy steroids are used. A special dye (fluorescan) may be used to check for the presence of foreign bodies or corneal abrasions if the inflammation fails to respond and irritation persists; the dye will stain selectively a corneal abrasion. Infection can easily be transmitted, especially via the fingers, if the cause is bacterial.

Chronic conjunctivitis is characterized by exacerbations and remissions that occur over months or years in people who seem to have especially sensitive conjunctiva. It is caused by the same things as acute conjunctivitis. Symptoms are similar but less severe: itching, smarting and the sensation that a foreign body is in the eye. Carefully monitored, frequent usage of topical steroids is beneficial in cases where the cause is plainly allergic, and some people have been helped by desensitization to pollens.

CONN'S SYNDROME

A rare condition due to over-secretion of the steroid hormone called aldosterone by the adrenal glands. Aldosterone is one of the salt (sodium) and water regulators of the body. Over-production causes an imbalance, resulting in muscle weakness with cramps, thirst and high blood pressure. Large amounts of urine are passed. The treatment of Conn's syndrome depends on the underlying cause. If the over-production is caused by a tumour of an adrenal gland, surgical removal is necessary; if it results from simple over-activity of the aldosterone-producing cells, drug treatment is required.

CONSTIPATION

Constipation means either the infrequent opening of the bowels or passing stools with difficulty. The range for normal bowel activity is between three times a day and three times a week.

It is thought that most people with constipation eat an insufficient amount of dietary fibre, so not enough bulk is passing to the colon (large bowel) to form a satisfactory mass of stools for propulsion along the bowel. This form of simple constipation is readily improved by eating a high-fibre diet, including wholemeal bread, a bran cereal, vegetables and fruit. Laxatives may be used to relieve constipation but may lose their effect if taken repeatedly.

The sudden onset of constipation in a middle-aged person needs review by a doctor, as it may be due to a blockage of the bowel.

Other causes of constipation can include a slimming diet, a painful anal lesion, persistently ignoring the body's signals to open the bowels, immobility, depression, underactivity of the thyroid gland (myxoedema), and certain drugs (narcotic analgesics, aluminium-containing antacids, and tricyclic antidepressants).

CONTRACEPTION

The prevention of conception, or pregnancy, by natural or artificial means. The different methods of contraception work in different ways:

- Barrier methods (sheath/condom, cap/diaphragm, sponge) present a mechanical barrier to the sperm reaching the ovum. They should be used with a spermicidal agent
- Hormonal methods (combined oral contraceptive and progestogen-only mini-pill, and injectable contraceptives) alter hormone levels in the female, either preventing ovulation or causing other changes that prevent implantation of the fertilized ovum in the womb

- The coil (intra-uterine contraceptive device or IUCD) prevents implantation
- Morning-after contraception works by preventing implantation and is achieved by a special dose pill or by insertion of a coil
- Sterilization permanently prevents sperm from reaching the ovum
- The safe period aims to prevent conception by avoiding intercourse at the time of ovulation
- Coitus interruptus, in which withdrawal of the penis from the vagina takes place before ejaculation, has a high failure rate due to difficulties in timing withdrawal.

No single method can be regarded

CONTRACEPTION METHODS

1 Combined pill: very reliable, regulates periods, possible side-effects; **2** Mini-pill: very reliable, irregular periods, possible side-effects; **3** Injectables: very reliable, last 2–3 months, irregular periods, can delay return of fertility; **4** Sponge: fairly reliable, effective for 24 hours, cannot be used during a period; **5** IUD: reliable, may cause heavier periods, requires professional fitting, causes pelvic infections; **6** Safe period: quite reliable, needs meticulous planning; **7, 8** Sterilization: very good reliability, irreversible; **9** Condom: quite reliable, protects against STDs and AIDS.

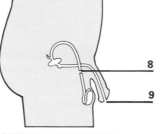

8

9

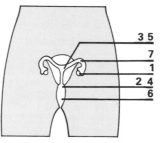

3 5
7
1
2 4
6

FITTING A DIAPHRAGM

The diaphragm, or cap, is reasonably reliable, has no side-effects and is easy to use. First cover the inside of the dome with a spermicidal agent, then fold it and, gripping the end between your fingers **(1)**, guide the

cap along the back wall of your vagina **(2)** and into position **(3)**. You should be able to feel your cervix through the dome of the cap **(4)**; this feels like a firm, round bump. To remove the cap **(5)**, hook one finger underneath the rim and pull downwards.

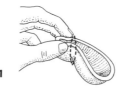

1

2

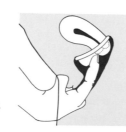

3

4

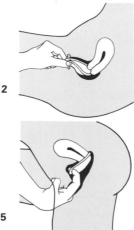

5

as 100 per cent effective: all methods have advantages and disadvantages and no one method will suit everyone.

Advice on contraception is available from your family doctor or from a family planning clinic. All forms of contraception are safe, but their effectiveness depends upon correct and careful usage.

SEE ALSO *Pill, Safe period, Sterilization*

CONTRACTURE

Contracture has two meanings in medicine. First, it may mean a prolonged, reversible contraction of skeletal muscle which may affect a part of the body, and in which no wave-like signals to initiate movement occur (see *Tetanus*).

Secondly, it describes a deformity due to permanent shortening of muscle, usually the result of fibrosis (the formation of fibrous tissue). Similar contractures of muscle also occur in the later stages of many neuromuscular diseases, such as muscular dystrophy and spinal muscular atrophy, or may follow muscle paralysis resulting from poliomyelitis. Volkmann's ischaemic contracture occurs when a fracture of the humerus, the bone in the upper arm, results in part of the broken bone impinging on the brachial artery (the main blood vessel in the arm), causing reduced blood flow and ischaemia. This contracture is preventable if the damaged vessel is promptly repaired.

SEE ALSO *Dupuytren's contracture*

CONVULSION

A fit or seizure. The most common cause is epilepsy (qv), in which abnormal electrical discharges in parts of the brain result in fits. Convulsions can also result from head injuries or strokes or have metabolic causes such as lack of oxygen, low blood sugar, high temperature in children (febrile convulsions) and during alcohol or drug withdrawal. Treatment is of the underlying cause.

CORNEAL GRAFTING

Replacing a diseased or damaged cornea with a healthy one from an organ donor. The cornea is the clear layer of skin in the front of the eye; the pupil and iris (the coloured part of the eye) lie immediately behind it. The function of the cornea is to help focus the light rays on to the retina (the light-sensitive membrane at the back of the eye). If the cornea is damaged, for example by scarring as a result of injury or chronic inflammation (keratitis), vision is impaired as the cornea becomes opaque. Initially there is blurring and cloudiness, and eventually blindness. A corneal transplant, or graft, can restore sight in these circumstances. The operation has a high success rate: the cornea is never rejected, as it has no blood vessels which the patient's immune cells (lymphocytes) can attack as 'foreign'. It is also straightforward: the old, damaged cornea is cut out and the new one lowered in like a manhole cover, and then stitched into place.

SEE ALSO *Transplantation*

CORONARY HEART DISEASE

Disease of the coronary arteries which supply blood to the heart muscle (myocardium); also known as ischaemic heart disease (see *Ischaemia*). Coronary heart disease has become the major health hazard in the Western world.

The cause is atherosclerosis (see *Atheroma*) of the coronary arteries which results in narrowing, irregularity and eventually blockage of the arteries, restricting blood supply to the heart muscle and so causing irreversible damage. Hereditary factors may play an important part in the development of coronary heart disease and there is often a strong family history of angina, heart attack, stroke, high blood pressure or sudden, unexpected death.

The first appearance of the disease is uncommon in men below 40 and rare in women of that age. In premenopausal women it is almost always associated with an underlying disease such as diabetes mellitus, high blood pressure or hypothyroidism. The highest incidence of heart disease occurs in those aged between 50 and 70 years; by this time men and women are equally affected.

Coronary heart disease may progress silently over many years with no symptoms, but eventually angina pectoris or heart attack will result. Heart failure may occur when the heart muscle has been irreversibly damaged.

Stopping smoking, reducing weight, and receiving treatment for underlying high blood pressure, high cholesterol levels and diabetes are important steps in the management of the disease. An ECG examination (see *Electrocardiography*) may show changes typical of ischaemia, indicating that the arteries are becoming critically narrowed. These changes may only appear when the person being examined is exercised on a treadmill or bicycle while the recording is made. Evidence of previous heart attacks may also be seen on the ECG, indicating that there has already been irreversible damage. The extent of the disease can be assessed by means of a coronary angiogram (see *Cardiac catheterization*). This is performed particularly if the patient is thought fit enough for coronary artery bypass surgery (see *Bypass*).

COR PULMONALE

Right-sided heart failure; also called pulmonary heart disease. In this condition restricted blood flow through the lungs causes back pressure on the right ventricle, which develops a thick wall (hypertrophies) to try to counter the increased pressure. Eventually, the right ventricle will cease to pump efficiently, resulting in heart failure. The main immediate cause of cor pulmonale is hypoxia (inadequate oxygen in the blood), which increases the resistance to blood flow in the lungs, as a consequence of chronic respiratory disease.

The heart failure of cor pulmonale is treated using digoxin, and diuretics and oxygen or even assisted ventilation may improve the hypoxia.

CORTICOSTEROID

Hormones also known as glucocorticoids, synthesized in the cortex of the adrenal glands; their production is closely regulated in turn by a hormone called ACTH, which is secreted by the pituitary gland at the base of the brain. They bring about metabolism in virtually all tissues, inhibiting glucose uptake and mobilizing fats and protein. The production of corticosteroids is normally increased at times of stress; levels fluctuate over 24 hours, being lowest at night.

Prolonged over-production of corticosteroids as a result of either an excess of ACTH or uncontrolled adrenal secretion produces Cushing's syndrome. Occasionally, malignant tumours of the lung can secrete an ACTH-like substance which increases the production of corticosteroids.

A deficiency of corticosteroid pro-

C

duction for any reason results in Addison's disease. Abnormalities of corticosteroid production and their origin may be determined by the identification of specific hormone metabolites (breakdown products) in the urine.

Synthetic substances which mimic naturally occurring corticosteroids are widely used for their anti-inflammatory and immuno-suppressive properties in the treatment of such diverse conditions as asthma, ulcerative colitis and rheumatoid arthritis.

COT DEATH

see *Sudden infant death syndrome*

COUGH

A reflex action which helps to remove harmful material from the vital lower airways where oxygen enters the bloodstream. Air is suddenly drawn in through the open upper part of the airway (glottis), which then closes causing substantial pressure to build up within the chest. When the glottis opens again, this pressure is released as a sharp burst of air, or cough, and carries with it phlegm and foreign bodies.

Coughing usually occurs in simple viral infections and in chronic bronchitis and should rarely be suppressed. Codeine or other narcotics are sometimes used to suppress coughing, but are only justified in some patients with advanced cancer or if sleep is being severely disrupted. All these drugs have adverse effects on breathing and require careful administration. Expectorants are the best method of easing a cough.

CRADLE CAP

see *Seborrhoeic dermatitis*

CREPITATION

A noise in the lungs which is heard through a stethoscope and sounds like hair being rubbed between the fingers. Usually it is an indication of abnormality, such as pneumonia in its early stage or fluid in the lungs (pulmonary oedema). A coarser type of crepitation may be heard in asthma and in some chronic disorders that cause fibrosis in the lungs, such as asbestosis.

CREPITUS

This term may be used to describe two distinct occurrences: the grating of the two ends of a bone in cases of fracture (splinting prevents this extremely painful phenomenon); and the sensation of air or gas under the skin, which crackles when it is pressed. The latter occurs as a result of some infections (for example, gas gangrene), or from a pneumothorax or occasionally from perforation of the oesophagus (gullet). The term surgical emphysema is also used to describe this type of crepitus.

CRETINISM

A condition arising from untreated congenital hypothyroidism (qv) (underactivity of the thyroid gland). The thyroid gland is responsible for producing the hormone thyroxine. If this hormone is lacking from birth and no treatment is given in the form of synthesized thyroxine, permanent brain damage may result and a characteristic expressionless face with coarse features will develop. In order to prevent cretinism, hypothyroidism is now routinely screened for in newborn babies. The screening method involves measuring the thyroid hormone in the blood, a sample of which is taken by pricking the heel.

CREUTZFELDT-JAKOB DISEASE

A brain condition so rare that it is identified in only 1 person in a million each year. It usually develops between the ages of 45 and 65, is worldwide in distribution, and causes dementia which progresses rapidly, advancing noticeably from day to day, to a fatal termination usually within a year. The dementia is accompanied by a variety of neurological symptoms such as ataxia (lack of coordination), paralysis, visual disturbances and jerking of the limbs and body.

Creutzfeldt-Jakob disease belongs to a group of uncommon diseases involving a complex chemical agent called a prion. A prion is an abnormal protein which, although not alive, is sometimes capable of being devastatingly infectious. The disease group includes scrapie, which produces the same symptoms in sheep; bovine spongiform encephalopathy, which affects cows; and kuru, once prevalent in tribes in Papua New Guinea. In all of these conditions the brain becomes riddled with tiny holes, giving the tissue the appearance of a sponge.

Creutzfeldt-Jakob disease may be transmitted by organ grafts and possibly by blood transfusions.

There is no treatment.

CROHN'S DISEASE

An inflammatory condition of the bowel which can affect any part of the intestine, ranging from the mouth to the anus; classically, the final part of the ileum (lower small bowel), the colon (large bowel), or the anus and rectum is involved.

The disease can be associated with a wide range of symptoms. Common symptoms include abdominal pain, diarrhoea, anaemia, loss of weight, mouth ulcers or various painful conditions around the anus.

The condition is diagnosed by the finding of patchy ulceration of the colon during either sigmoidoscopy or colonoscopy (see *Endoscopy*), by the finding of characteristic changes on either a barium meal enema or X-ray examination, or by characteristic changes on microscopic examination of biopsies taken from the bowel. The condition may also be associated with vitamin deficiency (particularly vitamin B_{12} and folic acid), and a low concentration of the protein albumin in the blood.

Treatment includes maintaining an adequate intake of calories and vitamins, the use of prednisolone and the other drugs prescribed for colitis, and the use of antibiotics (particularly metronidazole). The surgical removal of severely diseased bowel is often required for the complications of Crohn's disease — particularly if the bowel is narrowed (strictured), or if there is a diseased connection between the bowel and another part of the body (a fistula), or an abscess. Toxic megacolon is a rare feature of Crohn's disease in which the colon becomes extremely inflamed and blown up by intestinal gas. It requires intensive in-patient medical treatment; approximately one-third of patients require emergency surgery to remove the dilated bowel.

Despite the widespread inflammation that can be associated with Crohn's disease, most people with the condition are able to lead full and healthy lives.

CROUP

An acute childhood infection; also known as laryngo-tracheobronchitis. Croup is similar to laryngitis in the adult, where the infection particularly affects the vocal cords and voice-box (larynx). In young children, the infection also spreads to involve the windpipe (trachea) and larger airways in the lungs (bronchi). It is most common in the winter months and in the pre-school-age child, and is usually caused by the para-influenza virus.

Croup normally begins with the symptoms of a common cold; this progresses over a day or so to a cough which sounds remarkably like a seal barking, and sometimes to difficulty in breathing, with a whooping noise on breathing in. This noise (stridor) means inflammation has narrowed the upper airway, a situation made worse by crying. If stridor occurs when the child is breathing quietly, this means that the airways have narrowed significantly. Younger children, particularly babies under 1 year of age, are at more risk of obstruction to breathing because of their smaller airways.

The only treatment usually needed is to control the fever, and to keep the child calm. Steam inhalations are sometimes recommended. If stridor is worsening, the child may need to be observed in hospital, as in rare cases it is necessary to insert an artificial airway (an endotracheal tube) inside the windpipe to relieve the obstruction.

CT SCAN

A method of forming images from X-rays; it is also referred to as computerized axial tomography (CAT).

It requires specialized, highly sophisticated equipment known as a CT scanner. The scanner uses sensitive X-ray detectors and a rapid digital computer to evaluate the absorption of X-rays passing through the body, building up a cross-sectional image or slice. In this way, very much smaller differences in density can be distin-

guished than by conventional X-ray examinations and the depth of structures beneath the surface can be demonstrated. Images are displayed on a viewing monitor like a television screen and can be copied onto film.

The technique is invaluable for imaging the brain to detect strokes and tumours and to investigate possible brain damage after injury. It is also extremely useful in imaging the thorax (chest), abdomen and pelvis, particularly in the investigation of tumours, aneurysms (dilatation of the walls of blood vessels) and jaundice. Scanning of the spine has proved of value in the investigation of back pain.

So good is the anatomical detail obtained with CT that the technique can also be used to guide biopsy procedures, thus eliminating the need for open surgery in some cases.

CUSHING'S SYNDROME

A condition caused by excess steroid hormones in the circulation. Often this occurs as a result of steroid therapy – usually prednisolone tablets. The steroids concerned are all corticosteroids. In rare cases Cushing's syndrome develops as a result of a tumour (usually benign) of one of the adrenal glands or of the pituitary gland.

Symptoms include a puffy face, changes in the hair and skin, a tendency to easy bruising, ankle swelling, weight gain, and sometimes psychological changes.

Surgery (adrenalectomy, qv) is usually the best treatment for the tumour-related cases. If the syndrome is drug-related, the minimum dose of steroid needed to control the underlying condition is employed.

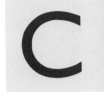

CYANOSIS

A bluish hue to the complexion due to the presence of significant amounts of deoxygenated haemoglobin in the circulating blood. Haemoglobin is the protein in red blood cells (erythrocytes) which picks up oxygen in the lungs and transports it to the tissues. Oxygenated haemoglobin is red. Deoxygenated haemoglobin is darker, hence the characteristic dusky appearance of patients with cyanosis. This appearance may simply be a normal response of the extremities to cold but usually it implies poor oxygenation of the blood in the arteries. Cyanosis may arise because of inefficient breathing due to lung disease or neurological damage. It is also seen in several congenital anomalies of the heart and great vessels. Certain acquired heart diseases are also associated with cyanosis, notably rheumatic fever damage to the mitral valve of the heart.

CYST

Derived from the Greek word meaning 'bladder', a cyst is a hollow, fluid-filled sac bounded by a wall. The fluid inside the cyst may be secreted by the cells lining the wall or derived from the surrounding tissue fluid or blood. The contents of the sac may either be clear and colourless or thick and cloudy.

Cysts are almost always benign and can be removed surgically.

CYSTIC FIBROSIS

An inherited (autosomal recessive) condition principally affecting the lungs and pancreas and sometimes the liver and kidneys; it is due to a defect in mucus secretion. It is first noticed in infancy and childhood. The usual symptoms are abdominal pain and repeated vomiting due to intestinal obstruction, repeated chest infections and failure to thrive (gain weight). The lungs eventually become scarred (bronchiectasis) and may be damaged further by infection.

The major treatment is physiotherapy and postural drainage (adopting an appropriate position to eliminate pockets of lung secretions which may become infected). In addition, pancreatic enzyme tablets and vitamins are given as supplements to prevent malabsorption. Death often occurs in adolescence, but survival to adulthood is now more common. Heart-lung transplantation in childhood is now being performed for many of these patients.

CYSTINURIA

A rare inherited defect in the transport of the amino acid, cystine, and occasionally of other amino acids, in the kidney and the small intestine which results in high urinary levels. (Amino acids are the building blocks of protein). The only outward sign of cystinuria is the production of kidney stones and 'sand' in the urine. Affected individuals are advised to take plenty of fluids to ensure a high urine output, the aim being to produce at least 3 litres ($5\frac{1}{4}$ pints) of urine in 24 hours to prevent the formation of stones (calculi). Drug treatment may dissolve the stones, but occasionally surgical removal is necessary.

CYSTITIS

Inflammation of the bladder. It is much more widely found in women than men. The most common symptom of cystitis is pain or a burning sensation when passing urine. Sufferers also experience a need to pass urine more frequently than usual, although when urine is passed the amounts are very small, and often have a strong urge to pass urine for fear of losing control. There may be fever, pain in the lower abdomen or back, and sometimes the urine looks cloudy or blood-stained.

Cystitis is often caused by bacterial infection but may be due to allergy to certain foods or chemicals. Non-bacterial vaginal infections, such as thrush (see *Candida*), and some sexually transmitted diseases, such as herpes simplex, may cause symptoms of cystitis. Some women develop cystitis after sexual intercourse ('honeymoon cystitis').

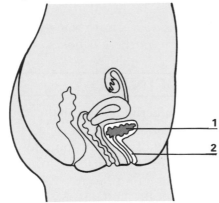

Cystitis can be a very distressing condition, although rarely a dangerous one. The bacteria usually responsible for cystitis enter the bladder (1) through the urethra (2).

The diagnosis is confirmed by testing a urine sample for infection. Antibiotics will be prescribed if the symptoms are caused by a bacterial infection. The symptoms may also be relieved by drinking large volumes of water, making the urine less acidic by taking bicarbonate of soda (one teaspoon in a glass of water), having a hot bath, and taking a mild painkiller such as paracetamol.

No significant abnormality is found in most women with recurrent cystitis. Simple preventative measures often help to stave off further attacks. These include drinking lots of fluids; avoiding antiseptics, talcum powder, perfumed deodorants and perfumed soap in the genital area; and not wearing tight trousers, nylon underwear or tights.

CYSTOSCOPY

One of the most specialized investigations used to examine patients who have trouble passing urine. Under a light general anaesthetic, the surgeon inserts an instrument called a cystoscope through the urethra (the small tube along which urine is carried away from the bladder) in order to examine the inside of the bladder. A cystoscope is a long narrow metal tube, about as thick as a pencil, through which light is passed. This enables the surgeon to examine the lining of the bladder and to inspect the tubes which drain urine from the kidneys (ureters). Various abnormalities, such as inflammation and tumours, can be seen through the cystoscope. Using special instruments, the surgeon can operate through the cystoscope and remove abnormal tissue, avoiding the necessity for major abdominal surgery in certain circumstances.

CYTOLOGY

The study of cells. In medicine cytology is used in the diagnosis of pre-cancerous and cancerous conditions and in the study of genetics. In the first of these applications a cytologist will examine the cells in a sample of tissue or fluid under a high-powered microscope.

In the second of the two applications, cytogeneticists examine the chromosomes in the nuclei of cells. Used in conjunction with amniocentesis, cytogenetics allows the prenatal diagnosis of conditions such as Down's syndrome.

CYTOMEGALOVIRUS (CMV)

A member of the herpes virus group. Blood tests would show that most adults have been infected with CMV, which generally causes a mild, non-specific illness. Occasionally an illness similar to glandular fever (infectious mononucleosis) occurs. In common with many other viruses, CMV causes more serious disease in people whose immune systems are weakened (such as premature babies and those treated for malignancy), and a fatal pneumonia may result.

After infection, the virus is slow to clear from the body, and may continue to be excreted in saliva, urine and faeces for many months or years, providing ample opportunity for cross-infection. More importantly, it may be passed from a pregnant mother to her fetus, especially if she acquires the infection for the first time during pregnancy. Serious fetal abnormality may result, with damage to the eyes, liver and developing brain. There is no effective treatment and, as yet, no immunization for prevention.

CYTOTOXIC

Drugs designed and used to kill cells. The term is employed almost exclusively for drugs used in cancer treatment (see *Chemotherapy*).

D & C (DILATATION AND CURETTAGE)

A procedure which involves scraping away the lining of the uterus or womb (endometrium) with a spoon-shaped instrument called a curette. The procedure is usually performed under a short general anaesthetic. It may be used to investigate abnormal bleeding from the uterus and to decide appropriate treatment, to stop heavy bleeding or to clean the uterus after a miscarriage.

DEAFNESS

The inability to hear sound. In most cases deafness is partial and sufferers are hard of hearing and not totally deaf. The disability may be conductive, sensorineural or neural in origin.

Conductive deafness occurs when sound is prevented from reaching the eardrum (for example, by wax), or when the drum is perforated, or the middle ear conducting mechanism is not functioning because of secretions or otosclerosis (spongy bone formation in the labyrinth of the ear). Mild conductive deafness caused by fluid in the middle ear is quite common, especially among children, and can be corrected by the insertion of a grommet (qv) to ventilate the affected part. In other cases, if the underlying cause cannot be corrected by an operation then a hearing aid can be of help.

By contrast, in sensorineural deafness the complex speech signal sent along the nerve to the brain is degraded, making amplification by means of a hearing aid very difficult because of the painful distortion of sound this brings; tinnitus (qv) is a common feature of sensorineural deafness. This type of deafness may be caused by damage to the cochlea as a result of excessive exposure to noise, drugs or infection (cochlear deafness). Neural deafness is caused by disease of the auditory nerve, such as a tumour. Most congenital causes of deafness (mal-development of the cochlea, for example) fall into the sensorineural pattern.

D

D

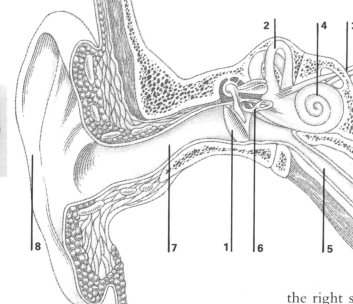

Structure of the ear: **1** eardrum; **2** semi-circular canals; **3** auditory nerve; **4** cochlea; **5** eustachian tube; **6** ossicles; **7** auditory canal; **8** auricle.

At present the treatment of both neural and sensorineural deafness is unsatisfactory. The use of hearing aids is only partially successful and it is only rarely possible to remove the underlying cause of deafness. However, currently new electrical methods of stimulating the auditory nerve are being developed and may prove of benefit to sufferers in the future.

DECOMPRESSION SICKNESS

see *Bends*

DEFIBRILLATION

An electric shock given to restore normal heart rhythm in a condition called ventricular fibrillation (chaotic twitching of the heart muscle of the ventricular wall). The machine used delivers a 200–400 joule shock of direct current lasting a fraction of a second through electrodes placed over the right side of the chest just to the side of the breast-bone (sternum) and over the left side of the chest below the armpit. Electrical contact is improved by using petroleum jelly or special electrode pads placed over the skin. The procedure is often effective but may cause skin burns.

DEHYDRATION

Water deficiency as a result of inadequate intake or excessive loss, or a combination of both factors. The commonest causes of dehydration are vomiting and diarrhoea, often due to gastroenteritis (qv), especially in infants. Patients with severe dehydration have a dry tongue, wrinkled skin and sunken eyes. Hypernatraemia (qv) is usual in severe cases. Prevention is important, as minor degrees of dehydration are common; an adult requires about 2 litres ($3\frac{1}{2}$ pints) of fluid per day.

Mildly dehydrated patients are rehydrated by fluids taken by mouth. More severe cases require intravenous fluid replacement. This is done slowly to prevent cerebral oedema, which is particularly likely in infants.

DELIRIUM

see *Confusion*

DELIRIUM TREMENS

Part of the spectrum of the alcohol withdrawal syndrome. It occurs when a physical dependence on alcohol has been established to such an extent that stopping alcohol during sleeping hours may produce symptoms of shakiness, malaise (a general feeling of being unwell) and vomiting in the morning. If alcohol is not taken, symptoms can progress to severe sweating, fever, visual hallucinations, convulsions and coma. Delirium tremens has a high mortality if it is not treated by sedative drugs in hospital. Treatment takes 1–2 weeks; sedation is tapered off over several days before symptoms disappear.
SEE ALSO *Alcoholism*

DELUSION

A false fixed belief out of keeping with a person's social and cultural background, and generally held with great intensity and conviction. A full delusion cannot be dispelled by argument, whereas a person with a partial delusion may admit to being mistaken when questioned or presented with evidence to the contrary.

Common types of delusion in severe psychiatric disorders concern outside interference with thinking through telepathy or mind-reading, interference by others with body function, a person incorrectly believing himself or herself to be ill, and believing that others may be trying to cause him or her harm. Delusions are a common symptom in schizophrenia and may also be found in severe affective disorders, dementia and confusion.

DEMENTIA

A chronic syndrome in which there is an irreversible deterioration in mental abilities and personality as a result of disease of the brain. It most commonly affects the elderly. In the early stages of dementia forgetfulness and difficulty in making simple calculations, perhaps in working out change when shopping, may be noticed by the sufferer or by others. Memory impairment gradually worsens, leading the affected person to buy repeatedly the same article, for example, or to mistake the time of day and so attempt daytime activities at night. Personality traits are accentuated and the sufferer becomes a caricature of his or her former self. Later the demented person will be unable to recognize familiar people and places, become emotionally unstable, sometimes deluded, and incontinent.

Dementias are often subdivided into pre-senile (occurring before the age of 65), and senile (with an onset after 65). The causes of pre-senile dementia include Alzheimer's disease (qv), Pick's disease (a rare inherited disease of the brain) and Huntington's chorea (qv).

DEMYELINATION

An abnormal process that causes the loss of a substance called myelin which surrounds nerve fibres. The myelin sheath normally surrounds the fibres in a spiral formation and is divided into short segments. Its function is to speed the transmission of nerve impulses along the fibre. Any disease process that primarily affects the myelin sheath and preserves the fibre itself will lead to a disturbance of nerve function. Multiple sclerosis is by far the most common demyelinating condition.

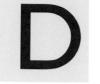

DENERVATION

The transection or severing of a nerve, leading to the immediate paralysis of muscles (if division is of a motor nerve), complete loss of sensation in an area of skin (if division is of a sensory nerve), or modification of function on internal organs and the skin. Many nerves contain both motor and sensory fibres. Denervated muscles will eventually die, causing profound structural, biochemical and physiological changes. This occurrence may be detected by electromyography (EMG), a recording of the electrical activity of muscle.

When an organ is partially denervated, any remaining nerve fibres may re-innervate the 'abandoned' structure and so lead at least to partial restoration of function. Reinnervation of completely denervated muscles depends on the success of microsurgery in restoring some continuity between the cut ends of the nerves, but rarely happens.

DENTITION

The arrangement of teeth in the upper

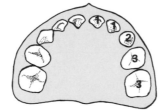

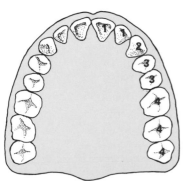

Above: Deciduous, or milk teeth, normally erupt at 6 months, beginning with the incisors (**1**), followed by the canines (**2**) and then the molars (**3**).

Left: Full permanent dentition consists of two incisors (**1**), a canine (**2**), two premolars (**3**) and three molars (**4**) on each side in both the upper and lower jaw.

(Maxillary) and lower (Mandibular) dental arches which form the jaw.

At birth the upper and lower gum pads have twenty segmental elevations marking the points at which the milk teeth will appear. These normally erupt at 6 months of age. The whole process is usually completed by the age of $2\frac{1}{2}$, though this can vary by six months either way.

At the age of 6 years the first permanent teeth erupt. The order and timing is variable, eighteen months either way being normal. The milk teeth begin to drop out, and during this time the dentition is said to be mixed. Permanent dentition is established when all the milk teeth have dropped out.

DEPRESSION

Refers both to a symptom found in psychiatric illness and a type of affective disorder in which it is the central symptom. Depression as a symptom refers to persistent and intense feelings of unhappiness. Depressive illness, on the other hand, describes a disorder in which many physical and psychological functions are disturbed.

Depressive illness usually occurs in episodes, sometimes after a precipitating event such as the loss of a partner or job. The sufferer usually experiences persistent feelings of unhappiness and despair. Associated symptoms are common, such as insomnia, loss of appetite, loss of interest in sex and in other activities normally enjoyed, persistent fatigue and difficulty in concentrating. In severe depression, a sufferer feels gloomy about life and the future and may have thoughts of suicide. He or she often has low self-esteem and may feel excessively guilty about previous actions. In the severest depressions delusions may develop, usually of a hypochondriacal kind, in which the person is convinced he or she is suffering with a serious illness.

Cases of severe depression are often treated in hospital, using various approaches, which may include antidepressants and electroconvulsive therapy (ECT). Psychotherapy is often used to treat milder depressions.

DERMATITIS

Synonymous with the word 'eczema', and meaning inflammation of the skin. There are many possible causes.

In infancy, nappy dermatitis is due to irritation of the skin in the genital area by faeces and urine. It is alleviated by frequent bathing; thick barrier creams should also be used.

In childhood, 'atopic' dermatitis (an inherited condition associated with asthma, hay fever and a family history of these problems) is extremely common. It waxes and wanes in severity but tends to improve gradually over a period of years.

In adults, contact dermatitis due either to allergy or irritation from a very wide variety of chemical substances found in the modern environment frequently affects exposed areas such as the hands or face. Avoidance of identified allergy-causing substances remains the basis of treatment.

Seborrheic dermatitis (qv) commonly affects the scalp, eyebrows, folds around the nose and lips, and areas over the breast-bone and may range from no more than excess dandruff to severe inflammation.

All forms of dermatitis respond to topical corticosteroids applied directly to the skin; these are prescribed with care because overuse can produce resistance in addition to side-effects such as atrophy (thinning) of the skin or systemic symptoms resembling those of Cushing's syndrome (qv).

DERMATOMYOSITIS

Inflammation of the skin, characteristically of the eyelids and backs of the fingers but which can affect anywhere, associated with muscle aching, tenderness and weakness, particularly around the shoulders and hips. There is a childhood form which can lead to calcium deposits in the soft tissues, with consequent contractures and deformity of the muscles or ligaments; this may be alleviated by physiotherapy. In the middle-aged or elderly adult, dermatomyositis may rarely be associated with an internal malignancy, and appropriate tests are usually made to investigate this possibility.

Treatment is directed at any underlying condition and thereafter consists largely of corticosteroids.

DESENSITIZATION

The abolition of sensitivity to a particular antigen (protein which causes the formation of antibodies).

Bee and wasp sting hypersensitivity is probably the only allergy in which desensitization has been found consistently useful. Sufferers are given injections of purified venom, starting with minute doses which are gradually increased over a period of time. The patient is observed for two hours after each injection because of the danger of anaphylaxis (qv).

In theory desensitization should be helpful for patients with allergic asthma and hay fever, and attempts to desensitize individuals by repeated injections of small doses of antigen have a long history. In practice, however, it is only in an unpredictable proportion of sufferers that a significant improvement in symptoms results. Also, the therapy is not without risk for the patient, who may suffer a violent reaction (anaphylaxis). For these reasons desensitization is not usually employed to control the symptoms of these allergies unless other therapy has failed.

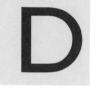

DEXTROCARDIA

Mirror-image orientation of the heart. In dextrocardia the heart lies to the right of the midline with the heart beat directed towards the right nipple. Dextrocardia alone does not cause any symptoms but in rare cases it can form part of a specific syndrome in which the spleen may be absent. In this case, the body is more susceptible to certain infections.

DIABETES INSIPIDUS

A rare disease of the posterior pituitary gland in which insufficient production of the hormone vasopressin leads to excessive urine production and thirst. It is caused by damage to the gland by local tumours, or conditions such as tuberculosis or sarcoidosis. Skull fractures and local surgery may also be causes.

The condition is usually noticed at an early stage. Urine production may be as much as 15 litres (26 pints) per day and the sufferer compensates by constant drinking in response to excessive thirst. Sleep is disturbed, although otherwise the person may look well.

Once diabetes mellitus, kidney failure, hypercalcaemia (high calcium levels in the blood) and hypokalaemia (low concentration of potassium in the plasma) are excluded as causes, the only problem is to differentiate the condition from voluntary over-drinking (psychogenic polydipsia). This may be done by appropriate tests of the function of the pituitary gland.

The condition responds rapidly to vasopressin replacement by means of injection or nasal spray.

DIABETES MELLITUS

A metabolic disease characterized by abnormally high levels of glucose in the blood (hyperglycaemia). The cause is unknown, but both genetic and environmental factors probably play a part. The disorder is primarily due to insulin deficiency, and may be divided into two main types, defined according to treatment. Type I (insulin-dependent) diabetes is probably auto-immune (qv) in origin, usually of early onset and requires insulin. Type II (non insulin dependent) usually develops in older patients who are often obese, and can usually be controlled by diet and/or oral hypoglycaemic agents.

The symptoms of hyperglycaemia include thirst, excessive urine production (polyuria) and weight loss, but abnormal though less high levels of blood glucose may be signalled by a malaise (a general feeling of being unwell), blurred vision or recurrent infection, particularly 'thrush' (candida albicans) infection in women. If untreated, patients may develop dehydration and ketoacidosis. Some patients are discovered on routine examination to have glucose in the urine (glycosuria); others are not recognized as diabetics until complications have become established. Although glycosuria suggests that diabetes may be the problem, an elevated blood glucose level is necessary to confirm it (see *Glucose tolerance test*).

The aim of treatment is to relieve symptoms, help the blood glucose to return to normal, prevent and treat complications, and educate the patient to look after himself or herself. Diet is the cornerstone of treatment for all patients. Adjustment of the amount and type of food (particularly carbohydrates) is necessary to prevent rapid swings in blood glucose. Calorie restriction is important in overweight patients as obesity reduces the action of insulin. Dietary treatment may need to be balanced with drug treatment and exercise.

Over-treatment may lead to low levels of blood glucose (hypoglycaemia), particularly if insulin is used. Both high levels of glucose due to inadequate administration of insulin and low levels due to excessive administration of insulin may result in coma. Both forms of coma can be effectively treated.

Many diabetics monitor themselves at home with blood glucose testing strips; if these are used in combination with more sophisticated laboratory tests many patients achieve near-normal blood glucose levels for long periods. However, some people cannot cope with self-monitoring.

Diabetic patients have an increased incidence of atherosclerotic disease (degenerative change within the arteries caused by fatty deposits), such as heart attack, stroke or claudication, and may develop specific, so-called microvascular complications. Microvascular disease primarily affects the eyes, leading to retinopathy (qv). Diabetics are regularly reviewed to detect any complications at an early stage, and to be offered appropriate treatment.

DIAGNOSIS

The naming of disease. The diagnosis is determined from the patient's history and/or from the doctor's examination, but additional investigations are often required; these may include blood or urine tests, X-rays, ECG (see *Electrocardiography*), endoscopy or biopsy.

The route to a diagnosis is indicated by the initial abnormalities. Many conditions with characteristic features and all emergencies are treated on the basis of a 'working' (that is the most likely) diagnosis; further investigations are performed as appropriate and particularly if there is no response to treatment.

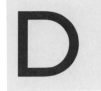

DIALYSIS

A procedure to remove waste products and fluid from the blood of patients with kidney failure. There are two types of dialysis: haemodialysis and peritoneal dialysis. Many patients learn to perform haemodialysis safely for themselves at home; it takes an average of five hours three times a week.

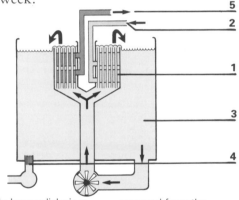

In haemodialysis a dialysis membrane (1) imitates kidney function. Blood from the artery (2) is pumped across the membrane. The waste products are removed from the blood by dialysis fluid (3) and drained off (4). The blood is then returned to the patient (5).

Continuous ambulatory peritoneal dialysis (CAPD) is performed at home by patients. Dialysis fluid sits in the peritoneal cavity for about six hours, and is then drained out; this is repeated four times a day so that dialysis is continuous. This technique is particularly suitable for children (in whom access to blood vessels for haemodialysis is often a problem) and the elderly. The main complication is infection (peritonitis), repeated

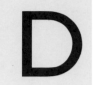

episodes of which may damage the peritoneal membrane and lead to failure of the technique.

Both haemodialysis and CAPD allow patients to survive for long periods (up to 20 years), but the quality of life they offer is generally inferior to that of kidney transplantation, which is the best treatment for chronic renal failure, especially in young people.

DIARRHOEA

The passing of either excessively frequent or liquid stools. The range for normal bowel action is between three times a day to three times a week.

Acute diarrhoea is usually due to some form of infection, such as food poisoning, traveller's diarrhoea or gastroenteritis. The illness usually settles within 48 hours without specific treatment, but the person needs to ensure an adequate intake of fluids, perhaps supplemented by small amounts of salt and sugar. The presence of a fever or blood in the stools may indicate a more serious form of infectious diarrhoea and medical help should be sought if either of these symptoms is present.

Chronic diarrhoea may also result from an infection, particularly infestation of the colon by parasites. Alternatively it may be due to failure to absorb or digest food completely (malabsorption), to inflammation of the bowel (Crohn's disease or ulcerative colitis), or to some irritation within the lower bowel (cancer of the colon). A person with persistent diarrhoea should always seek expert medical advice and investigation.

DIATHERMY

The heating of tissues by means of a high-frequency electric current or by electromagnetic radiation. Diathermy has two main applications. In surgery it is used to destroy abnormal tissues while controlling bleeding or to cut tissues in a bloodless fashion. The heat, which is conducted by the forceps holding the tissue, effectively coagulates the small blood vessels to prevent bleeding. In physiotherapy diathermy is used in the form of high-frequency electromagnetic radiation and applied to localized areas of the body to promote healing in various rheumatic disorders or injuries affecting soft tissues and joints.

DIGOXIN

A drug derived from the foxglove (*digitalis*). It improves the efficiency of heart pumping (increases cardiac output), though probably only temporarily, and controls the excessively rapid heart rate of atrial fibrillation. Until recently it was one of the most valuable drugs in cardiology and is still very widely used. Unfortunately, it is also toxic and can itself cause arrhythmias, nausea, vomiting, and visual disturbances, particularly in the elderly. In heart failure it is gradually being replaced by vasodilator drugs which, by dilating the blood vessels, reduce the amount of work the heart has to do. Atrial fibrillation is increasingly being controlled by other, safer, antiarrhythmics such as amiodarone.

DIPHTHERIA

A serious and highly infectious disease mainly affecting children and young adults. Due to widespread immunization diphtheria has become a very rare disease in most developed countries. It is caused by the diphtheria bacillus (*Corynebacterium diphtheria*) and is spread by droplet infection in sneezing and coughing and by direct contact. The incubation period is 2–5 days. Diphtheria is usually signalled by a sore throat accompanied by a 'false' greyish membrane over the tonsils and the throat. This 'false' membrane may spread to the larynx (voice-box), leading to serious complications such as croup and difficulty in breathing. The toxin produced by diphtheria can enter the bloodstream and cause damage to the heart and nerves. Diphtheria can sometimes also infect wounds of the skin or genitalia. Diagnosis is by laboratory examination of a swab from the nose and throat or other infected area.

Diphtheria patients are treated in strict isolation with antitoxin and antibiotics. All contacts have to be investigated and may require antibiotics.

DIPLOPIA

Double vision. Diplopia is caused by disease affecting the extra-ocular muscles that move the eyeball, the nerves that send impulses to them, or central control of eye movement. The defect may be present and constant all the time, or may only occur in certain directions of gaze; it is a feature of paralytic squint (qv).

Many diseases of the eye-socket can distort the eyeball and extraocular muscles, including injury, tumour and infection. Treatment is directed at the underlying cause.

DISLOCATION

A joint between two bones has a fibrous covering (the capsule) to link the two moving surfaces as well as the muscles acting over the joint. If one of the bones is forced out of the joint capsule it is dislocated. This can be caused by falls, fractures and abnormal forces acting on the bones. The shoulder and the hip are particularly prone to 'coming out of joint'. If the capsule of the shoulder is damaged it can result in weakness of the joint so that repeated dislocation is a problem (known as habitual or recurrent dislocation). Dislocation is remedied by manipulation usually under anaesthetic. SEE ALSO *Congenital dislocation of the hip*

DIURETIC

A drug which increases the production of urine and the excretion of salt by the kidneys. The many different types of diuretic available are used in the treatment of fluid retention, which is often found in association with heart failure. A common type of diuretic used for this purpose is the group known as thiazides, examples being bendrofluazide and chlorothiazide. This type is also useful in treating high blood pressure (hypertension), often in association with other drugs such as beta-blockers.

Diuretics may give rise to a number of side-effects: a particular complication of thiazides is the tendency for excess loss of potassium from the body; this may be counteracted by taking a potassium supplement to help the body retain potassium or combining the drug with another type of diuretic.

DIVERTICULITIS

The inflammation involved in diverticular disease of the large bowel (colon). The symptoms of this disease are often similar to those of irritable bowel syndrome (qv), with diverticulitis as an additional complication. Most people in the Western world have mild symptoms of diverticular

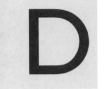

disease, which is associated with a low fibre diet. This diet produces a characteristic ageing process of the bowel which involves the development of small pockets or sacs (diverticula) in the wall of the colon. Diverticulitis occurs when one or more of these pockets becomes infected and inflamed. The illness it produces is sudden and very like appendicitis, with severe pain, fever and tenderness; however, the tenderness is felt in the lower left side of the abdomen. In some cases the diverticular inflammation may irritate the colon, causing it to contract, or spasm, excessively. Untreated, such an infection may produce severe illness. Acute diverticulitis often requires hospital admission for treatment with a combination of antibiotics, and some patients may require surgery to remove the diseased segment of the colon.

DIVERTICULUM

A blind sac or pocket leading from an organ — characteristically affecting the large bowel (colon); see preceding entry. Less commonly, one diverticulum or many diverticula may arise from the small intestine (diverticular disease of the small intestine), causing bacteria to collect within the normally sterile small bowel; these bacteria may interfere with the normal absorption and digestion of foods to produce malabsorption and associated diarrhoea.

DNA (DEOXYRIBO-NUCLEIC ACID)

A complex substance found in the nuclei of all plant and animal cells. The molecule consists of purine bases (thymidine and adenine) and pyrimidine bases (guanine and cytosine) linked to sugar molecules. Two chains of these bases are bound together and wrapped round each other in a spiral configuration (double helix). The chains of DNA are further tightly coiled to form the chromosomes of an individual, of which there are 23 pairs in each cell (except spermatozoa and ova, where chromosomes are not paired). A chromosome is made up of many genes; a gene is the segment of a DNA that codes for a particular protein. The molecules of DNA carry all the information necessary for the cell to produce proteins, and form the genetic basis for heredity, as a child inherits half (one of each pair) of his or her chromosomes (and hence DNA) from each parent.

DOMINANT (PATTERN OF INHERITANCE)

Inherited characteristics are determined by information stored on genes and may be passed from generation to generation in one of three manners: dominant, recessive or sex-linked. An individual affected by an autosomal dominant disease (for example, Huntington's chorea or adult polycystic kidney disease), will carry an abnormal gene (inherited from the

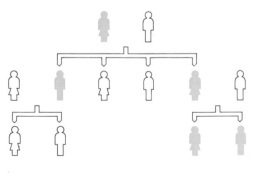

Affected individual

Normal individual

affected parent) and a normal copy of the gene (inherited from the unaffected parent). Therefore, each of his or her children will have a 50 per cent risk of inheriting the gene, irrespective of the sex of the parent or child.

DOWN'S SYNDROME

A congenital disorder characterized by mental retardation and a variety of physical abnormalities which gave the condition its other name of mongolism. These include a round skull with a flattened face, oblique eyes, a small mouth, a short broad neck, short broad hands with abnormal skin creases, and slow developmental progress. Other physical abnormalities are common, including some involving the heart and bowel.

Around 95 per cent of cases are caused by an abnormal egg (oocyte) or sperm being produced with an extra chromosome 21. The chance of this occurring increases with maternal age, being around 1 in 1,000 below the age of 30, but over 1 in 50 at the age of 45. The risk of it happening more than once to the same couple is no greater than in any people of an equivalent age. In the remaining 5 per cent of cases the condition is inherited from the parents, and the chance of recurrence can be as high as 25 per cent at any age. It is recommended that women who have had a child with Down's syndrome and those over the age of 35 have an amniocentesis (qv) in subsequent pregnancies to check the chromosomes of the fetus.

In general, people with Down's syndrome are severely retarded and need special education. As adults they require supervision either within the family or in an institution. No male is known to have fathered children, but females have borne children, half of whom are also mongols. Life expectancy of Down's syndrome sufferers is shorter than that of a normal person.
SEE ALSO *Gene*

DROWNING

In most fatal cases of drowning, death is caused by asphyxia after a struggle. A small number of people die immediately from asphyxia due to a reflex spasm of the larynx (voice-box) or cardiac arrest. As the human body is slightly heavier than water, it sinks when it is first immersed. The person then struggles up to the surface only to go down again; this may be repeated several times. During the struggle water mixed with air is drawn into the air passages and churned up with mucus into a froth, which then stops air from entering the lungs and leads to asphyxia. Death is said to occur within 2–5 minutes of drowning in fresh water and 7–10 minutes in sea water. In a few cases submersion for up to 40 minutes in very cold water has been followed by recovery.

A drowning person who has been rescued requires urgent first aid treatment.

DRUG DEPENDENCE

Drug dependence refers to the state in which a person feels compelled, for psychological or physical reasons, to take a drug repeatedly in order to experience its effect or to avoid withdrawal symptoms. Drug addiction implies that a person is physically dependent and will experience physical symptoms when he or she ceases to take the particular drug. Drug abuse implies neither psychological nor physical dependence, but that the use of a drug has brought about harmful effects on a person's psychological, physical or social function. Smoking

D

and alcoholism are the commonest forms of drug dependence in the Western world.

Heroin, the commonest opiate or narcotic causing dependency, may be taken by injection or inhalation. It leads to both physical and psychological dependence. During withdrawal, which may begin a few hours after the last dose, a person experiences a craving for the drug, agitation, sweating, diarrhoea, and abdominal pain. Heroin addiction is commonest in young men and there is evidence that it has increased. Methadone (a morphine-like drug) is commonly used to aid withdrawal. There is a high rate of HIV and hepatitis infections in intravenous opiate users, largely as a result of sharing needles for injection.

Cocaine is usually taken by sniffing and causes a strong psychological dependence. Withdrawal symptoms are usually mild. Amphetamines may be taken by mouth or injection. They probably cause both physical and psychological dependence, as do the new 'designer drugs' such as 'ecstasy'. The withdrawal symptoms of amphetamines include depression, fatigue and headache. LSD, cannabis (hashish, marijuana) and solvents are not associated with physical dependence. More common than dependency on illicit drugs is dependence on minor tranquillizers, which include benzodiazepines and barbiturates. Common withdrawal symptoms from these are insomnia, anxiety, headache, tremor and, occasionally, fits.

DRUG OVERDOSE

Intentional drug overdoses are a very common cause of admission to casualty departments. If a drug overdose is suspected, it is important to establish quickly which drug has been consumed, and in what quantity. This information is sought by hospital staff from prescriptions or tablet bottles. Analysis of specimens of blood or urine is often helpful in identifying the substance.

Early measures include the administration of an emetic or gastric lavage (qv). General measures include supporting vital functions by establishing and maintaining a clear airway for respiration. Specific antidotes exist for some poisons. Naloxone, for example, is a specific antidote for morphine and related drugs like heroin. N-acetylcysteine is used as an antidote to paracetamol.

DTs

see *Delirium tremens*

DUCTUS ARTERIOSUS

A blood vessel which is open during the development of a baby in the womb. It connects the main artery (the aorta) to the artery supplying the lungs (pulmonary artery), as the lungs do not function in the womb. The ductus usually closes off spontaneously after birth when the lungs expand. If it does not do this, then a heart murmur is present which, if undetected, can lead to heart failure in later life. An open (patent) ductus arteriosus can be induced to close by treatment with anti-prostaglandin drugs. Surgical closure is therefore less commonly used than in the past.

DUMBNESS

The lifelong inability to speak. As the dumb individual has never learnt to speak, dumbness is distinct from acquired speech problems such as a phasia (the most severe form of dysphasia, qv), or the result of surgery for a tumour of the larynx. Most dumb individuals are also deaf. There is not necessarily any deficiency of intelligence in the dumb, and careful training by speech therapists may allow the development of near-normal speech in people who are born deaf.

DUODENAL ULCER

A duodenal ulcer characteristically occurs in the first part of the duodenum, the first part of the intestine. Duodenal ulceration is probably the end result of a number of factors, including excessive acid secretion, family background, the use of aspirin-like drugs, cigarette smoking, and possibly infection by the organism *Campylobacter pylori*.

The pain (indigestion) felt with a duodenal ulcer characteristically occurs in the upper part of the abdomen, is relieved by eating but usually recurs during the night. More rarely, the ulcer may penetrate deeper into the wall of the duodenum to produce either a haemorrhage (haematemesis and melaena) or perforation right through the full thickness of the bowel wall to bring on peritonitis. Many years of inflammation may block the outlet of the stomach (pyloric stenosis).

Duodenal ulcers are diagnosed by either endoscopy (qv) or a barium meal (qv). Most ulcer patients are now managed using drugs such as cimetidine or rantidine, or less commonly using a compound containing bismuth, which is a heavy metal. Ulcer patients should stop smoking and avoid aspirin–like compounds. No special diet is required. Long-term medical treatment is offered to some people with either aggressive ulceration or other medical problems.

DUPUYTREN'S CONTRACTURE

A disorder of the hands. It usually, but not always, occurs in males and involves shortening, thickening and fibrosis of the connective tissue in the palm of the hand which produce a gradual and progressive deformity of, first, the ring finger and then the little fingers. In the early stages the thickening takes the form of one or more nodules in the palm of the hand; when the fingers are extended fully, a dimple is seen in the palm. The fingers gradually become curled towards the palm of the hand and cannot be straightened. The condition affects both hands, although it may be more advanced in one.

The cause of the contracture is unknown, but the condition may be associated with liver disease, notably alcoholism and cirrhosis. More often, however, there is no underlying illness. Dupuytren's contracture is treated by surgery to cut out the fibrous scar tissue; the operation usually has good results.

The term may also be used to describe a similar condition affecting the feet.

DWARFISM

A term usually applied to individuals with a defect of bone development known as achondroplasia (qv) (hence achondroplastic dwarf). This condition is inherited in dominant fashion, and so there is a 50 per cent chance that the children of a dwarf will also be dwarfs, and a 75 per cent chance if both parents are dwarfs. As the condition affects predominantly the long bones, dwarfs usually have very short arms and legs; the skull and trunk are comparatively normal. Intelligence and physical health are generally

D

normal in dwarfs but there is an increased risk of arthritis and paraplegia.

DYSARTHRIA

Imperfect articulation of speech. Mechanical problems may result in dysarthria — for example, cleft palate or badly fitting false teeth. Damage to the muscles of the face or to the nerves supplying the lips, tongue or palate as, for example, in motor neurone disease or stroke may also cause dysarthria. Impaired hearing early on may cause a child to have difficulty in learning how to speak, resulting in dysarthria.

DYSENTERY

Bloody diarrhoea resulting from gastro-intestinal infection. In most cases the organisms responsible are bacteria such as *Shigella* (bacillary dysentery) and amoebae (see *Amoebiases*), usually *Entamoeba histolytica* (amoebic dysentery). Dysentery is usually of sudden onset, and is characterized by very frequent bowel actions often with accompanying abdominal pain. Individuals most commonly affected are those exposed to poor sanitary conditions.

Treatment often requires admission to hospital and comprises oral fluid replacement, called oral rehydration therapy (rarely, rehydration is carried out by intravenous infusion or drip), and antibiotics to fight the infecting organism once this has been identified from laboratory examination of the stool. The patient is usually cured but is not then immune to recurrent attacks.

Bloody diarrhoea can also be a feature of ulcerative colitis, Crohn's disease and tumours of the bowel, and so tests may be needed to exclude these conditions in some patients.

DYSLEXIA

Difficulty in learning to read. It is sometimes known as word blindness, which implies a serious form of the disorder. General causes of reading retardation include educational difficulties (such as truancy) and intellectual impairment. Specific dyslexia may occur as an inherited defect, sometimes following delay in learning to speak, or as a result of brain damage in infancy or later childhood. The problem lies in the dominant cerebral hemisphere. (In right-handed people this is the left side of the brain, in left-handed, the right.)

The severity of dyslexia is variable. Rarely there may be complete word blindness. More commonly there are difficulties with the identification of letters, with substitutions of similar-sounding groups of letters, a tendency to guess according to the shape or context of a word, or reversal of a word (saw/was). There is often associated difficulty with spelling and writing. Remedial teaching is usually effective from the age of about 7 years, so that many dyslexic children are able to read adequately for purposes of secondary education.

DYSMENORRHOEA

The medical term for painful periods. If periods are painful right from the start it is termed primary dysmenorrhoea. Almost 50 per cent of women experience some kind of discomfort with their periods. The cause is thought to be excessive production of prostaglandins (substances normally present in many tissues in the body), which are known to increase the uterine contractions. Progesterone (a hormone produced in the second half of the cycle after the release of an egg from the ovary) probably also plays a part though the mechanism is uncertain. Symptoms often improve after a woman has borne children.

If periods become painful in a woman who has had painless periods in the past, it is called secondary dysmenorrhoea. The likely cause is an underlying gynaecological disease.

Treatment of primary dysmenorrhoea depends upon the severity of the symptoms. Simple painkillers (analgesics) will help some sufferers. Some drugs suppress the production of prostaglandins and are effective in relieving symptoms in almost 80 per cent of patients. Oral contraceptives can be used to suppress ovulation and thus prevent the onset of the pain that is known to only accompany ovulatory periods. Treatment of secondary dysmenorrhoea depends upon the underlying cause.

DYSPEPSIA

Simple dyspepsia may be due to overeating, rich or fatty food, or excess alcohol. However, dyspepsia may also be due to inflammation of the lower oesophagus (oesophagitis), peptic ulcer (either gastric or duodenal), gallstones or, more rarely, either cancer of the stomach or disease of the pancreas.

It is very difficult for a doctor to distinguish the different causes of dyspepsia without arranging additional tests — ideally a barium meal or endoscopy to examine the oesophagus (gullet) and stomach (first part of the intestine), and either an ultrasound examination or CT scan of the abdomen to examine the gall-bladder and pancreas.

DYSPHAGIA

Difficulty in swallowing. Dysphagia is usually described as 'food sticking', particularly bread and meat. The most common causes are narrowing due to scarring of the gullet (oesophagus) caused by stomach acid or a cancer of the gullet or stomach. A rarer cause, which also makes the swallowing of liquids difficult, is achalasia; this is brought only by a defect in muscular relaxation of the gullet. Dysphagia can also occur as a rare consequence of stroke or can be due to neuromuscular diseases such as myasthenia gravis.

Treatment is of the underlying cause.

DYSPHASIA

A disorder of both written and spoken language, usually following a stroke (cerebrovascular accident) and affecting the dominant side of the brain. (In right-handed people this is the left side of the brain; in left-handed people, usually the right.) Dysphasia can be sub-divided into motor (expressive or Broca's) dysphasia and sensory (receptive or Wernicke's) dysphasia. In motor dysphasia it is the production of speech that is affected. The patient is unable to produce one or more words spontaneously, although he or she will recognize the correct ones on prompting. In sensory dysphasia there is a disorder of comprehension of the spoken word, but spontaneous speech is fluent, though often consisting of jargon. Pure motor or sensory dysphasia is uncommon and most patients suffer from a mixture of both types.

Treatment with speech therapy usually brings some improvement but complete recovery is uncommon in severe cases.

DYSPNOEA

Difficulty with breathing; the feeling

of breathlessness, at first experienced on exertion and later at rest if the underlying disease worsens.

Dyspnoea is due to disease of the heart and/or lungs. In heart failure the lungs become overloaded with fluid, gas exchange across the pulmonary alveolar membrane is impaired, and the patient experiences shortness of breath, especially when lying flat. As cardiac failure worsens fluid leaks into the air spaces so that in effect the patient is drowning. Some congenital heart defects shunt deoxygenated blood from the veins into the arterial tree, bypassing the lungs to produce cyanosis (blueness) and dyspnoea (see Shunt).

There are many diseases of the lung which may cause breathlessness. In emphysema the gas-exhanging alveoli are destroyed and the small peripheral air spaces are enlarged; thus the areas where blood and fresh air meet are reduced. In embolic disease (see *Embolism*) some of the pulmonary arteries are blocked, thus pulmonary blood flow and ventilation (oxygenation) become 'mismatched'. In fibrosis of the lung, as occurs in some pneumoconioses (qv), the ability of the lung to expand is limited, impairing ventilation. Diseases affecting the major airways (bronchi), such as asthma, also impair ventilation of the lungs.

DYSURIA

Pain on passing urine. Dysuria is usually described as a stinging sensation and is associated with an increased frequency of passing urine. The most common cause is an infection in the urine. The condition is much more common in women, in whom infection is usually confined to the bladder, and is easily treated by antibiotics. Dysuria in men should always be investigated as there is usually another cause, such as an enlarged or inflamed prostate. Infection of the urethra (the tube leading from the bladder to the outside) can also cause dysuria.

EATING DISORDERS

see *Anorexia nervosa, Bulimia nervosa*

ECCHYMOSIS

The medical term for bruising. It tends to be used in cases where bruising is disproportionate to the injury sustained. Sometimes the patient may be unaware of any injury at all. So-called 'simple bruising' is often seen in healthy young individuals (usually women) where trivial injury has caused obvious bruising. There is no treatment for the condition which, though unsightly, is harmless. Ecchymosis is particularly common in patients with skin fragility (for example, the elderly and those on steroids) and in patients with disorders or reduced numbers of platelets (such as in chronic liver disease or splenomegaly). In these cases the underlying condition is treated.

ECG

see *Electrocardiography*

ECHINOCOCCUS

see *Hydatid disease*

ECHOCARDIO-GRAPHY

A technique using ultrasound waves to examine the structure and function of the heart from outside the body. It can assess the efficiency of ventricular contraction (the ventricles are the lower chambers of the heart), heart valve defects, infection of the heart valves and 'holes' in the heart. Recent developments mean that assessment of the direction of flow and turbulence of the blood in the heart can be carried out using a technique called colour flow doppler echocardiography. This non-invasive technique has made diagnosis and monitoring of heart lesions much easier, with less resort to cardiac catheterization (qv).

ECLAMPSIA

A term applied to convulsions occurring in pregnancy; about 50 per cent of cases arise during the second half of the antenatal period, 30 per cent during labour and 20 per cent within a few days of delivery. Eclampsia is more common during a first pregnancy or the first with a new partner. Its cause is unknown.

Eclampsia is usually preceded by pre-eclampsia (previously known as toxaemia of pregnancy), which is characterized by high blood pressure and protein in the urine (proteinuria). If these signs go unchecked eclampsia may develop, with convulsions accompanied by swelling of the face and limbs (oedema) as well as severe headache, blurring of vision or upper abdominal pain. Left untreated eclampsia can lead to death of the fetus and also of the mother, usually from a brain haemorrhage or kidney/heart failure. Only delivery of the baby will help the condition.

ECT

see *Electroconvulsive therapy*

ECTOPIC BEAT

A premature contraction of the heart that is independent of the normal rhythm and arises in response to an impulse in some part of the heart other than the sinuatrial node, the natural pacemaker (see *Arrhythmia*). It is also called an extrasystole or premature beat.

The impulses may arise from an area or areas in the atrium, atrioventricular node or ventricle. The commonest irregularity is the atrial ectopic beat. After the abnormal beat there is usually a pause followed by a stronger beat than normal while the pacemaker is 'reset'. This may produce the symptom of a skipped beat or palpitation. In elderly patients, atrial ectopic beats may indicate ischaemic heart disease and may precede more serious disorders of rhythm such as atrial fibrillation (qv) or ventricular tachycardia (qv).

Ventricular ectopic beats or extrasystoles are more common than atrial ectopic beats in patients with structural cardiac disease. They are more serious if they occur in pairs or groups as they may then precede ventricular tachycardia or fibrillation. Both atrial and vertricular ectopic beats are quite common in normal individuals and may be caused by excessive use of stimulants such as tobacco, coffee, tea and alcohol.

An ECG (see *Electrocardiography*) is usually necessary to distinguish between atrial and ventricular types. Drugs such as betablockers or calcium antagonists may be needed in some cases.

ECTOPIC PREGNANCY

When a fertilized egg, instead of developing in the uterus (womb), starts developing in another site, usually the Fallopian tube. There is a higher risk of ectopic pregnancy if

E

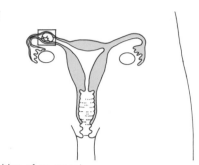

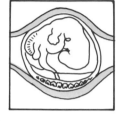

The position of an ectopic pregnancy. Once the pregnancy starts to develop in the Fallopian tube the placenta burrows into the surrounding tissue. The tube cannot enlarge — as the uterus does — to accommodate the growing fetus and may rupture, leading to internal bleeding.

there has been previous infection, or surgery to the tubes has been performed.

Symptoms occur in early pregnancy with abdominal pains due to stretching of the tube and internal bleeding; slight vaginal bleeding occurs in some cases. The tiny fetus inevitably dies.

Diagnosis cannot always be confirmed by clinical examination or by an ultrasound scan; laparoscopy (qv) may have to be carried out under a general anaesthetic to be sure.

Treatment consists of replacing the lost blood by transfusion, if required, and by removing (or repairing if possible) the affected portion of the tube.

ECTROPION

Outward folding or retraction of

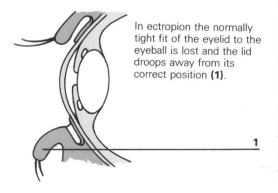

In ectropion the normally tight fit of the eyelid to the eyeball is lost and the lid droops away from its correct position (1).

1

the eyelid. This frequently leads to inflammation of the exposed conjunctiva (the membrane covering the front of the eye and eyelid) and predisposes to bacterial conjunctivitis. Ectropion is commonly seen as a feature of the lax facial skin found in the very elderly, in whom the natural elasticity of the tissues has been lost. There are a variety of other causes including acute or chronic inflammation of the skin around the eyes. Surgery around the eye may also lead to the development of ectropion, because all scars have a tendency to contract with the passage of time.

Treatment is directed at any underlying inflammatory cause, but surgical correction of the redundant tissue or refashioning of a retracted scar may be required.

ECZEMA

see *Dermatitis*

EEG

see *Electroencephalography*

EFFUSION

A collection of fluid in a cavity or potential cavity in the body. The term is not used in cases where the fluid is infected; that is called empyema (qv). An effusion occurs most commonly between the two layers of the pleura of the lungs (pleural effusion) or in the peritoneal space of the abdomen (ascites), and less frequently in the pericardium which sheathes the heart, where it may cause an obstruction (see *Tamponade*). Effusions may be transudates, when the fluid leaks out from capillaries or tiny blood vessels because of increased pressure within them (as in heart failure); or they may be exudates, when an inflammatory process involving the surface of the particular space causes fluid to leak into it.

The most frequent causes of pleural effusion are pneumonia, heart failure, pulmonary infarction due to embolism (death of lung tissue due to arterial blockage), and malignant disease. Effusions usually cause symptoms by exerting pressure on other organs; for example, dyspnoea (breathlessness) due to lung compression is the commonest symptom of pleural effusion.

Aspiration is the favoured treatment for the effusion itself, but the underlying condition has to be sought and then treated appropriately.

EISENMENGER'S SYNDROME

A rare complication of some forms of congenital heart disease which involves an abnormal shunt or communication (such as ventricular septal defect) between the high-pressure left-sided circulation which supplies the body, and the low-pressure right-sided circulation which supplies the lungs. If this left-to-right shunt is large, the extra blood flow to the lungs causes a reaction in the arteries, which become narrower, leading to a rise in right-sided pressure. If left untreated over many years, the right-sided pressure may come to equal or exceed that of the left, leading to reversal of the shunt and the development of cyanosis (qv). By this stage it is too late for a corrective operation, and the only hope for a cure is a heart-lung transplantation.

ELECTRIC SHOCK

The passage through the body of a high-voltage electrical current by contact with a live wire or lightning.

Fright, tingling and cramp occur in mild cases and soon pass without treatment. In serious cases, skin and deep tissue burns, convulsions, fractures, loss of consciousness and death, due to the stoppage of breathing and heart beat, may occur. The shock is greater with AC current and if the skin is wet.

In serious cases the first action should be to turn the electric switch to off. If the victim is still in contact with the live wire, he or she should be pulled away by someone wearing rubber gloves or shoes, or whose hands are wrapped in a thick layer of dry cloth. Mouth-to-mouth respiration and cardiac massage may be necessary to revive the victim.

ELECTRO-CARDIOGRAPHY

The study of the electrical activity of the heart using electrodes which are placed externally on the limbs and across the chest. The electro-cardiograph (ECG) allows diagnosis of abnormal types of heart rhythm (arrhythmia), abnormalities of the conducting system of the heart (the system of electrical pulses which control heart rate and contraction), and abnormalities of the heart muscle, particularly after a heart attack.

Electrocardiograms are of particular value in the emergency diagnosis of the cause of chest pain or unexplained

An ECG reading is taken by strapping electrodes to both arms and both legs. An additional electrode is placed over the heart itself.

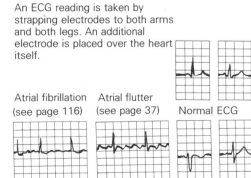

Atrial fibrillation (see page 116) Atrial flutter (see page 37) Normal ECG

collapse. Recently, technology for monitoring the ECG for 24 hours without the need to restrict patients from moving around has become available and may become a valuable tool in the diagnosis of transient abnormalities of heart rhythm.

ELECTRO-CONVULSIVE THERAPY (ECT)

A form of treatment usually only employed in cases of very severe depression, where other treatments (such as antidepressants) have been ineffective or are unsafe. A typical course consists of between six and twelve treatments administered twice-weekly. Each treatment takes place under general anaesthetic and entails the placing of electrodes on the head to deliver sufficient shock to induce a fit. Unilateral ECT, where shocks are delivered to the non-dominant cerebral hemisphere (in a right-handed person, the right half of the brain; in a left-handed person, the left side), causes less memory disturbance and is often used in preference to bilateral ECT.

ECT has been surrounded by controversy, some critics holding it to be an invasive treatment which may lead to brain damage. While patients may describe a headache and amnesia, there is little evidence that ECT is anything other than a safe and effective treatment for depression.

ELECTROENCEPHA-LOGRAPHY (EEG)

A technique for measuring the electrical activity of the brain. A set of electrodes is placed over the scalp to pick up changes in electrical impulses (brain potentials), which are recorded as brain waves. With alterations in consciousness, for example in sleep, the pattern of the brain waves changes: the EEG had identified four distinct stages of sleep. The EEG is commonly used as a diagnostic instrument by neurologists and psychiatrists to detect abnormal electrical activity in cases of epilepsy and of brain disease.

ELECTRO-MYOGRAPHY (EMG)

A recording of the electrical activity of muscle. An EMG is produced by inserting a fine needle electrode into the muscle under study and recording electrical activity at rest and during contraction. This procedure is helpful in determining whether there is an abnormality in the muscle itself, in its supplying nerve, or in the junction between the nerve and muscle. Normal muscle is electrically silent at rest, and produces characteristic patterns on contraction. Different disease processes will produce differing abnormal electrical patterns. Electromyography is particularly useful in investigating the causes of polyneuritis and in distinguishing between myopathies such as muscular dystrophy on the one hand and denervating disorders such as motor neurone disease on the other.

EMBOLISM

The scattering of particles (emboli) of clot, fat, air or tumour from one site in the circulation to other blood vessels. The most common cause of embolism is a clot from a thrombosis in a leg vein travelling to vessels in the lung (pulmonary embolus). This causes a block in the blood vessels and the death of the part of the lung tissue that they supply. Treatment with anticoagulant drugs usually prevents further thrombosis. Severe injury may result in fat embolism, when particles of bone marrow fat are scattered and usually lodge in the lung and brain, causing coma.

EMETIC

A substance which causes vomiting, used for medicinal purposes. Emetics act through the vomiting centre in the brain and were commonly used to induce vomiting after ingestion of poisons; ipecacuanha syrup is an example. Nowadays stomach wash-outs (lavage) are preferred to emetics because the induction of vomiting in unconscious patients and in cases of poisoning with corrosives is always dangerous.

EMG

see *Electromyography*

EMPHYSEMA

A progressive condition of the lungs which involves the generalized destruction of the walls of the alveoli (the smallest parts of the airways involved in gas transfer with the blood). It is often associated with chronic bronchitis and disability will depend to an extent on the severity of this accompanying disease. The major cause of emphysema is cigarette smoking; the smoke damages cells in the lungs, leading to the release of enzymes which destroy the lung tissue. Patients develop shortness of breath, initially only on exertion but later also at rest. Emphysema eventually leads to respiratory failure; this occurs because the alveoli or air sacs rupture and enlarge so that there is insufficient air in contact with the capillaries between them to oxygenate the blood. Heart failure may develop;

asthma and bronchiectasis are also sometimes associated with emphysema.

There is no specific remedy for emphysema and treatment is directed to improving the general health of the patient and ensuring that likely aggravators of the condition, such as cigarette smoking or obesity, are avoided. Treatment of the accompanying chronic bronchitis or other condition will be required. Oxygen administration may be needed during severe attacks of breathlessness.

EMPYEMA

The accumulation of pus in the pleural space (the potential cavity between the outside of the lung and the chest wall). This is usually brought about by infection in an adjacent structure, commonly the lung, as a result of conditions such as pneumonia or tuberculosis. Less commonly, empyema may follow a deep chest wound. Symptoms include fever, often with severe sweating attacks (rigors), malaise (a general feeling of being unwell), weight loss, chest pain and breathlessness, with a productive cough if there is underlying chest infection.

In the acute stage, when the pus is thin in consistency, drainage of the fluid through the chest wall and the administering of appropriate antibiotics may be sufficient to clear up the problem; if the empyema is chronic, more extensive surgical procedures may be required to eradicate the infection. Pulmonary infections have become more easily treatable with antibiotics, so empyema is now comparatively rare.

ENCEPHALITIS

Inflammation of the brain, usually caused by a virus. Mumps, measles

E

and chickenpox are frequently to blame, although many other viruses may cause the condition. Indeed, encephalitis is a very rare complication of these common childhood illnesses. The symptoms are headache, confusion, irritability, impaired consciousness and, in severe cases, coma. The disease usually runs a benign course to complete recovery, but occasionally it is very severe, even fatal, and leaves permanent brain damage. When the spinal cord as well as the brain is involved the condition is called encephalomyelitis; in this complication the limbs may be paralysed.

There is no specific treatment for viral encephalitis, and this is an important reason for vaccination.

Encephalitis is sometimes associated with meningitis, and in cases in which the two co-exist the term meningoencephalitis is used to describe the condition. Bacterial in origin, meningoencephalitis is caused by the organism *Neisserai meningitidis* or the *Mycobacterium tuberculosis*. It behaves in much the same way as meningitis (qv), although survivors are more likely to suffer epilepsy in the future. Unlike viral encephalitis, bacterial meningoencephalitis can respond to antibiotics.

ENCEPHALOPATHY

A reversible abnormality of brain function as a result of non-neurological disease. Encephalopathy will always clear up completely when the underlying cause is removed (if this is possible). Mild encephalopathy is characterized by drowsiness and reversal of the normal sleeping pattern. With progressive severity, especially in cases where the condition is due to toxic or metabolic causes, the patient becomes more confused and dis-

orientated and ultimately falls into a coma.

The commonest form of encephalopathy is that associated with sedative drugs, such as diazepam and other tranquillizers. These may have been used during medical procedures (to treat amnesia, for example), or in self-poisoning. As the drug is cleared from the body the encephalopathy resolves. It is more usual, though, for patients to be termed encephalopathic when the cause is metabolic in origin, such as uncontrolled diabetes mellitus, liver failure, severe kidney failure, hypercalcaemia (high levels of calcium in the blood) and (perhaps most importantly) infection (usually septicaemia).

ENDARTERECTOMY

A special operation to unblock the larger arteries (particularly the carotid arteries) and so normalize blood supply and prevent stroke. The surgeon removes the blockage, caused by atheroma (qv), by carefully stripping off the innermost lining of the blood vessel, which contains the atheromatous deposit. The thick fibres in the rest of the arterial wall will then allow the blood to flow unimpeded to the organs. Endarterectomy is also employed in other operations on arteries when grafts (qv) are used to bypass the blockage. SEE ALSO *Claudication*

ENDOCARDITIS

see *Infective endocarditis*

ENDOCRINOLOGY

The study of the endocrine or hormone-producing glands of the body, such as the thyroid, adrenals (suprarenals), parathyroids, pancreas and gonads (ovaries and testes). These glands are under the overall control of the principal endocrine gland, the pituitary, which is found in the base of the brain.

Endocrinological tests often involve measurement of the level of the appropriate hormone in the blood, and studies of the structure and function of the gland responsible for producing the hormone.
SEE ALSO *illustration on page 144*

ENDOMETRIOSIS

In this condition specialized tissue (epithelium) normally only found lining the uterine cavity (endometrium) is also present in other areas of the body. The most common abnormal site is the ovary, followed by the Fallopian tubes (the ligaments that support the uterus, or womb) and then the muscle of the uterus (this last condition is called adenomyosis). The tissue can also be found on the bowel and bladder and more rarely in the lungs. Like endometrium it grows in a cyclical manner under the influence of hormones produced by the ovary and, as in the uterine lining, it disintegrates and bleeds if pregnancy does not occur. Unlike normally sited endometrium, however, it has no natural outflow tract and therefore blood and breakdown products accumulate in the tissues, leading to pain, inflammation and damage to surrounding structures. This can cause intense scarring and is one cause of infertility in women.

The treatment of endometriosis depends upon how severe the condition is and whether there is a need or desire to preserve fertility. Medical treatment involves the use of drugs to prevent hormones stimulating endometrial growth; surgical management can range from removing affected tissues to removing all the pelvic organs (uterus, tubes and ovaries).

ENDOSCOPY

A technique involving the use of fibre-optic instruments to obtain a clear view in colour of the oesophagus, stomach and duodenum (gastroscopy), or colon (colonoscopy), or lungs (bronchoscopy). The great majority of endoscopy procedures are performed on outpatients, who receive mild sedation.

Endoscopy can be used either for making a diagnosis (when the endoscopist may be able to see signs of disease) or to take samples for later analysis under the microscope. Endoscopy may also be used for certain forms of treatment; for example, removing small tumours or polyps from the colon (polypectomy) or dealing with more complicated diseases of the biliary system or pancreas during a technique called ERCP (endoscopic retrograde cholangiopancreatography).

ENDOTRACHEAL TUBE

A tube inserted into the trachea (windpipe), via the nose or mouth, for the purpose of assisting ventilation (see *Artificial respiration*). A laryngoscope is used to guide the tube through the vocal cords and into the trachea. The patient is unconscious, anaesthetized or heavily sedated while this is done.

When the tube is in position an inflatable cuff near the tip is filled to ensure an airtight fit in the trachea.

ENEMA

Instillation of liquid into the rectum

E

and large bowel through a tube inserted via the anus. Enemata (plural) may be performed to aid diagnosis or as a form of treatment. Water, possibly with a mild irritant added, may be used in order to wash out the colon, prior to endoscopy or a barium enema. Steroid enemata are used to control ulcerative colitis during periods of acute inflammation.

ENZYME

A protein made within living cells which speeds up or triggers a very wide variety of chemical reactions in the body, particularly in the blood and gut, without itself being used up in the reaction. There are many different types of enzyme, each type responsible for a limited range of chemical reactions. For example, enzymes manufactured by the pancreas are responsible for digestion. Specific enzyme defects − for example, phenylketonuria (see *Inborn errors of metabolism*) in cells and lactase deficiency in the gut − can lead to disease.

EOSINOPHILIA

An increase in number of a type of circulating white blood cell called eosinophils. Eosinophilia occurs in allergic disease (such as asthma), parasitic infestations, rare medical conditions and as a result of sensitivity to drugs. The eosinophil count is obtained from the percentage of eosinophils seen on a blood film.

EPIDURAL ANAESTHESIA

An injection into the lumbar region of the back to relieve pain. It is most frequently employed to relieve the pain associated with labour and childbirth, although it can also be used to

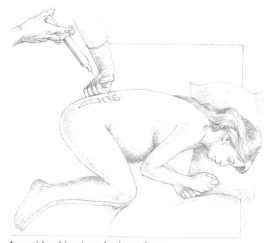

An epidural is given by inserting a fine tube (cannula) into the epidural space surrounding the spinal cord and then bathing the sensory nerves with local anaesthetic drugs.

relieve chronic back pain or pain during abdominal and pelvic surgery.

The effect of 'blocking' the nerves in this way gradually wears off, depending on the amount and type of drug used. When used to maintain pain relief in women in labour, repeated doses of drug can be administered down the same cannula. (The drug does not enter the fetal circulation, so it has no effect on the baby.) The anaesthesia extends to cause some numbness over the lower abdomen and legs and can temporarily lead to weakness in the muscles and limit the mother's ability to push. Also, as pain is abolished so is the desire to push and there is an increased chance of a forceps delivery. In experienced hands an epidural is safe and effective, allowing the mother to be comfortable and alert during labour.

EPILEPSY

A disease in which an abnormal electrical discharge in one or other part of the brain triggers a range of physical and sensory disturbances. In most types of epilepsy, the cause of this discharge is not found. However, the condition can be associated with a brain tumour, abscess or abnormal blood vessels, or may follow head or birth injury or strokes.

The principal types of epilepsy are termed grand mal, petit mal, temporal lobe, and focal. In grand mal, or major epilepsy, fits are accompanied by loss of consciousness. In about half of these cases the fit is preceded by an aura, a type of premonition which the patient recognizes well as a sign that an attack is imminent. There are two phases to a fit. In the first (the tonic phase) the muscles are permanently contracted, including those used for breathing and so the patient may turn blue due to lack of oxygen. In the second, or clonic, phase there is jerking of the limbs, loss of bladder control and tongue biting. Sleep then often ensues. Emergency care involves protecting the patient from injury during the fit and wedging the jaw open with a soft instrument to prevent tongue biting.

Petit mal almost always begins in children, with very brief periods of 'mental blankness'; very occasionally the patient also has major fits. This type of epilepsy rarely arises in, or continues into, adult life. Temporal lobe epilepsy (also called complex partial epilepsy) causes disturbances of the interpretation of visual, smell or taste stimuli; automation (movements or activities carried out spontaneously without voluntary control) may be associated with this form of epilepsy. In focal (Jacksonian) epilepsy, convulsive movement starts in only one part of the body and may proceed to involve that side of the body and then the whole of the body. Paralysis after a focal fit may last for up to three days (Todd's paralysis).

Diagnosis is based on the patient's history and is often assisted by investigations with EEG, which measures the electrical rhythms of the brain. Treatment involves regular medication with anti-convulsant drugs to suppress the abnormal elec-trical activity. Intractable cases of temporal lobe epilepsy sometimes can be helped by surgical removal of part of the temporal lobe in the brain.

EPISIOTOMY

A deliberate incision of the skin around the vulva (perineum) and vagina made during delivery by a midwife to enlarge the outlet of the birth canal and prevent extensive tearing.

Episiotomy can also be employed to help hasten delivery if the baby is distressed and is nearly always needed to prevent tearing in forceps-assisted deliveries. After delivery the episiotomy is quickly repaired under local anaesthetic, using sutures which dissolve in a matter of weeks and do not require removal.

ERYSIPELAS

An acute infection caused by bacteria, usually streptococci, and sometimes staphylococci, of the facial skin. The symptoms are swelling of the skin around the cheeks and eyes, together with tenderness, redness, heat, systemic upset and fever. The condition usually appears over a matter of hours, reaching a peak perhaps one or two days after onset. Treatment is with antibiotics directed against the suspected organisms.

ERYTHEMA

Red discoloration of the skin. This results from dilatation of the underlying blood vessels and is almost universally present during the course of any inflammatory skin disorder such as psoriasis or dermatitis. Erythema is the result of the release of a variety of active substances into the skin during the course of the disorder.

E

Blood vessels may also dilate and induce erythema in response to other stimuli, such as emotion (blushing), heat or cold wind.

ERYTHEMA MULTIFORME

A widespread skin eruption which characteristically involves the extremities, with lesions on the forearms, lower legs, hands and feet. The classic sign of erythema multiforme is the 'target lesion', so called because the two or three concentric rings of alternating erythema and pallor may resemble the bull's-eye of an archery or darts target. Large areas of skin usually remain entirely unaffected but in severe cases lesions may be widespread, in some instances affecting the membranes of the mouth and eyes. Sometimes the lesions may take the form of blisters and frequently this indicates a severe form of the disease.

The exact cause of erythema multiforme is unknown but precipitating events include the administration of almost any drug, and a variety of infections (typically herpes simplex or cold sores); very rarely it may be a sign of some systemic disorder.

It usually clears up without treatment, in most cases within a few days or weeks.

ERYTHROCYTE

The red blood cell which is produced in the bone marrow, contains haemoglobin, and carries oxygen to the cells of the body. It does not possess a nucleus but generates its own energy from glucose. It is estimated that there are about 5 million erythrocytes per cubic millimetre of blood. Each erythrocyte is a flexible biconcave disc which has a life of 120 days.

In medicine the size and shape of erythrocytes are studied for the information they give about certain conditions. Different types of anaemia may be distinguished in this way: small red cells occur in iron deficiency, and large red cells in vitamin B_{12} deficiency. Disease activity can be assessed by the rate at which red cells sink in a sample of blood.

EXOPHTHALMOS

Prominence or protrusion of the eyeball due to disease so that the eyelid will not cover it. Exophthalmos is caused by fluid and lymphocytes (a type of white blood cell) infiltrating the retrobulbar tissues behind the eye, together with a retraction or spasm of the upper eyelid. The result is a widening of the corners of the eye, so that the white of the eye (sclera) protrudes above the upper edge of the iris and cornea.

Exophthalmos is found in Graves' disease (see *Hyperthyroidism*, *Thyrotoxicosis*). In malignant exophthalmos (not a cancerous condition) corneal ulceration occurs, with destruction of the eye. Ophthalmoplegia is the term used to describe the inability to move the eye which sometimes accompanies exophthalmos; this is known as exophthalmic ophthalmoplegia or ophthalmic Graves' disease.

Exophthalmos is usually self-limiting and may regress a little even before treatment is given. Sleeping propped up and having the eyelids partially sewn up (lateral tarsorrhaphy) are measures that help to protect the eye but not to prevent the condition getting worse. Steroids and, in severe cases, orbital decompression (making a surgical hole to relieve pressure), are used to treat ophthalmoplegia, and are in addition to the treatment given for the thyrotoxicosis (qv).

EXOSTOSIS

A childhood condition in which a small bony swelling sticks out from the surface of a bone. This extra growth of bone occurs near a joint, and stops after adolescence. It is quite harmless and only rarely causes pressure on a tendon, necessitating treatment.

EXPECTORANT

A compound given to patients with a productive cough (with phlegm) to loosen secretions from the respiratory tract. Such compounds act by a reflex from the stomach to stimulate coughing and may also cause an increase in watery secretions from the airways.

Expectorants include compounds such as iodides, chlorides, bicarbonates, acetates, ipecacuanha, creosotes, volatile oils and guiaicols. They are usually given in the form of cough mixtures, sometimes mixed with antihistamines which may also stimulate the stomach and reduce unnecessary coughing by their sedative effect.

EXTRADURAL HAEMORRHAGE

Bleeding outside the main covering of the brain (dura mater), but within the skull. It is caused by injury to the middle meningeal artery as it passes on the inside of the temporal bone of the skull, which is on either side of the head. There may be a transient loss of consciousness, followed by recovery for a few days, but unless early surgery is performed to remove the clot (when recovery may be complete) death occurs because of the increasing pressure exerted by the clot on the soft brain. Fractures of the temporal bone should always be investigated in hospital to exclude an extradural haemorrhage.

SEE ALSO *illustration on page 49*

EXTRASYSTOLE

see *Ectopic beat*

EXTRINSIC ALLERGIC ALVEOLITIS

A group of uncommon diseases in which the inhalation of a range of organic dusts gives rise to a diffuse allergic reaction in the lungs. Among this group is farmer's lung, which is caused by exposure to the fungal spores of *Micro polyspora faeni*, found in mouldy hay. Other diseases in the group include mushroom picker's lung (caused by mushroom dust) and malt worker's lung (caused by mouldy barley and malt dust).

All of these diseases share the same symptoms. Four to six hours after exposure, the patient will feel generally unwell, with a fever, breathlessness, dry cough and aches and pains. The symptoms usually subside in 2−3 days. Treatment involves avoiding the causative agent; sometimes steroids are prescribed.

Fibrosis (scar tissue) may occur in the lungs with clubbing of the fingers, respiratory failure and cor pulmonale (pulmonary heart disease).

FALLOPIAN TUBE

In the normally developed female there are two Fallopian tubes. These are small fibromuscular structures, approximately 10 cm (4 inches) long, which provide a conduit between the ovaries and the uterine cavity. The tubes have relatively wide openings (ostia) at each ovarian end which contain finger-like projections called

F

F

fimbria: these assist the egg to enter the tube at the time of ovulation.

After intercourse sperm enter the cavity of the uterus (womb) through the cervical canal and after traversing the uterine cavity enter the uterine ends of the tubes. They then pass through the tubes where fertilization of the recently ovulated egg may occur.

Each tube has a specialized lining containing cells with small hair-like structures (cilia) that assist the passage of sperm and egg respectively. The tubes also produce special fluids that provide the correct environment for fertilization to take place and maintain the viability of the early embryo before it implants in the lining of the uterus.

Damage to the tubes can occur either as a result of disease, such as infections, or deliberately, as in sterilization operations. If the tubes become completely blocked then the woman will be infertile; then pregnancy may still occur if the tubes are only partially damaged although there is an increased risk of an ectopic pregnancy as a result of the fertilized egg failing to reach the uterus and therefore continuing to develop in the tube.

SEE ALSO *illustration on page 212*

FALLOT'S TETRALOGY

A form of congenital heart disease in which there is abnormal development of the partition (septum) between the ventricles (lower chambers of the heart). This has four consequences (hence tetralogy, from the Greek for 'four'): a deficiency of the upper part of the septum (ventricular septal defect); an overriding aorta; thickening of the muscle of the outlet of the right ventricle (subpulmonary stenosis) and of the ventricle itself.

In Fallot's tetralogy the narrowed pulmonary valve **(1)** causes a reduction in the blood flow to the pulmonary artery. The hole in the partition between the two ventricles **(2)** (ventricular septal defect) allows blood from both left and right ventricles to enter the aorta.

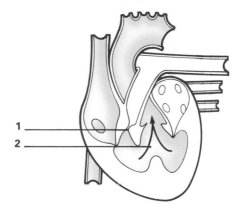

The cause of Fallot's tetralogy is unknown and there may be no signs of the disease at birth, though some babies have a heart murmur. Symptoms start to develop after 1 month of age, consisting of attacks of cyanosis (blue spells — hence the lay term 'blue baby'), particularly on exertion; some older children gain relief by squatting when they begin to feel breathless. The diagnosis is made by ultrasound. Open-heart surgery may be effective in correcting the abnormality.

FAMILY PLANNING

see *Contraception*

FARMER'S LUNG

see *Extrinsic allergic alveolitis*

FASCICULATION

Spontaneous and random contractions of groups of muscle fibres comprising part of a single muscle. When enough of these fibres are involved simultaneously, the contractions are visible.

Benign fasciculation occurs as a

result of tiredness in an otherwise healthy individual, who may experience it as coarse ripples of the calves or twitches of the lower eyelids. Abnormal fasciculation is often associated with diseases of the nervous system. It is, for example, a principal feature of motor neurone disease.

FEBRILE CONVULSIONS

Fits associated with fever; fits without fever suggest a different diagnosis. Febrile convulsions occur in 3 per cent of children aged between 6 months and 5 years. In many cases, other members of the family have had similar fits. Febrile convulsions are not associated with epilepsy and do not occur unless the child has a high temperature.

During a fit the affected child loses consciousness and then jerks all over. Such fits are usually shortlived and do not last longer than 15 minutes. Prevention involves keeping the feverish child cool and treating the underlying condition (tonsillitis, for example). The child must be examined by a doctor after the initial fit to make sure there is no sign of meningitis; in some cases it may be necessary to carry out tests. Drug treatment may be necessary if the fits recur frequently.

FEMINIZATION

The process whereby female characteristics are acquired by the male. Feminization may occur as a result of drug use (oestrogen, for example) or may be an inherited defect. If it is inherited, the fetus may be a genetic male (XY — see *Chromosome*) and have testicles, but because there is an inherited resistance to the effects of

the male sex hormone (testosterone) the bodily appearance is that of a female. At birth the baby looks like a female, the penis is small and like a clitoris and the testes are recessed. The genitalia look female, so the condition may only be recognized when periods do not start at puberty. This is because there is no uterus and no ovaries. The vagina is also absent.

FERTILITY DRUG

A drug given to infertile women in order to induce ovulation. One such drug, clomiphene, acts on part of the brain and increases the production of hormones that stimulate the ovaries. It is given as a course of tablets for five days each month. Of those women who conceive as a result of the treatment, around 10 per cent have twins. If clomiphene is unsuccessful, natural hormones in concentrated form are given by injection. These are obtained from post-menopausal women who produce them in large quantities. The preparation contains follicle-stimulating hormone (FSH) and luteinizing hormone (LH), a combination known as human menopausal gonadotrophin or pergonal. This is very potent and treatment with it requires careful monitoring by means of ultrasound and urine tests to avoid multiple pregnancies.

FETOSCOPY

A specialized procedure during which a very thin telescope (fetoscope) 1.7 mm in diameter is inserted through the abdominal wall and into the uterus (womb) to obtain a direct view of the fetus. Fetoscopy can be performed under a local anaesthetic at a gestation of 16–18 weeks; beyond this time it becomes progressively more difficult to visualize important fetal structures.

F

F

It can be used to diagnose structural congenital abnormalities such as defects of limbs, hands and feet, and also to diagnose rare inherited conditions affecting the skin of the fetus. Another form of fetoscopy can detect some inherited blood conditions (thalassaemia, haemophilia and sickle cell disease, for example) and involves using a thin needle to obtain fetal blood specimens from the umbilical cord for analysis. However, fetoscopy has now largely been superseded by chorionic villus biopsy or sampling and by improved ultrasound techniques, both of which are safer for the fetus and more acceptable to the mother.

FEVER

An increase in body temperature, known medically as pyrexia. The hypothalamus, located just above the pituitary gland in the brain, is primarily responsible for the maintenance of a stable body temperature, between 36°C and 37°C (96.8°F and 98.6°F). It may vary slightly during the day, being lowest in early hours of the morning. Body temperature may be measured with a thermometer placed under the tongue, in the groin, under the arm, or in the rectum. Prior to use, a thermometer should be cleaned with alcohol to kill bacteria and the mercury column should be shaken down. The thermometer should be left in place for at least one minute. Glass thermometers should not be placed in the mouths of children or unconscious patients.

The commonest cause of an increase in body temperature is infection with bacteria or viruses. In young children a rapid rise in body temperature may produce febrile convulsions (qv).

Aspirin and paracetamol are good antipyretics, but aspirin should not be given to children. Sponging with tepid water is beneficial in cases of high fever.

FIBRILLATION

Contraction of single muscle fibres. It is a sign of damage to or disease of the nerve supply of the muscle. Fibrillation cannot be seen with the naked eye but can be recorded by means of an electromyogram (see *Electromyography*). The same term is used in cardiology to signify uncoordinated contractions of cardiac muscle so that effective action is lost: hence atrial fibrillation (fibrillation of the atria — the two receiving chambers of the heart) and ventricular fibrillation (fibrillation of the two main muscles constituting the pumps which sustain the circulation).

Atrial fibrillation (an exaggerated form of atrial flutter, qv), is a common condition, particularly in elderly people with coronary artery disease or previous rheumatic fever-associated heart valve disease. Because the atrial muscle contraction is unco-ordinated, blood is less efficiently passed into the ventricles and the overall pump action of the heart is therefore diminished; there is a tendency to heart failure. Digoxin is often used to treat atrial fibrillation, although it is increasingly being replaced by other anti-arrhythmics such as amiodarone. Patients at particular risk of forming clots in the circulation are usually given an anticoagulant, such as warfarin.

Ventricular fibrillation (qv) causes the ventricles to twitch continuously but with no significant output of blood to maintain the circulation; it is therefore one of the commonest causes of sudden death from cardiac arrest.

SEE ALSO *illustration page 138*

FIBROADENOMA

In women the breast contains fat and muscular, fibrous and glandular tissue to make milk. Occasionally there is excessive growth of the fibrous and glandular tissue, particularly in younger women, which results in a firmer area in the breast. This has a fibrous covering which makes the lump very mobile. The fibroadenoma is benign, but requires surgical biopsy to distinguish it from the uncommon breast cancer that feels like a fibroadenoma.

FIBROID

A tumour of the uterine muscle; also called a fibromyoma. The cause is unknown. Fibroids are relatively common and the vast majority of them are benign. They can be found in different areas of the uterus and originate from the external surface (subserosal fibroids), the internal surface (submucus fibroids) or from the muscle wall itself (intramural fibroids). Whatever their size, which varies, fibroids usually result in an enlarged uterus (womb). Although there may be no symptoms, fibroids are usually noticed because of a painless swelling in the abdomin-opelvic region, heavy periods (see *Menorrhagia*), and occasionally pain due to disintegration of their internal tissues (known as degeneration). Fibroids may also be a cause of infertility.

Treatment is essentially surgical and either involves removing the fibroid (known as a myomectomy) or the entire uterus. The former operation is usually attempted, but unfortunately it is not always possible to conserve the uterus, especially if the fibroids are large.

Women between the ages of 35 and 45 are most commonly affected by fibroids, which tend to regress spontaneously after the menopause.

FIBROSIS

The formation of fibrous or scar tissue; it is caused by an increase in the amount of collagen fibres. (Collagen is a protein, and the main component of connective tissue.) The area of fibrosis is firmer to the touch than the surrounding tissues. Fibrosis is common when the tissue repairs itself after inflammation or lack of blood supply, but occasionally no cause can be found. A good example of fibrosis is the scar that is left after a surgical wound has healed. The inhalation of certain noxious dust particles can sometimes result in fibrosis of the lungs.

FILARIASIS

An infection caused by the filaria worm; the commonest type is found in many tropical and subtropical areas across the world, and is spread by mosquito bites. The adult worm lies in the lymphatic system, blocking the flow of lymph fluid. This results in the thickening of the legs and genitals, hydrocoele (qv) and milky urine. Fever, a cough and asthma may also be symptoms.

Another form of filariasis occurs in West Africa and Latin America, near fast-flowing rivers. It is spread by a type of fly. The filaria worm lives beneath the skin and causes blindness (river blindness).

A third type of filariasis is caused by loa loa or eyeworm in West Africa. In this condition small swellings are seen in the skin (calabar swellings).

Effective drug treatment for filariasis exists, but depends on the form of the infection.

F

F

FISSURE

A term applied to a groove, cleft or furrow, or to a small narrow ulcer. The first meaning refers specifically to natural anatomical structures of the body, such as fissurae cerebelli (the curved fissures running across the surfaces of the cerebellum in the brain). The most common example of an abnormal fissure or ulcer is the anal fissure, or fissure-in-ano. Small, and exceedingly painful, this ulcer is found in the anal canal where it usually causes spasm of the anal sphincter. Constipation and straining at stool may contribute to the formation of an anal fissure.

Treatment is by application of a local anaesthetic together with laxatives and, if necessary, anal dilatation or division of the sphincter by surgical means.

FISTULA

An abnormal passageway between two parts of the body which allows any type of body fluid (such as blood, bile, urine and bowel contents) to travel to an abnormal location. Most fistulas are caused either by disease or injury. The fistula may be internal (between two cavities) or it may lead from a natural cavity to the surface of the body. The effect of the fluid in the abnormal location produces symptoms that vary according to the type of fistula. One type of internal fistula, called a gastrocolic fistula, is in effect the body's attempt to bypass an obstruction (stricture) caused by a stomach growth. In some cases the fistula is formed as a result of the distended stomach rupturing into the colon. Examples of fistulae to the external surface of the body are fistula-in-ano (qv), the most important type, and biliary fistula. The latter is caused by bile leaking through the skin of the abdominal wall after an operation on the bile duct or gall bladder. Fistulas are often narrow and difficult to treat. They are usually operated on surgically.

FISTULA-IN-ANO

This term means fistula from the rectum and refers to an abnormal passageway, lined by raw or healing tissue, which opens deeply in the anal canal and leads to the exterior of the body, near the anus. It usually occurs as a result of an abscess of the anus or rectum. The fistula continually discharges faeces and sometimes pus and seldom closes spontaneously because of constant re-infection from the rectum. Low-level fistula-in-ano (where the internal opening is below the junction of the anus and rectum) is treated surgically by laying the fistula tract open, cutting out the raw or healing tissue and packing the wound daily until it heals. Higher-level fistulas cannot be laid open (incontinence due to sphincter division would result) and are consequently somewhat more difficult to treat.

FIXATION

The orthopaedic term for pinning bones together. Fixation is used in cases of unstable fracture or in those that are slow, or unlikely, to heal in plaster. Either an internal or external method may be employed. Nailing and plating are internal techniques. In the first, a metal rod is passed down the inside of a long bone, such as the femur (thigh-bone). In plating, the alternative technique, a metal plate is screwed into the bone on either side of the fracture.

The external method is particularly useful for fractures in the lower leg or if there is risk of infection in the fracture. In this method, a metal frame is pinned to the outside of the limb, the pins passing through the skin and into the bone.

Fixation is performed under anaesthesia and allows the healthy individual almost normal activity straightaway after the operation.

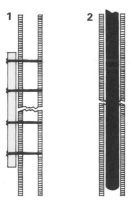

Two methods of fixation: **1** bone grafted to the outside of the fractured bone and held in position by screws; **2** passing a nail down the inside of a long bone — this technique is especially suitable for fractures near the middle of the shaft.

FLOPPY INFANT SYNDROME

A term used to describe infants who soon after birth have poor muscle tone and reduced activity. Normal muscle power and tone depend on an intact neurological system consisting of brain, spinal cord, nerves and muscles. Disease of any of these components may cause floppiness, and includes chromosome abnormalities, structural and metabolic brain disease, damage to the spinal cord during delivery, inherited degeneration of the nerves, and congenital myopathies (muscle wasting diseases). A battery of tests is required to find the cause. There remains a small group of floppy babies in whom a cause is not established; they gradually improve in tone and activity as they mature, and appear normal by 1 or 2 years of age (benign congenital hypotonia).

'FLU

see *Influenza*

FLUKE

A small flatworm which mainly infests animals such as sheep and cattle but can occasionally cause disease in man. Fluke infections are more common in the Far East. Different types of fluke infect the liver, lungs and intestines.

People become infected by eating undercooked or raw fish or wild water-cress. Infection causes jaundice and liver disease. Treatment is with drugs.

FOLIC ACID

A constituent of the Vitamin B complex. An insufficiency of this essential vitamin causes anaemia. Fats, sugar and spirits excepted, folic acid is present in all foods, though in varying amounts. Rich sources of folic acid include dark green vegetables, liver, kidney, wholegrain cereals and yeast extracts. Malabsorption, particularly in coeliac disease, causes a deficiency of folic acid, as does increased use of the vitamin by the body (in haemolytic anaemia, for example). During pregnancy too the body requires increased amounts of folic acid, and in order to avoid insufficiency the vitamin is often prescribed as a supplement together with iron.

FOLLICULITIS

Inflammation or infection of the hair follicle (the passage through which each shaft of hair reaches the surface of the skin). Folliculitis may occur

F

F

as part of the process of acne, or may occur independently to cause common isolated 'spots'. It can arise anywhere on the body but is commoner in moist areas (the armpits and groin, for example) as well as in the beard area in men. A particular susceptibility to folliculitis may suggest the presence of some disorder associated with a predisposition to infection, such as diabetes mellitus. It is more likely, though, to be an indication of infection elsewhere in the body, such as with *Staphylococcus aureus*, the usual causative organism.

Treatment of folliculitis usually involves simple antiseptics applied to the skin and only sometimes are antibiotics necessary. If, however, the skin around the genital area is affected, surgical treatment may be required to repair the chronic cavities (sinuses) that sometimes occur.

SEE ALSO *illustration on page 265*

FOOD ADDITIVES

Substances which help to preserve food, enhance their flavour or colour them. The evidence suggests that although the vast majority of permitted additives are harmless some of these substances cause an intolerance to the foods in which they are used. For example, sulphites (preservatives found in red wine and many other foods) can cause attacks of tightness in the throat, and asthma; the flavour enhancer monosodium glutamate can cause asthma; and the food colouring agent tartrazine and the preservative benzoate may be associated with an allergic rash. There has been considerable interest too in the possible link between certain additives and behavioural, intellectual and emotional disorders in children. Diets excluding colourings are sometimes tried as treatment for hyperactivity.

FOOD POISONING

Generally the result of eating food that has been contaminated by certain bacteria or their toxins. It usually tends to cause short-lived diarrhoea and vomiting which clear up without any treatment. Food poisoning may also be due to chemicals like monosodium glutamate in food or may be the result of eating poisonous fish or mushrooms. Inadequate cooking, unsatisfactory storage of cooked food and cross-contamination between raw and uncooked food due to poor food hygiene may also result in food poisoning.

Food poisoning due to salmonella bacteria is common worldwide and is on the increase. The bacteria themselves are found in all foods of animal origin as a result of modern poultry farming and animal husbandry methods. Commonly involved foods include chicken, turkey, eggs and meat. Most cases of salmonella poisoning are caused by inadequate thawing of deep-frozen poultry which are then not cooked through properly. Salmonella bacteria are not resistant to heat so this type of food poisoning is easily avoided. Poisoning with the bacteria usually leads to abdominal pain, moderate diarrhoea and fever starting about 12 hours after the contaminated food is eaten; it lasts for 2–3 days.

The micro-organism *Clostridium welchii* is another common cause of food poisoning. Outbreaks of this type mainly occur in institutions where meat dishes are pre-cooked and then inadequately stored and reheated.

Bacterial food poisoning is sometimes caused by toxins created by the bacteria and not the bacteria themselves. In staphylococcal food poisoning, for example, the staphylococci produce an enterotoxin which rapidly produces symptoms after ingestion (1—6 hours). This type of food poisoning is most often found in meat and dairy products (such as cold meats, pies and milk), usually as a result of poor hygiene on the part of food handlers. Unlike salmonella bacteria, this toxin is heat-resistant and no amount of heating or re-cooking will render it harmless. Toxins also arise in *Bacillus cereus* poisoning (caused by eating reheated, unrefrigerated rice) and in one of the rarest types of food poisoning, botulism (qv), as a result of food being incorrectly preserved.

Food poisoning is a notifiable disease and all serious cases must be reported to the public health authority. SEE ALSO *Listeriosis*

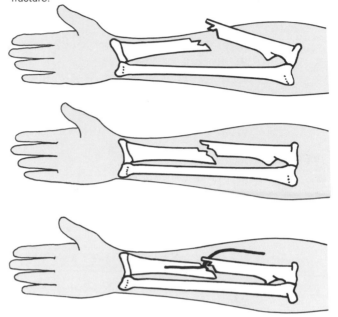

Types of fracture: **Top**, simple fracture; **middle**, complex simple fracture; **bottom**, compound fracture.

FRACTURE

A break in the continuity of bone. A fracture is caused by injury but may also occur in diseased bone.

There are several types of fracture. A simple fracture is a clean break in bone. In comminuted fractures multiple bony fragments are present. Complex simple fractures indicate damage to the surrounding structures (usually to a blood vessel or nerve) as well as to the bone. In a compound fracture the skin overlying the fracture is breached. Bacterial organisms may enter, causing a wound infection and possibly osteomyelitis (inflammation of bone marrow). Greenstick fractures occur in children. If the fracture line enters a joint, this is referred to as an intra-articular fracture; in this type early mobilization at the joint is essential to reduce joint stiffness. Wedge fractures due to loss of calcium with bony softening occur in the vertebral bodies of the spine in elderly patients taking steroids.

Fractures are treated by immobiliz-ing the bone ends, so that movement at the fracture is prevented. This allows callus formation and bone healing (6—12 weeks). Depending on the site and type of fracture, immobilization can be achieved by a plaster of Paris cast, external splints or traction devices, and by a range of fixation techniques (qv).

FROZEN SHOULDER

Pain and stiffness over the shoulder and upper arm as a result of swelling of the main muscle that lifts the arm away from the body. A minor injury usually starts off this painful condition, which is often also called pericapsulitis of the shoulder. Movement of the affected part is limited. The condition gets worse over several months before the pain subsides, leaving a stiff (or frozen) shoulder. It takes several more months with physiotherapy or local hydrocortisone (steroid) injections to restore full movement, particularly that of raising the arm above the head.

F

FUGUE

An abnormal state of awareness usually lasting for several hours but sometimes longer. Fugues may accur in association with depression, hysteria and epilepsy. During a fugue sufferers often wander away from their normal surroundings and are unable to state their identity. They may carry out complex activities and yet will often seem dazed and incoherent. Afterwards they will have no recollection of what occurred during the abnormal state.

FUNGAL INFECTION

Infection with microscopic fungi is uncommon compared to bacterial infection, but its incidence is on the increase as a result of the use of broad-spectrum antibiotics, steroids and other drugs causing immunosuppression. In patients suffering from diabetes mellitus or cancer, for example, fungal infections are more common than in non-sufferers.

Most cases of fungal infection involve superficial areas of the body such as the skin. Candida (qv) and ringworm are the two most common fungal diseases of this type. Ringworm infection is contracted either indirectly from other people (perhaps from gymnasium floors or baths) or from animals. The commonest form is 'athlete's foot', which usually occurs in-between the clefts of the toes. Ring-worm may occur on the trunk, in the groin, causing itchy patches, and also the scalp, causing localized hair loss. The diagnosis is confirmed by microscopic examination of skin scrapings.

Certain fungi can invade the lungs via contaminated dust and spread through the blood to other organs such as the brain and liver; in rare cases this can lead to death (see *Extrinsic allergic alveolitis*). Other inhaled fungi can cause allergy and give rise to asthma–like symptoms.

Effective anti-fungal drugs exist to combat all types of fungal disease.

FUNGAL POISONING

Fungal poisoning is caused by the inadvertent gathering and eating of poisonous field mushrooms instead of edible ones. Fortunately, most mushroom poisoning only gives rise to indigestion and serious illness is rare. The most poisonous fungus is the 'death cap' mushroom (one in three cases is fatal). It is about 11 cm ($4\frac{1}{2}$ inches) tall and has a 9 cm ($3\frac{1}{2}$ inch) wide, yellowish-green cap with white gills and a cup at the base of the stem. 'Fly agaric' is another highly poisonous mushroom, about 25 cm (10 inches) high, which has a 18 cm (7 inch) wide red cap with white patches.

Symptoms will occur within a few hours of eating highly poisonous mushrooms and will comprise nausea, vomiting and diarrhoea. In severe cases this may be followed by excitement, hallucination and delirium. Death may follow, due to liver or kidney failure. If the poisoning is discovered before symptoms arise, bits of the mushroom may be removed from the stomach by inducing vomiting with an emetic. Once the symptoms occur, hospital treatment is vital and includes stomach and bowel washouts, intravenous fluid replacement and removal of the toxin from the body by dialysis.

GALACTORRHOEA

Excessive or inappropriate secretion of milk from the breasts. Secretion may be gross and spontaneous or so slight that it only becomes evident when the breasts are manually compressed. Galactorrhoea may occur in non-pregnant women and in men, as well as in pregnant women. The condition is usually caused by a raised level of the hormone prolactin (which is produced by the pituitary gland in the brain) in the blood but in some cases, for reasons which are not understood, the breasts themselves seem abnormally sensitive to normal blood levels of prolactin. Around 50 per cent of women with raised prolactin levels experience galactorrhoea. Causes of raised prolactin levels include overactivity of the pituitary, pituitary tumours, and underactive thyroid gland (see *Hypothyroidism*) and various drugs.

Treatment is usually with the drug bromocriptine.

GALLSTONE

A stone in the gall-bladder or bile ducts. Gallstones vary in composition and size. They mainly consist of cholesterol (fat), calcium bilirubinate, calcium carbonate and calcium phosphate. Most stones comprise a mixture of these. They are facetted by pressure or friction and if cut open can be seen to be made of concentric layers. The centre of the stone is usually composed of debris or bacteria on which alternating layers of cholesterol and calcium carbonate and/or bilirubinate are deposited. Mixed stones nearly always occur in tens or hundreds, whereas cholesterol stones are usually solitary. Rounded and light in weight and colour, cholesterol stones may exceed 1.25 cm ($\frac{1}{2}$ inch) in diameter; often these contain deposits of bile pigment. Pigment stones (calcium bilirubinate) are black and come in varying shapes.

The 'fat, fertile, flatulent female of fifty' was once regarded as the classic sufferer from gallstones. Today gallstones are common in both men and women and, increasingly, in young women who take the contraceptive pill.

The main symptoms of gallstones are flatulent indigestion (dyspepsia) and intolerance of fatty food. If their presence is unrecognized or if they are left untreated, gallstones may lead to cholecystitis (inflammation of the gall-bladder), cholangitis (inflammation of the bile ducts), biliary colic (see *Calculus*), jaundice and pancreatitis; see individual entries.

Treatment involves surgical removal of the gall-bladder (cholecystectomy) and the removal of any stones within the bile ducts. Certain types of stone may dissolve with long courses of drug therapy, but the recurrence rate is high. Some centres treat gallstones by lithotripsy (crushing them), a technique that is still in the early stages of development.

GANGLION

This term usually refers to a fluid-filled sac or diverticulum formed on top of a synovial sheath. The normal function of such sheaths is to protect tendons as they pass across joints. Ganglia are common in young people, especially around the wrist, and appear as smooth, soft swellings about the size of a grape. Their cause is unknown. The old-fashioned treatment was to squash them but because ganglia usually recur it is best to remove them surgically.

'Ganglion' has a second specialized meaning which refers to the location of a collection of nerve cells that share a common function; examples are the basal ganglia of the brain or the sensory ganglia of the spinal nerves.

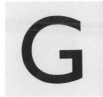

G

GANGRENE

Death (necrosis) and putrefaction of tissue, most often a limb, as a result of complete blockage of an artery cutting off the blood supply. Emboli (fragments of a clot), atherosclerosis (see *Atheroma*) or traumatic thrombosis (physical injury to a blood vessel causing a clot to form) may be responsible for this blockage. There are several different types of gangrene: dry, wet, diabetic and gas. In dry gangrene the skin becomes shrunken and blackened and there is a clear divide between necrotic and viable tissue. Bacterial growth is minimal in this type, which does not spread.

In wet gangrene inflammation is usually present, together with obstruction of the veins as well as the arteries. The tissue becomes swollen, soggy and infected with numerous organisms. This type of gangrene spreads widely.

Diabetic gangrene is due to arterial blockages in a person with diabetes mellitus, infection usually being an important complication. Gas gangrene is a classic battlefield infection, the treatment of which was revolutionized by the introduction of penicillin during the Second World War. In this type, anaerobic bacteria (especially *Clostridium welchii*), which multiply in the absence of oxygen, infect wounds and cause spreading oedema (fluid beneath the skin) and necrosis as well as gas formation.

Dry, wet and diabetic gangrene do not respond well to antibiotics, unlike gas gangrene, and usually require amputation of the affected part.

GASTRECTOMY

Surgical removal of all or part of the stomach. Total gastrectomy is usually reserved for a large gastric cancer or ulcer, and cases of Zollinger-Ellison syndrome (qv). In subtotal gastrectomy most of the stomach is removed, leaving a small part behind. In each case continuity of the gastro-intestinal tract is achieved by suturing or stitching the small intestine to the oesophagus (gullet) or the part of the stomach left behind.

Gastrectomy is performed through a vertical incision in the middle of the upper abdomen. For the first 3—6 days after the operation the person is usually given nothing to eat while receiving intravenous fluids. Normal food is slowly re-introduced thereafter.

A number of well-recognized complications occur after gastrectomy including weight loss, malabsorption, diarrhoea, dumping syndrome (feeling unwell after eating), a form of anaemia, vitamin B deficiency and calcium deficiency. The anaemia, vitamin and calcium deficiencies usually respond to replacement therapy either by mouth or injection, but other consequences are often only partially controlled by dietary adjustment.

GASTRITIS

Inflammation of the lining of the stomach. Gastritis may be present without symptoms, but it may also produce upper abdominal discomfort, nausea or bleeding. The condition may be acute or chronic. Diagnosis can only be made by microscopic examination of a biopsy of the stomach taken by means of fibre-optic endoscopy. Acute gastritis is produced by various drugs, especially aspirin, anti-inflammatory drugs and alcohol; this type of gastritis usually clears up after withdrawal of the offending agent, but drug treatment may be needed.

There are several types of persistent or chronic gastritis. Atrophic gastritis is associated with a lack of acid secretion by the stomach and vitamin B_{12} deficiency (pernicious anaemia); people with this condition require life-long regular vitamin B_{12} injections. Chronic active gastritis is caused by a bacterium (*Campylobacter pylori*) infecting the layer of mucus that lines the stomach; patients with gastric or duodenal ulcers usually have this type of gastritis. *C. pylori* is eliminated using a bismuth-containing compound (bismuth is a heavy metal) together with antibiotics.

GASTRO-ENTERITIS

An acute illness due to inflammation of the gastro-intestinal tract. Bacteria or viruses are the usual causative agents. Gastro-enteritis is common in infants under 2 years of age, mainly as a result of a rotavirus (qv); more cases occur in this group during the cooler months, but for what reason remains obscure. In adults, infection is often acquired during travel abroad, common causes being cholera (endemic in parts of India) and *Escherichia coli* bacteria (so-called travellers' diarrhoea, more descriptively known as the 'Aztec two-step' or 'Delhi belly'). The contamination of food with bacteria or their toxins before, during or after cooking may also cause gastro-enteritis. Various types of salmonella are often responsible, particularly in poultry.

Mild cases of gastro-enteritis do not usually cause problems so long as the fluid lost through diarrhoea can be made up by an increase in intake. Most adults are able to withstand moderate fluid loss, but the elderly and especially babies are at increased risk of serious dehydration, especially if diarrhoea is accompanied by vomiting. When these symptoms coincide dehydration may arise because, even with increases in fluid, intake may be insufficient. In the elderly, dehydration is treated by giving fluid intravenously, by means of a 'drip'. In the case of infants, an electrolyte-containing drink (oral rehydration fluid) is given. If dehydration is more severe or vomiting persists, fluids may be given intravenously until symptoms improve. Most infants begin to improve after 24–48 hours of oral rehydration, and normal feeds are gradually reintroduced.

G

GENE

The basic unit of heredity; each human cell has a nucleus which contains approximately 100,000 genes arranged on 23 pairs of chromosomes, which together determine all the inherited characteristics of an individual. Each gene consists of a sequence of DNA (qv) which codes for a particular protein. The genetic code of DNA consists of components which each specify an amino acid, the building block of proteins. Each cell contains two copies of a gene, one inherited from the mother and the other from the father. Genetic mutations cause the gene to produce abnormal amounts or an abnormal form of the protein by disrupting the genetic code. Inherited diseases result from the transmission of genetic mutations from parents to children and may show dominant, recessive or sex-linked patterns of inheritance (see individual entries for discussion of these patterns). Recent advances in recombinant DNA technology (see *Genetic engineering*) have enabled the genetic mutation responsible for an increasing number of inherited diseases to be identified, and have offered the chance of antenatal diagnosis and, in some cases, the possibility of corrective treatment.

GENETIC ENGINEERING

The technique of manipulating genetic material, made possible by a method called recombinant DNA technology. The most important advance in recombinant DNA technology was the discovery of a class of enzymes, known as restriction endonucleases, which cut strands of DNA at specific sites. In DNA cloning experiments a restriction endonuclease is used to cut out a sequence of DNA (a gene, for example) which is then copied to produce multiple examples of the sequence in question. Other recombinant DNA techniques allow specific sequences of DNA to be identified, gene structure to be analyzed and genes to be sequenced. These techniques have revolutionized the diagnosis of genetic diseases, and an ever-increasing number of genes are being mapped to specific locations on chromosomes. The identification of a gene, or a marker DNA sequence close to the gene, for an inherited disease will allow pre-symptomatic and antenatal diagnosis by analysis of DNA from blood, by chorionic villus biopsy or amniocentesis. The genetic mutation and the protein abnormality responsible for the disease may then be identified, so providing a basis for understanding the cause of the disease and offering a possibility of treatment. The technique of gene therapy — that is, treating a genetic disease by replacing an abnormal gene with the correct DNA sequence — may be possible in the future. Recombinant DNA techniques can also be used to produce proteins such as insulin, growth hormone and factor VIII.

GERMAN MEASLES

see *Rubella*

GIARDIA LAMBLIA

A single-cell parasite which causes infection of the small intestine. It is spread by contaminated water and food and is not infrequently found in travellers and in patients who have undergone immunosuppressive treatment. *Giardia lamblia* is distributed throughout the world, and in certain areas (USSR, India and Nepal, for example), it is endemic. Its incubation period is about fourteen days. The illness it causes usually takes the form of abdominal discomfort, wind and diarrhoea. These symptoms often subside spontaneously. Sometimes the infection becomes chronic and causes lethargy, weight loss and fatty diarrhoea.

Diagnosis can usually be made by microscopic examination of the faeces. The condition responds to treatment with the drug metronidozole.

GIGANTISM

A condition caused by the over-secretion of growth hormone before normal growth has ceased (compare acromegaly). A considerable increase in height, sometimes to over 2.4 m (8 feet), may result. The bones are not only long but thick. The cause of excess growth hormone is almost always a benign tumour (adenoma) of the pituitary gland at the base of the brain. Headache and visual disturbances (bitemporal hemianopia) may also arise as a result of this.

Treatment is aimed at reducing the levels of growth hormone by eliminating the pituitary gland by surgery or irradiation.

GINGIVITIS

A gingival or gum inflammation produced by accumulation of bacteria next to the edge of the gums. Soft deposits of non-calcified material containing bacteria called plaque accumulate naturally on the surfaces of teeth. The plaque bacteria do not appear to invade the gum but chemicals produced by them accumulate as irritants. The result is inflammation, with the symptoms of gum soreness and bleeding, an objectionable taste in the mouth and bad breath. Gingivitis is an important cause of loss of teeth, after caries. It is prevented by good dental hygiene.

GLANDULAR FEVER

An acute infection caused by the Epstein-Barr virus; also known as infectious mononucleosis. It occurs chiefly in children and young adults and may occur in epidemics. The incubation period is between 5 and 10 days. Common symptoms are malaise (a general feeling of being unwell), tiredness, generalized muscle pains, headache, fever and enlargement of the lymph glands. There may be a sore throat and, in the early stages of the disease, a skin rash. The spleen may become enlarged and rarely other complications, such as hepatitis, ensue. The condition may be diagnosed by means of a blood test which detects antibodies against the virus and characteristic changes in the appearance of the lymphocytes (a type of white blood cell), which may be increased in number.

There is no specific treatment for the condition though the patient may need to stay in bed during the period of fever. Recovery takes place in all cases but the duration of the illness is very variable, some individuals being unwell for weeks or months with intermittent fever, sweats and malaise.

GLAUCOMA

Raised pressure within the eyeball. In most cases glaucoma is acquired; rarely it is congenital, occurring in association with neurofibromatosis (qv) or the Sturge-Weber syndrome (qv). Acquired glaucoma may be acute or chronic and is the result of inadequate drainage in the forward chamber of the eye, which causes fluid to accumulate and block the drainage canals. Acute glaucoma occurs chiefly in long-sighted, elderly women and is a medical emergency; treatment must be started at once if the sight is not to be lost (see below). The blockage of the drainage canals may be exacerbated by dilatation of the pupil. Affected individuals complain of pain in the eye, sensitivity to bright light (photophobia), haloes around bright objects and loss of vision. The conjunctiva (the membrane covering the inside of the eyelid and the front of the eye) may be reddened.

Chronic glaucoma is a common cause of blindness in the elderly. Its onset is insidious without pain or conjunctival reddening; only in the late stages does the individual notice restriction of the visual field and loss of acuity or sharpness of vision. For this reason, regular eye checks are advisable, especially for the elderly, in order to detect this serious condition at an early stage when effective treatment is available. The early signs will be picked up by an optician.

Treatment in all cases consists of reducing pressure within the eye by using drugs (in the form of eyedrops or tablets) prior to surgery or laser therapy to improve drainage of the forward chamber. Acute glaucoma may affect both eyes in turn and con-

G

sequently surgery is often performed on the unaffected eye at the same time.

GLOMERULONEPH-RITIS

A kidney disease primarily affecting the glomeruli, coils of specialized capillaries (tiny blood vessels) which filter waste products from the blood into the urine. Glomerulonephritis can take the form of an acute disease with nephrotic syndrome, haematuria (blood in the urine), high blood pressure or acute kidney failure; or the onset may be insidious and the diagnosis made after tests have been done for asymptomatic proteinuria (protein in the urine), haematuria, high blood pressure or chronic kidney failure. Glomerulonephritis can be primary, when the disease process is restricted to the kidney, or secondary to systemic diseases such as systemic lupus erythematosus, diabetes mellitus, arteritis, infections (streptococcal throat infections or malaria, for example), amyloidosis or malignant disease.

The diagnosis of primary glomerulonephritis usually requires a kidney biopsy and tests to exclude possible systemic causes. The best guide to outlook and treatment in primary glomerulonephritis is the result of the biopsy, as patients with similar clinical features may have very different risks of developing kidney failure. Symptoms such as hypertension or nephrotic syndrome may require specific drug treatment; many types of primary glomerulonephritis are thought to be examples of auto-immune disease, and corticosteroids or other immunosuppressive drugs (azathioprine, cyclophosphamide) may be administered, depending on the results of the biopsy. In secondary glomerulonephritis the emphasis is on treatment of the underlying systemic disease.

SEE ALSO *illustration on page 171*, and *Nephrotic syndrome*

GLOSSITIS

Inflammation of the tongue, resulting in a painful, red, swollen tongue. It may be caused by lack of certain vitamins, including vitamin B_{12}, iron or folic acid. It is treated by vitamin replacement.

GLUCOCORTICOIDS

see *Corticosteroids*

GLUCOSE TOLERANCE TEST

A test used primarily to confirm diabetes mellitus. A single instance of elevated glucose in the plasma (the fluid component of blood) is considered diagnostic of diabetes mellitus in a person who has symptoms of the disease, whereas two raised levels are required in a person with no symptoms. Before taking the test, the patient has to maintain a certain daily carbohydrate intake, and then fast for twelve hours immediately prior to the test. A glucose solution is then dissolved in water and taken by the patient. The level of plasma is recorded before the test and every half hour up to two hours afterwards. Some people who record intermediate values are diagnosed as having 'impaired glucose tolerance'. A normal fasting level, with a return to normal two hours after glucose has been given but with very high intermediate levels, may be found in patients with thyrotoxicosis (qv) and in some patients with impaired gastro-intestinal function as a result of gastrectomy (qv).

GLUE SNIFFING

The repeated inhalation of volatile gases from adhesives and other chemicals in order to induce a state of euphoria; also known as solvent abuse. Glues containing toluene, acetone and xylene, paint varnishes, lacquers, cleaning fluids and butane are commonly abused. Intoxication occurs within minutes and the euphoric effects will continue for minutes to hours. During this state a person may experience hallucinations and blurring of vision, and become disinhibited, drowsy and uncoordinated. The euphoria is typically followed by a hangover and depression lasting for several hours.

Although physical dependence on solvents is uncommon, there are significant dangers associated with their abuse, such as brain damage, or death as a result of asphyxia, poisoning, inhalation of vomit or accidents taking place while the person is intoxicated.

GLYCOSURIA

The presence of glucose in the urine. Diabetes mellitus (qv) is the most common cause of glycosuria, although some patients with kidney disorders may also develop it as a result of having a low 'renal threshold' for sugar. Glycosuria is detected by means of either dipstick or tablet testing. (In dipstick testing a paper stick is dipped in urine for a few seconds. If glucose is present the dye of the stick will change colour. Similarly, in tablet testing a tablet is dropped in urine and a colour change is looked for.) Used as a method of diagnosing diabetes mellitus, glycosuria testing is unreliable; some people, especially the elderly, have high 'renal thresholds' and diabetes mellitus may be present without glycosuria being detected. Also, agents such as lactose (in pregnancy or lactation) or fructose and galactose (in rare genetic disorders) may give positive results. Testing for glycosuria is also inadequate as a monitor of diabetes; blood testing strips are far more accurate.

GOITRE

Enlargement of the thyroid gland. This causes a noticeable swelling in the neck. The condition is usually associated with under- or overproduction of thyroid hormones (hypo- and hyperthyroidism respectively) and is either non-toxic or toxic. Non-toxic goitre caused by hypothyroidism (qv) is commonly found in women and often develops at puberty. The enlarged gland is thought to be caused by increased secretion of thyroid stimulating hormone (TSH). This is brought about by an underlying disturbance in iodine metabolism which leads to reduced secretion of thyroid hormones and a corresponding increase in TSH from the pituitary gland. In some parts of the world, non-toxic goitre commonly arises as a result of iodine deficiency (in food or water, for example); it can be prevented by iodine supplements such as iodized salt. Toxic goitres occur as a result of hyperthyroidism (qv), cancer of the thyroid or autoimmune disease (see *Thyrotoxicosis*).

Non-toxic goitre can only be treated by surgery, whatever its cause. Surgery (thyroidectomy, qv) is indicated if the size of the swelling causes compression of the trachea or windpipe (leading to difficulty in breathing), jugular veins in the neck (facial congestion) or nerves of the larynx or voice-box (hoarseness). It may also be required for cosmetic

G

reasons. Treatment in cases of toxic goitre is directed at the underlying cause.

GONORRHOEA

A sexually transmitted disease caused by the bacterium *Neisseria gonorrhoea*, which can infect the genital tract, rectum, throat and eyes. In heterosexual men the urethra (the tube which drains the bladder) is the commonest site of the infection, causing a discharge from the penis and a burning sensation when passing urine. In women the condition may be symptomless if, as is usual, the cervix (neck of the womb) is the only infected site; in others a vaginal discharge may be present, or the infection may involve the urethra or rectum. In couples practising oral sex gonorrhoea may infect the throat. In homosexual men rectal gonorrhoea predominates. Babies born to mothers with gonorrhoea can develop an eye infection which can, if untreated, lead to blindness. Gonorrhoea can progress to epididymitis (inflammation of the delicate tube which leads from the testis to the urethra) in men, and to infection of the Fallopian tubes (salpingitis) in women; both are important causes of infertility. Rarely, rashes and arthritis can occur. Treatment consists of penicillin injections, although some bacteria have now become resistant to this. The sexual contacts of patients with gonorrhoea are traced to prevent further spread of the disease.

GOUT

A disorder in which uric acid crystals are deposited in joints, particularly around the cartilage lining, and the surrounding soft tissues. The condition is associated with high circulating levels of uric acid; this may be due to an excess of it in the diet, metabolic abnormalities associated with increased production, or abnormalities of the kidneys resulting in reduced excretion. Not all individuals with raised uric acid levels will, however, develop gout.

Gout is more common in men who are typically obese and have a family history of the condition, raised blood pressure and a high alcoholic intake. An acute attack of gout is sudden in onset and is excruciatingly painful. It usually occurs in the big toe, which becomes red, hot and swollen within a few hours. Pain is at a peak after around 24 hours. Both big toes may be involved and sometimes other joints as well. Chronic forms of gout exist and the condition may sometimes be associated with kidney damage.

Treatment of acute attacks involves rest and anti-inflammatory medication (see *NSAID*); in some individuals drug treatment (allopurinol, for example) to reduce circulating uric acid concentrations may be necessary.

GRAFT

Tissue used in a site other than that of its origin. There are many types of graft. Skin, organs (see *Transplantation*), bone marrow (see *Bone marrow transplants*), heart valves and veins may all be referred to as grafts when they are used in this way. Skin grafts (qv) are frequently used to aid healing and minimize scarring in severe cases of burns or ulcers. They may be taken from other species (particularly pigs) or from healthy areas on the patient's own body. The whole thickness of skin ('full-thickness' graft) may be used or just the superficial layers ('split-skin' graft), depending on the severity of the injury being treated.

The term 'graft' is applied to heart valve replacements particularly when pig valves are used. Coronary artery bypass grafting refers to using veins obtained from the patient's own legs and is now a routine operation in cardiac surgery units. Similarly obtained vein grafts may also be used by surgeons to reconstruct or bypass severely arteriosclerotic arteries (see *Atheroma*), though at some sites artificial grafts are preferred.

GRAFT-VERSUS-HOST DISEASE (GVHD)

Rejection of the patient by the graft in cases of transplant. This problem is almost unique to bone marrow transplantation but may also occur in organ transplants. It is caused when the T lymphocytes (cells important to immunity) present in the transplant attack the patient. Symptoms are severe skin disease, abnormality of the liver and very severe diarrhoea. The drug cyclosporin A is used to stop rejection of transplanted organs such as the kidneys and heart.

GVHD is non-existent in the majority of cases of bone marrow transplantation but where it does exist severity ranges from extremely mild to fatal. The removal of the T lymphocytes from the bone marrow by means of special antibody treatment has been very effective in stopping GVHD. Interestingly, the disease itself probably has some anti-leukaemic effect and may contribute to cure when bone marrow transplantation is performed for leukaemia.

GRANULOMA

A term which is loosely used to describe a localized area of chronic inflammation (composed of granulation tissue) which, because it is in the form of a lump, bears some resemblance to a tumour (hence the suffix –oma). An example of this is the granuloma of the skin seen in leprosy and some fungal infections.

There is now an increasing tendency to use the term to describe a microscopic inflammatory lesion composed mainly of macrophages (a type of scavenger white cell), such as is found in tuberculosis or sarcoidosis, for example.

GROMMET

A hollow, bobbin-like 2–3 mm tube which can be inserted through an incision made in the eardrum, and held there to allow air to enter the

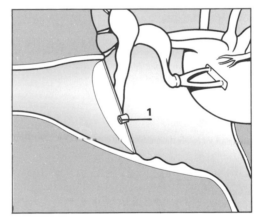

A grommet (**1**) is usually inserted with the aid of a microscope under general anaesthesia. It stays in place for about six months after which time it is spontaneously rejected.

middle ear space.

A grommet is required when the Eustachian tube is not ventilating the middle ear adequately, usually as a result of an obstruction caused by the adenoids. The anatomical shape of a child's Eustachian tube also predisposes to this problem. Lack of air in the middle ear causes fluid to be secreted, causing 'glue ear' and temporary deafness.

G

GUILLAIN-BARRÉ SYNDROME

This condition is the result of inflammation of the nerves shortly after they have left the spinal cord; also called acute idiopathic polyneuritis. The cause of the Guillain-Barré syndrome is unknown but it is thought to be precipitated by certain viral infections and is probably autoimmune. The condition usually begins acutely, sometimes with pain and tingling in the lower limbs, and sometimes with headache and fever. After an interval of hours or days, weakness sets in; it may progress to cause paralysis of muscles in the limbs. The muscles of the trunk, respiratory muscles and muscles of the face may also be affected. If respiratory paralysis occurs, mechanical ventilation may be required. Maximum weakness is usually within 3–4 weeks of onset of the condition. Recovery without any significant disability occurs in 80 per cent of cases, but relapses may occur in a few.

Treatment involves supportive care, assisted ventilation (when necessary), avoidance of respiratory infection, physiotherapy and, sometimes, antibiotics.

GUTHRIE TEST

see *Inborn errors of metabolism*

GYNAECOMASTIA

Enlargement of the male breasts, a main feature of feminization (qv). In some cases either or both the male breasts enlarge at puberty, no obvious cause being found and no ill-effects observed. Most cases resolve spontaneously but in some the enlargement persists. Other cases are caused by an excess in the production or administration of the female hormone oestrogen. Some varieties of testicular, lung and adrenal tumours occasionally produce oestrogens or other hormones, and can lead to gynaecomastia as a relatively harmless sign of a serious condition. Oestrogens such as stilboestrol are used in large doses to treat cancer of the prostate gland and almost invariably produce gynaecomastia. A variety of drugs can cause the condition, including digoxin, marijuana (cannabis), heroin, cimetidine, spironolactone and some cytotoxic drugs used in the treatment of cancer. Liver disease and, because of its effect on the liver, alcoholism can lead to gynaecomastia, as can an overactive thyroid (hyperthyroidism), leprosy and Klinefelter's syndrome, in which men possess an extra female chromosome.

HAEMANGIOMA

An abnormal development of blood vessels which may appear as a discoloration of an area of skin, or as a red or blue lump. Though most obvious on the skin, haemangiomas may be found in other sites, such as the brain, liver, bowel and respiratory system, where symptoms may occur if the vessels bleed, or if the lump causes obstruction. The common visible types are the flat, pink capillary haemangioma (of the tiny blood vessels) and the raised red strawberry mark, often called a naevus. This appears shortly after birth, grows over the first year, then gradually disappears to leave a white scar by 5 years of age.
SEE ALSO *Angioma, Birth mark*

HAEMATEMESIS

Vomiting up blood. This can vary from a small amount of old blood, which appears like coffee grounds, to a large amount of fresh red blood clots. There is often no warning, except for faintness or even collapse. Emergency admission to hospital is needed to set up an intravenous infusion (or 'drip') and prepare the patient for an emergency operation in case the bleeding continues.

Diagnosis of the cause is made by endoscopy as soon as practicable. Most cases are due to ulcers in the stomach or duodenum, related to the use of NSAIDs or excessive production of gastric acid. Rarer causes are dilated veins in the lower oesophagus (varices) with underlying liver disease, gastric cancer and the Mallory Weiss syndrome. In the last condition the haematemesis is due to a small tear in the lower oesophagus caused by profuse vomiting.

A good proportion of cases will settle with blood transfusion and powerful antacids to lower the gastric acidity. Severe or repeated haematemesis requires an operation: ulcers are stitched over to close the bleeding vessel, or part of the stomach is removed (gastrectomy). In patients over 60 years of age an early operation is more likely, since waiting increases the risk of complications.

HAEMATOMA

A collection of blood within tissue, such as muscle, or within a body cavity. It may occur after an operation or injury or spontaneously because of an underlying abnormality of coagulation. The blood is often absorbed gradually, but large haematomas may have to be evacuated surgically, as for instance in the subdural space within the skull and there is always the risk of a secondary infection. The underlying cause (a disorder of coagulation, for example) should be investigated.

HAEMATURIA

The presence of blood in the urine. With large amounts of blood the urine appears red; with smaller amounts, a dusky grey; and with minute amounts the urine may not be coloured at all (microscopic haematuria). Haematuria may be confirmed by dipping a testing strip into the urine; the strip changes colour by varying degrees, depending on the presence of blood.

Haematuria may be painful or painless. Painful haematuria suggests an infection of the bladder (cystitis) or kidney stones (urolithiasis). Painless haematuria is considered to be due to a tumour of the genito-urinary tract until proven otherwise. First, microscopic confirmation is required (certain dyes and foodstuffs cause red urine). The two investigations commonly performed are cystoscopy and intravenous urography. Cystoscopy will reveal any bladder tumours or benign papillomatas. Urography will highlight any tumours of the kidney and ureters (which lead from the kidney to the bladder), outline any kidney stones (calculi) and also give some indication of bladder abnormalities. Where a renal tumour is suspected, ultrasound imaging of the kidneys may be used to help in diagnosis.

Renal injury and pelvic fractures often cause traumatic haematuria.

HAEMOCHROMA-TOSIS

Haemochromatosis, also known as bronze diabetes, is a rare disease, usually inherited (in the autosomal recessive pattern), in which excessive amounts of iron are absorbed and deposited in the tissues of the body. This results in the eventual damage and loss of function of the organs involved.

The liver is usually the first organ to be damaged; initially it becomes large, but may then become fibrotic and shrunken. Liver cancer develops in about 35 per cent of patients and is a common cause of death. Excessive skin pigmentation, giving a bronzed appearance, is present in about 90 per cent of patients. This is due to the deposition of the dark brown pigment melanin, but excess iron may also be present in the skin. Diabetes develops in about 60 per cent of patients, due to damage of the pancreas by iron. In 20 to 50 per cent of cases, patients develop arthritis; the relationship of this to iron metabolism is not known. Heart disease is common and arrythmias may also occur.

There are other non-hereditary forms of haemochromatosis. One may be seen in patients with thalassaemia and similar disorders who have increased iron absorption and who also have frequent blood transfusions as part of their treatment.

Excessive iron ingestion over many years may result in haemochromatosis in certain circumstances. The disease is seen, for example, in the Bantu tribe of South Africa who brew alcohol in iron vessels, and in people who take an excessive quantity of iron in the form of tonics or multi-vitamin preparations. There is no treatment.

HAEMOGLOBINURIA

The presence of haemoglobin (the red blood cell pigment) in the urine, which acquires a red colour. Haemoglobinuria is distinguished from haematuria (qv) (red blood cells in the urine) by putting the urine in a centrifuge: if haematuria is present the red cells will form a sediment. The condition is caused by the breakdown of red cells releasing haemoglobin (haemolysis qv) and occurs either as a result of a mismatched blood transfusion or damage to the red cells due to physical distress. The latter was first described in 1888 in a Prussian soldier with badly fitting boots, and has been noted since in marathon runners, karate practitioners and demented patients who purposely knock their heads.

Paroxysmal cold haemoglobinuria describes bouts of haemoglobinuria upon exposure to cold. This was formerly very common in patients suffering from syphilis, but is now rare.

HAEMOLYSIS

Increased destruction of red blood cells. Normally a red cell survives 120 days, but when haemolysis occurs the cell's life is shortened to a variable degree. To compensate for this, the bone marrow produces more red cells (reticulocytes), which then increase in the bloodstream. Anaemia may result if the marrow cannot produce enough red cells to compensate for the increased destruction. The breakdown product of haemoglobin, bilirubin, increases in the blood.

Haemolysis has a variety of causes. Within the red cell there may be abnormal haemoglobin (as in sickle cell disease) or a lack of enzymes which generate energy for the red cell. Outside the red cell, antibodies may be produced which react with proteins on the red cell surface; this may occur after treatment with drugs or blood transfusions, or in rare autoimmune medical conditions. Haemolysis is treated by removing the cause; sometimes steroids are given when the condition is autoimmune in origin. Folic acid tablets usually form part of the treatment as the increased red cell production by the bone marrow may result in a shortage of this vitamin.

HAEMOLYTIC DISEASE OF THE NEWBORN

A serious disease of the newborn characterized by severe haemolytic anaemia and jaundice. It is due to anti-bodies from a rhesus negative mother crossing the placenta to her rhesus positive baby where they react with and destroy red blood cells in the fetal circulation (see *Rhesus factor*). Occasionally, HDN is caused by the antibodies of other blood group systems.

Severe haemolytic disease may kill the baby in the womb. A moderately affected baby will be born with anaemia and jaundice. Treatment of a baby born with HDN involves an exchange transfusion, in which all the baby's blood is exchanged, to prevent the jaundice causing brain damage.

Fortunately, HDN is now preventable by injecting the mother with rhesus antibody immediately after the birth of her first or any subsequent rhesus positive baby, or after any invasive procedure in pregnancy (such as amniocentesis). (A rhesus negative mother will only develop these antibodies after the birth of her first rhesus positive child.)

The rhesus antibody is specially made by injecting volunteer rhesus negative men with rhesus positive red cells after which the antibody produced is harvested from their blood.

HAEMOPHILIA

An inherited disorder of blood coagulation, affecting 1 in 10,000 males. (Females are affected extremely rarely.) The bleeding tendency results from a congenital deficiency of factor VIII in the blood, a protein normally made in the liver and essential for normal blood clotting. The principal symptom is repeated and spontaneous bleeding into joints (haemarthrosis), especially the knees. Less common symptoms include gastro-intestinal haemorrhage and haematuria (blood in the urine). The disease is usually inherited from a female carrier who shows no symptoms of the disorder (see *Sex-linked pattern of inheritance*), but one-third of cases appear as new mutations. The son of a female carrier has a 50 per cent chance of inheriting haemophilia and each daughter a 50 per cent chance of being a carrier. Sons of male haemophiliacs do not inherit the disease, but all their daughters will be carriers. Antenatal diagnosis of haemophilia is now possible.

Treatment consists of giving infusions of factor VIII concentrates prepared from donated blood in order to prevent and stop haemorrhaging. Before the AIDS epidemic, life expectancy for haemophiliacs was almost as high as that for normal males; AIDS is now the commonest cause of death among haemophiliacs. Although all donated blood is now screened for the AIDS virus, only when genetically engineered factor VIII becomes available, in a few years' time, will the risk of transmission of this and other viruses be reduced to nil.

HAEMOPTYSIS

The coughing up of blood from the lungs. Until fifty years ago the commonest cause of haemoptysis was tuberculosis, but the incidence of this condition has declined and today haemoptysis is more likely to be a symptom of pneumonia, lung abscesses and chronic bronchitis, especially with repeated coughing. Bronchial cancer is a major cause of haemoptysis. The repeated occurrence of bloodstained phlegm, especially in an older person

H

who is a smoker, requires a chest X-ray and usually bronchoscopy (qv) to detect the underlying cause. Pulmonary embolism (a clot in the lungs) and the death of lung tissue that it typically results in produce symptoms of chest pain and haemoptysis. A history of deep vein thrombosis, recent surgery or use of the contraceptive pill can also suggest this diagnosis. However, not all haemoptysis is the result of lung abnormalities. Mitral stenosis (narrowing of the mitral valve in the heart), for example, can lead to blood being coughed up by causing a rise in blood pressure in the lungs.

Blood loss due to local lesions in the nose or pharynx is sometimes mistaken for haemoptysis.

HAEMORRHAGE

Bleeding; this can be acute or chronic. Acute haemorrhage causes shock with low blood pressure, fast pulse and cold extremities. It is life-threatening unless a blood transfusion is given and the underlying cause remedied. Chronic haemorrhage results in iron deficiency anaemia and tiredness.

Haemorrhage most commonly occurs from the gut, with the vomiting of blood (haematemesis) or blood in the stools (melaema, which has a black tar-like appearance). Haemorrhage from the lungs is haemoptysis. Haemorrhage from the urinary tract is seen as blood in the urine (haematuria). Excessive menstrual bleeding is menorrhagia. Haemorrhage can also occur internally after an operation, or if there is an underlying disorder of coagulation. A localized collection of blood is known as a haematoma.

HAEMORRHOIDS

Also known as piles, haemorrhoids occur when the pads of blood vessels which help maintain continence in the anus become flooded with blood. Constipation and straining to pass hard stools causes them to enlarge and bleed and often to become painful. Eventually they prolapse through the anus, and are then known as 'prolapsing piles'. An 'acute attack of piles' is a very painful condition. It can be due to strangulation of a prolapsed pile, or bleeding into an external pile which is trapped under the skin outside the anus.

The treatment of piles consists of increasing the dietary fibre, and local injections to shrink their size. If itching, bleeding or the associated mucous discharge is severe, the piles can be removed surgically. (The operation is called haemorrhoidectomy.)

HAEMOSTASIS

The response to blood vessel injury, which involves interaction of the blood vessel wall, circulating platelets and blood coagulation factors. The damaged blood vessel first constricts to prevent further blood flowing to the injured area. The platelets are activated and stick to the blood vessel wall. The contents of granules within the platelet are also released, resulting in further platelets sticking together. Tissue factors are released which stimulate production of a fibrin clot.

Haemostasis can result from an abnormality of platelets or clotting factors. Haemophilia, for example, is an inherited disorder of coagulation. There are several tests of haemostasis to reveal such abnormality. They include: measuring how long the skin takes to stop bleeding after a small cut (bleeding time) and clotting tests performed in the laboratory (the prothrombin time and activated partial thromboplastin time).

HAIR LOSS

see *Alopecia*

HALLUCINATION

True hallucinations are perceptions which may occur through any of the senses in the absence of external stimuli and are viewed by the person as originating outside of him or her. They occur alongside normal perceptions and cannot be conjured up or dismissed at will. Hallucinations may occur in acute confusion, epilepsy, delirium tremens and drug intoxication and in psychiatric disorders such as schizophrenia and depression. They are commonly classified by the sense through which they are perceived; for example auditory hallucinations (hearing voices).

Hypnagogic hallucinations occur at times of transition from wakefulness to sleep. Hallucinations occurring from sleep to wakefulness are called hypnapompic.

HAMARTOMA

A tumour-like mass present at birth or appearing shortly afterwards. It can be any size but grows at the same rate as the individual, ceasing when normal growth stops. Hamartomas can occur singly or be multiple, and may be found in any organ or tissue of the body (see *Tuberous sclerosis*). Complications are rare and depend on the site and number. Hamartomas are made of normal tissues and are not malignant. They only require surgical removal if they compress or severely impair the function of normal tissue.

HARE LIP

Also known as cleft lip. Facial clefts are present very early in fetal development and normally close by 9 weeks as the components of the nose and upper jaw come together. Failure of complete fusion leaves a cleft which varies in severity from a notch on the upper lip to a gap extending from the upper lip to the nostril. It may affect one or both sides of the lip. One in 1,000 babies has hare lip, and two-thirds of cases are associated with cleft palate. Surgery to repair the defect may be performed soon after birth, or be delayed until 3 months of age.

HAY FEVER

Seasonal allergic rhinitis and allergic conjunctivitis, caused by an allergy to pollen. After exposure to pollen, the affected individual develops itching eyes, nose and throat with a watery discharge, repeated sneezing and nasal obstruction. The development of hay fever depends on an inherited hypersensitivity to pollen (see *Atopy*) and on the degree of exposure. Major pollen sources are trees, grasses and weeds, which have seasons in spring, summer and autumn respectively.

Hay fever often starts in childhood, is most frequent in adolescence, improves in middle age and is rare in the elderly. Asthma sufferers may have hay fever as well at the peak of the season. Diagnosis is usually easily made from the patient's symptoms and skin tests.

Treatment consists of avoiding excessive exposure to pollen, together with taking antihistamine medication and, in some cases, inhaled steroids or the drug sodium cromoglycate. Desensitization (qv) is rarely necessary and should only be done under strict medical supervision.

HEADACHE

A very common and often harmless

complaint. Headaches are usually caused by tense muscles, and described medically as tension headaches. The discomfort may be felt at the front, crown or back of the head and often affects both sides. Relief may be obtained from gentle pressure, massage, altered posture or simple painkillers such as paracetamol. The headache of migraine (qv) initially affects only one side of the head and is often associated with other symptoms such as visual disturbances and vomiting. So-called 'cluster headaches' (also called periodic migrainous neuralgia) also tend to be one-sided, affecting the same part of the head at the same time of day for several days in a row but then ceasing for weeks or months before recurring. They have no sinister implications and can be pre-empted by treatment given prior to the expected time of onset. It is very rarely necessary for patients with any of these common forms of headache to need special tests or scans.

Other forms of headache are relatively rare apart from those due to jaw or dental disease. A severe one-sided headache associated with tenderness over the temple in the elderly may indicate temporal arteritis (qv). A sudden onset of severe headache associated with pain and stiffness of the neck suggests subarachnoid haemorrhage (qv) or, less commonly, meningitis (qv). Brain tumours (qv) may first come to light because of headaches that tend to be throbbing in character, often worse in the mornings and sometimes associated with vomiting.

HEART ATTACK

Known medically as myocardial infarction; during a heart attack part of the heart muscle dies because of a lack of sufficient oxygen in the blood carried to the heart muscle by the coronary arteries. The usual cause of heart attack is a blood clot forming on damaged lining (atheroma) in these arteries. Pain, often extremely severe, is the commonest sign and is typically described as 'crushing', located centrally in the chest or top part of the abdomen and, in 25 per cent of cases, radiating down the left arm. The pain does not extend above the cheek-bone or below the umbilicus (navel). The pain may occur during exertion but, in contrast to angina, does not go away with rest. However, in 20 per cent of cases there is no pain, particularly in the elderly, in whom the symptoms may be breathlessness, heart failure, a confused state or an

Structure of the normal heart: **1** systemic vein (from body tissues); **2** aorta (to body tissues); **3** pulmonary artery (to lungs); **4** right atrium; **5** pulmonary valve; **6** tricuspid valve; **7** right ventricle; **8** septum; **9** left ventricle; **10** mitral valve; **11** aortic valve; **12** left atrium; **13** pulmonary veins (from lungs).

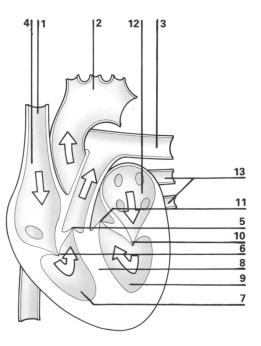

abnormal heart rhythm. Diagnosis is confirmed by changes in the ECG (see *Electrocardiography*) and enzyme values in the blood during the first few days after the attack; the enzymes are those released by dead muscle cells.

Intensive nursing care and monitoring are required in the first few days after an attack. Specific treatment is directed at dissolving the blockage of the coronary arteries, using thrombolytic agents if the patient is being treated soon after the onset of pain; these agents are much less effective if given later. Narcotic analgesia, oxygen and sedation are the other emergency treatments. Abnormal heart rhythms are treated with a temporary pacemaker or drugs. Heart failure requires vasodilator drugs to dilate the blood vessels, sometimes diuretics and sometimes drugs which stimulate the heart if there is a 'pump failure' due to a massive infarct (death of tissue).

HEART BLOCK

Heart block occurs when some areas of the heart receive electrical impulses much later than other areas or not at all. Normal electrical activity in the heart produces a sequence of contractions of the muscle of the different heart chambers, resulting in a pumping action. It originates in a specialized area, the sino-atrial node, and is transmitted by conducting tissue throughout the heart.

Heart block can be present at birth (congenital heart block), but more commonly it occurs after a heart attack, when it may be temporary or permanent. There are three types:

- In first degree heart block there is merely a delay in conduction between the atria (the upper chambers of the heart) and the ventricles (the lower chambers). It

is only detected on an ECG (see *Electrocardiography*)

- In second degree heart block there is an intermittent failure of the impulse to reach the ventricles
- In third degree or complete heart block no electrical impulses pass from the atria to the ventricles at all. This type of heart block may also be seen in the elderly in whom it is possibly caused by chronic ischaemia (a decrease in blood supply and oxygen delivery) due to scarring of the conducting tissue.

Although the ventricles can initiate an electrical impulse to cause them to contract when none comes from the atria, the rate is much slower than that generated in the sino-atrial node and consequently the pulse is slow and Stokes-Adams (qv) attacks can occur.

First and second degree heart block rarely require treatment but patients with third degree heart block invariably need a cardiac pacemaker.

HEARTBURN

A burning sensation felt in the upper abdomen and chest (behind the sternum or breast-bone), produced by gastric juices regurgitating (refluxing) from the stomach into the oesophagus (gullet). Waterbrash (gastric fluid in the throat causing a bitter or acid taste) may accompany heartburn. The condition is very common and is usually caused by stooping or lying down flat after large meals, smoking, coffee, tight clothing or being overweight; all increase the reflux of acid. Some severe cases of heartburn may be caused by a defect in the one-way valve that normally prevents reflux (see *Reflux oesophagitis*).

In the majority of cases heartburn is easily avoided by giving up smoking or eating small meals. Treatment may involve the use of antacids.

H

HEART FAILURE

A condition in which the heart cannot pump sufficient blood to meet the needs of the body. Heart failure may be due to many underlying diseases, most commonly coronary artery disease (causing damage to the heart muscle), longstanding high blood pressure (hypertension), heart valve abnormalities, lung disease or disease of the heart muscle itself (cardiomyopathy).

When heart failure occurs, fluid accumulates in the lungs (causing breathlessness, especially with exercise and when lying flat) and in the limbs (causing the ankles to swell). Severe heart failure, especially of sudden onset, can cause very poor circulation to the vital organs of the body such as the kidney and brain, and can result in death.

Treatment measures include reducing the body fluid and salt with a diuretic medication to increase the amount of urine passed by the kidneys; use of the drug digoxin to increase cardiac output and, increasingly, vasodilator drugs, to dilate the blood vessels and so reduce the amount of work the heart has to do. Some patients are suitable for surgery, which may involve replacing damaged heart valves and reestablishing blood flow to diseased coronary arteries by by-pass grafting or heart transplantation.

HEAT STROKE

Also termed hyperpyrexia. Heat stroke is due to a rise in body temperature after exposure to intense heat over a period usually lasting for several hours. The normal sweating mechanisms usually fail when the body temperature exceeds 41°C (106°F), so that the skin is dry. Heat stroke with the development of a coma may come on suddenly in severe cases, although some individuals may have symptoms of thirst, headache, dizziness and progressive confusion for a few hours beforehand. After coma sets in, there may be other signs of brain involvement, such as convulsions. The condition is associated with a fast heart and respiration rate; in severe cases there may be disorders of heart rhythm and the patient may suffer from shock.

Treatment involves effective cooling to about 39°C (102°F) within an hour. The patient may also require total immersion in re-cooled water or spraying with cold water, and fanning to promote evaporation. The outlook depends on the duration and degree of hyperpyrexia: if untreated, the condition is fatal.

HEMIANOPIA

Blindness in one half of each visual field. The term homonymous hemianopia (right or left) is used if blindness occurs in the same half of each field;

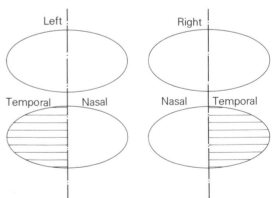

Bitemporal hemianopia

this may result from a stroke. If the right side of one visual field and the left of the other are affected, the resulting visual defect is known as crossed or heteronymous hemianopia. This in turn may be subdivided: bitemporal hemianopia affects the outer halves of each visual field and binasal hemianopia affects the inner halves. The latter is not infrequently associated with a tumour of the pituitary gland compressing the optic nerves that carry signals from the eye to the brain. In quadrantic hemianopia the visual field is restricted by one-quarter.

HEMIPLEGIA

Paralysis of one side of the body involving the muscles of the leg, arm and sometimes also the face. This usually arises as a consequence of a lesion in the part of the brain where the nerve fibres which control the movements of one side of the body run closely together (the area known as the internal capsule). These nerve fibres cross over before entering the spinal cord and so a lesion in the internal capsule on one side will cause a hemiplegia on the opposite side of the body. The commonest cause of hemiplegia is a stroke; examples of other causes are brain damage at birth, abnormalities of blood vessels in the brain, or any structural lesions in the brain such as abscesses or tumours.

The outlook depends on the cause and duration of hemiplegia. After a stroke improvement may begin within a few days and progress may be helped by physiotherapy. No improvement may be expected in cases of irreversible brain damage.

HEPATITIS

Inflammation of the liver. Hepatitis produces symptoms of tiredness, nausea, loss of appetite, jaundice (yellow eyes and skin), dark urine and upper abdominal pain. The skin may become itchy. The inflammation may range in severity from very mild (and producing no symptoms) to so severe as to cause death. The inflammation may be acute and short-lived or chronic and lasting for many years. It may be caused by viruses, drugs, immune attack, or alcohol. In some cases the cause is not known.

The most common cause of hepatitis is a virus called hepatitis A, transmitted via contaminated food or water (the highly infective virus is passed in the faeces). Most people with hepatitis A make a full recovery after bed-rest, a high carbohydrate diet and adequate fluids but with total prohibition of alcohol, usually for six months.

Hepatitis B is sometimes called serum hepatitis. Infection is by contact with blood or body fluids either at birth, sexually or via the intravenous route (for example, infected blood transfusion or drug users sharing needles). The majority of adults recover completely from hepatitis B infection. Some may become carriers of the virus: their blood and body fluids are infectious over many years and they may develop a long-lasting or chronic illness that can progress to cirrhosis or liver cancer. Vaccines are now available to prevent hepatitis B.

Drug-induced hepatitis usually clears up when the patient stops taking the drug. Alcohol-induced hepatitis can be fatal and complete abstention from alcohol in those who recover is essential. Chronic active hepatitis is an autoimmune illness in which the body's own immune system causes the damage to the liver; the drug prednisolone may be given to curb this inflammation.

HERNIA

Protrusion of an internal organ through a defect in the wall of the cavity in which it lies.

Inguinal hernia is the commonest externally visible type; it is first noticed as a lump or swelling in the groin and may result from heavy straining or

H

lifting. The intestine protrudes through a small defect in the muscle of the inguinal canal (where the testes originally descended to the scrotum) but often disappears when the patient lies flat. It is repaired surgically, except in the very unfit patient when a truss may be worn. A femoral hernia is a less common type of groin hernia; it too is repaired surgically.

Umbilical hernias (at the navel) are seen in infants and commonly disappear by the age of 6 years.

Incisional hernias are found at the site of a previous surgical incision where the muscle layer is deficient, allowing the deeper organs to protrude and give rise to a swelling beneath the skin. This type of hernia is particularly common in the abdomen.

In hiatus hernia part of the stomach slips through the diaphragmatic hiatus (the gap in the diaphragm where the oesophagus passes through) and lies in the chest. The condition gives rise to acid regurgitation into the oesophagus (reflux oesophagitis) and heartburn. Treatment consists of antacids and other acid-reducing drugs. Surgery is used as a last resort in resistant cases.

Obstruction or strangulation are fairly common complications, particularly of femoral hernias. In an obstructed hernia the contents of the bowel cannot pass through the intestine, causing vomiting and abdominal distension. In a strangulated hernia the veins draining blood from the bowel, or arteries supplying blood to it, are constricted by pressure from the surrounding ring of tissue where the hernia passes through the abdominal wall. This cuts off the blood supply to the bowel, which dies and turns gangrenous if the pressure is not rapidly relieved. Both of these complications require urgent surgery.

HEROIN

Heroin is a synthetic derivative of morphine, which is derived from the opium poppy. Heroin and the other opiate analgesics bind to specific sites in the brain, grouped around the cerebral ventricles (cavities). These receptor sites usually play host to chemicals called encephalins and endorphins which produce analgesia (kill pain) and allow the individual to cope better with physical and emotional stress. The medical uses of heroin are for analgesia, especially in the acutely injured and terminally ill, in the management of severe breathlessness due to heart failure and, very rarely nowadays, as pre-medication prior to general anaesthesia.
SEE ALSO *Drug dependence*

HERPES SIMPLEX

A member of the herpes virus family. The most frequent infections it causes are cold sores and infection of the cervix. The latter causes inflammation and is associated with an increased risk of cervical cancer. Antiviral drugs such as idoxuridine (for topical administration) or cytarabine (which can be given by injection) may help to control the infection.

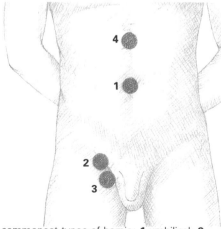

The commonest types of hernia: **1** umbilical; **2** inguinal; **3** femoral; **4** incisional or epigastric.

HERPES ZOSTER

Shingles, caused by the *Varicella zoster* virus which also causes chickenpox. In this condition inflammation of some of the spinal nerves or those in the head (particularly the nerve supplying the cornea of the eye) causes the skin to erupt painfully with blisters along the pathways of the affected nerves. The virus can be isolated from vesicle fluid during the few days in which the blisters contain fluid (and the patient can transmit the infection) but not when these dry up to form crusting lesions or scabs. The disease occurs because of reactivation of the herpes virus which has remained dormant in the cell bodies of the nerves. Herpes of the eye must be seen by an ophthalmologist in the hope of preventing corneal scarring.

Treatment is with locally applied idoxuridine or systemic cytarabine anti-viral agents which reduce the severity of pain after the infection (post-herpetic neuralgia). Herpes zoster and post-herpetic neuralgia are both more common in the elderly.

HIRSCHSPRUNG'S DISEASE

A congenital disorder of the large bowel (colon) caused by the absence of nerve cells in the lower bowel wall (megacolon). It produces constipation and dilatation of the bowel and usually becomes evident in infancy. The diagnosis is made by microscopic examination of a biopsy sample taken from the rectum. The usual treatment is an operation to remove the segment of abnormal bowel and so allow the normal passage of faeces.

HIRSUTISM

Excessive hair growth which, in af-fected women, may occur in a pattern characteristic of men. It has many causes, some of them due to endocrine disorders. Hirsutism may also be a side-effect of certain drugs (phenytoin, for example). Minoxidil, a drug first used to control high blood pressure, is now used to treat certain forms of baldness (alopecia) and may cause increased hair growth elsewhere on the body. Virilizing syndromes (see *Virilism*) are another important cause, usually due to dysfunction of the ovaries or adrenal glands. However, in many cases no specific cause can be found and the individuals concerned simply have a tendency to more hair than might normally be expected.

HISTOLOGY

see *Cytology*

HIV

see *AIDS*

HIVES

see *Urticaria*

HOLE IN THE HEART

see *Congenital heart disease, Ventricular septal defect*

HORMONE

The term 'hormone' was originally coined to describe substances that are secreted into the bloodstream and act on tissues distant from their site of origin — thyroid hormone, for example. However, some hormones act on the tissue that produces them (such as insulin) and some are found only in particular circuits (such as the blood circuit of the hypothalamus in the

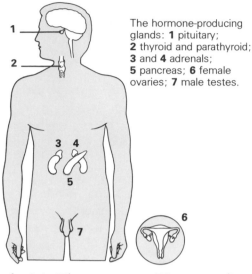

The hormone-producing glands: **1** pituitary; **2** thyroid and parathyroid; **3** and **4** adrenals; **5** pancreas; **6** female ovaries; **7** male testes.

H

brain). There are over 50 mammalian hormones of three general types: peptides, steroids and amines. Tissues that make hormones cannot store very large quantities so that there is a constant manufacture. The control of hormone release is still poorly understood, whereas how they work is clearer. Hormones may latch on to molecules (receptors) on the surface of cells, as insulin does, or to receptors inside the cell, as thyroxine and steroids do. The clinical branch of medicine involved with disordered hormone function is endocrinology.

HORMONE REPLACEMENT THERAPY

The replacement of the body's naturally produced hormones by hormones from an outside source. This may be necessary because of natural failure or certain diseases, when the body either no longer produces any hormone or does not produce it or them in sufficient quantities. The term is now generally applied specifically to oestrogen replacement in women at the time of the menopause when the production of oestrogen by the ovaries starts to decline. This is a natural process, but it can be associated with symptoms such as hot flushes, night sweats and vaginal dryness (which may make sexual intercourse uncomfortable). Treatment with supplementary or replacement oestrogens can abolish these symptoms and reduce the risk of osteoporosis (qv), a condition which weakens the bones and is associated with oestrogen withdrawal. Prevention of osteoporosis is the principal reason for giving HRT to young women in whom ovarian function has ceased (naturally or as a result of surgery).

Hormone replacement therapy can be continued over a period of months or more often for years. It can be given in several ways: in tablet form, as an implant (a special hormone pellet placed in the fatty layer under the skin), or transdermally (a special skin plaster applied twice a week).

All women receiving hormone replacement therapy require careful supervision by a doctor. In patients who have not had a hysterectomy, it can cause vaginal bleeding similar to a light period; heavy or irregular bleeding should be reported immediately to the doctor. There is also, statistically, a slightly increased risk of uterine cancer in later life in patients receiving such treatment.

HORSESHOE KIDNEY

A congenital abnormality in which there is a bridge of tissue between the lower poles of two normally positioned kidneys, giving a horseshoe appearance. Horseshoe kidneys usually cause no symptoms and often do not present a problem; they may be an incidental finding during investigation of another condition. However, if the horseshoe kidney is associated with abnormalities or malposition of the ureters, then infection, obstruction

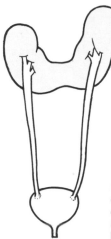

Horseshoe kidney. The connecting segment may consist of functioning kidney tissue or of a fibrous band.

(hydronephrosis) and stones (urolithiasis) may occur. It may then require surgical treatment to correct the malformation.

HUNTINGTON'S CHOREA

see *Chorea*

HYALINE MEMBRANE DISEASE

see *Respiratory distress syndrome*

HYDATID DISEASE

Hydatid disease in man is found in sheep-shearing areas of the world and is caused by the echinococcus tapeworm to which both dogs and sheep play host. The eggs of the tapeworm are found in the stools of these animals and man becomes infected by accidentally ingesting them through contaminated feeding utensils and hands. The eggs hatch into larvae in the stomach and then pierce the stomach wall to enter the bloodstream. They then lodge in various organs, most commonly the liver and lungs, to form hydatid cysts which may grow quite large. The symptoms of hydatid disease, such as breath-lessness (cysts in the lung), abdominal pain, and swelling (in the liver), are caused by pressure or rupture of the cyst and allergic reaction.

Treatment involves the surgical removal of the cyst.

HYDATIDIFORM MOLE

A benign tumour of the placenta (afterbirth) diagnosed early in pregnancy. A hydatidiform mole occurs as a result of incorrect tissue development; instead of a normal placenta, multiple small cysts form resembling a bunch of grapes. In most cases a fetus cannot be found; this is termed a complete mole. In a minority of cases some fetal tissue can be found and this is called a partial mole. There is a 3–5 per cent risk of the tissue undergoing malignant change and resulting in choriocarcinoma (qv).

The condition is usually discovered when pregnancy has been diagnosed (on the basis of the presence of hormones in the urine) but the uterus (womb) is larger than expected for the period of gestation, there is excessive vomiting or small grape-like structures are passed down the vagina.

Treatment involves emptying the uterus by a special suction curette (see *D & C*) and following up the patient carefully using special blood and urine tests to detect a hormone called human chorionic gonadotrophin (HCG). This hormone is produced by normal pregnancies and by both malign and benign pregnancies involving hydatidiform moles. Monitoring the levels of HCG may lead to early detection of recurrence and/or malignant change, either of which may rarely occur even when it has been thought that the mole had been completely removed.

H

HYDROCEPHALUS

An increase in the amount of cerebrospinal fluid (CSF) in the internal spaces of the brain (ventricular system), and often also within the covering of the brain and spinal cord (subarachnoid space). Hydrocephalus is usually caused by obstruction to CSF flow somewhere between its site of production (in cells in the ventricular system) and its absorption from the subarachnoid space into the blood. It occurs for a variety of reasons: as a result of congenital malformation of the ventricular system, pressure on the ventricular system from an enlarging brain tumour, haemorrhage into the ventricular system in a pre-term baby causing an obstruction with blood clot, or meningitis damaging the absorption sites within the subarachnoid space. The condition may also be associated with spina bifida.

Depending on the cause, hydrocephalus may be present at birth or develop later. The symptoms of hydrocephalus are due to the excess of CSF increasing pressure within the skull. When the condition occurs in the fetus or in early infancy, this pressure leads to abnormally rapid head growth as the incompletely formed skull bones allow the head to enlarge unchecked; in the fetus this leads to difficulty with delivery. In older children and adults, where head expansion is not possible because fusion of the skull bones has occurred, the pressure causes headache, vomiting and neurological abnormality such as fits or progressive paralysis.

The diagnosis is made by ultrasound in infancy, or by computerized tomography (CT scan) in older children and adults. If possible the cause is treated. Most cases, however, require a shunt to bypass the blockage and a permanent tubing system with a valve is inserted to divert CSF from the ventricular system to the peritoneal cavity in the abdomen.

HYDROCOELE

A swelling in the scrotum resulting from a collection of fluid around one or both testicles. Hydrocoele usually occurs in middle age but may occur in childhood. The type seen in infancy is often accompanied by an inguinal hernia (in the groin). The fluid may occasionally be able to flow between the hydrocoele and the peritoneal cavity within the abdomen, leading to a variation in the size of the swelling. In adults, rapid and painful accumulation of fluid may occur as a result of injury, twisting or infection of the testis. More gradual, painless swelling may accompany a testicular tumour but more often there is no obvious cause.

Surgical removal of the sac is the most effective treatment. In the elderly, the fluid is drawn out with a needle and syringe, in order to avoid an operation; removal of the sac is the preferred treatment in younger patients, as aspiration of fluid is almost always followed by recurrence.

HYDRONEPHROSIS

Dilatation of the pelvis of the kidney, usually caused by an obstruction to the flow of urine from the kidney. Urine flows from the kidney tubules into the kidney pelvis, down the ureters into the bladder and then out through the urethra. Obstruction at any point will increase the pressure in the system above the blockage and then usually produce dilatation. Common causes of obstruction include stones (urolithiasis), tumours, enlarged prostate and fibrous constriction in the ureters or urethra. Urinary obstruction does not, however, invariably cause the urinary tract to dilate and in a few cases of hydronephrosis no obstruction can be found and the underlying problem remains obscure.

Symptoms include dull flank pain and difficulty in passing and retaining urine. High blood pressure and kidney failure are the principal complications of the condition.

Hydronephrosis is easily detected by an ultrasound scan, but other more invasive tests may be necessary to define the site and cause of obstruction. Treatment depends on the cause; it may involve removing the obstruction (perhaps a stone) or bypassing or relieving it by inserting catheters (through the urethra) from above or below the obstruction.
SEE ALSO illustration on page 171

HYPERACTIVITY

Abnormal behaviour in children in the first 6 years of life; sometimes known as attention deficit disorder. Hyperactivity may be a symptom of underlying neurological disease, when it is often associated with mental handicap, or of emotional or psychiatric disturbance. There is considerable overlap between hyperactivity and so-called conduct disorder such as anti-social or aggressive behaviour. Whether a child is labelled hyperactive therefore depends on how strictly the term is defined.

Psychological and drug treatments are of short-term benefit in treating hyperactivity. Various diets have been tried, but a relationship to food allergy is not proved. Some believe that food additives, such as colouring materials, play a part and diets excluding such additives are sometimes recommended.

HYPERBARIC OXYGEN

Oxygen therapy under high pressure; it is unquestionably of value in carbon monoxide poisoning and essential for the treatment of 'bends' in divers. Trials have not confirmed its value in MS, and its use is not now recommended. Hyperbaric oxygen has also been claimed, but not proven, to be of value in heart attack, gas gangrene and peripheral vascular disease. Hyperbaric oxygen is also effective in treating neonatal asphyxia but is not the preferred therapy, intermittent positive pressure ventilation (in which pressure is raised as a person breathes in) being less dangerous and cheaper.

HYPERCALCAEMIA

Increased calcium in the blood. There are many causes, including hyperparathyroidism (qv), malignant disease, myeloma (qv), sarcoidosis (qv) and excess intake of vitamin D. Specialized investigation, including biochemical, radiological and hormone tests, is usually necessary to identify the cause.

If hypercalcaemia is acute and severe, symptoms include thirst, nausea, vomiting, weakness and mental disturbance. Kidney failure can also occur. If hypercalcaemia is chronic and mild, the symptoms are less pronounced (or may be absent) and the patient only becomes aware of the condition when a complication develops, such as a stone in the kidney (nephrolithiasis) or the urinary tract (urolithiasis), peptic ulcer or bone disease.

Treatment depends on the underlying disease: for example, removal of the parathyroid glands in hyperthyroidism or the giving of corticosteroids in sarcoidosis. A number of

H

drugs may be tried to control hyper-calcaemia in patients with malignant disease; they include corticosteroids, calcitonin, diphosphanates and mithramycin.

HYPERKALAEMIA

High concentrations of potassium in the plasma (the fluid component of blood). Hyperkalaemia is rarely seen, except in patients whose ability to secrete potassium is reduced (for instance, in kidney failure or Addison's disease). It may also occur in otherwise normal individuals, especially infants, in whom a rapid intravenous infusion of potassium (stored blood, for instance) may overload the kidneys' ability to excrete it. Hyperkalaemia produces restless-ness, muscle weakness and, if un-treated, cardiac arrest. The ECG (see *Electrocardiography*) may show a characteristically abnormal pattern.

Treatment is directed at eliminating potassium from the diet, promoting its excretion with resins or dialysis, or promoting its absorption by cells by either bicarbonate (if acidosis co-exists) or insulin and glucose infusion, together with specific treatment of the underlying cause, if possible.

HYPERMETROPIA

Hypermetropia, or long-sightedness, is a condition in which the parallel light rays entering the eye do not focus clearly on the retina but at a point behind it. As a result, images falling on the retina are out of focus and appear blurred. The condition occurs either because the eyeball axis is too short or the refractive power of the lens is too weak. Corrective glasses or contact lenses can compen-sate for this. A convex (plus) lens increases the refraction of light and brings the point of focus further forward.

A similar condition which occurs with advancing age is presbyopia (qv).

HYPERNATRAEMIA

A concentration of sodium in the blood higher than the top of the normal range (150 millimols per litre). The principal cause is lack of body water relative to total sodium content as a result of simple dehydration; this may be due to insufficient intake of water, excessive sweating or loss of water through the kidneys, as in diabetes insipidus, diuretic treatment or when blood sugar is very high in diabetes mellitus. If the balance is not restored, hypernatraemia can result in disturbances of the brain, with clouding of consciousness, coma and convulsions because of loss of water from the brain cells.

Treatment is by slow replacement of water; rapid correction can result in brain disturbances as the brain cells re-adapt to normal water content.

HYPERPARA-THYROIDISM

Overactivity of one or more of the four parathyroid glands which produces excessive amounts of parathyroid hormone and leads to an increase in calcium in the blood (hypercalcaemia). The commonest cause is an adenoma (a benign tumour) of the gland, but apparently identical problems can arise in some patients with malignant tumours, particularly of the lung. In these cases substances very similar to parathyroid hormone are produced by the tumour and released into the circulation. Para-thyroid hormone plays an important role in controlling the level of calcium in the body, and an excess of it (or the substance similar to it in cases of malignancy) is the commonest cause of hypercalcaemia. Symptoms other than those due to chronic hyper-calcaemia (qv) are unusual, but the bones, particularly of the hands, may be affected. Pain may be felt in both bones and joints. The bones are also prone to fracture as calcium is withdrawn from them to increase the levels in the blood. The increase in blood calcium can lead to the development of stones in the kidney. Grumbling abdominal pain and mental disturbance may also be symptoms.

Hyperparathyroidism is usually treated by surgical removal of the affected parathyroid gland(s).

HYPERPLASIA

An increase in size of an organ or tissue due to an increase in the number of its cells. This is often accompanied by a corresponding increase in its functions. Hyperplasia can occur as a result of external stimulus from a hormone, an antibody or an irritant. For example, in many cases of thryotoxicosis there is hyperplasia of the thyroid gland due to an antibody against thyroid hormone in the blood; enlargement of the breast during pregnancy is due to hyperplasia caused by some hormones; or chronic skin irritation by ill-fitting shoes results in skin hyperplasia (a corn). In such cases, the hyperplasia tends to regress once the stimulus is removed.

HYPERTENSION

Abnormally high blood pressure. Normal blood pressure is usually stated as 120/80 mmHg, but no precise figures can be given for the upper limit of normal because the range in the population is so wide; even in an individual it varies considerably, being lowest during sleep and reaching its highest levels during periods of anxiety or excitement. However, below 60 years of age sustained levels greater than 150/90 mmHg may need treatment. Blood pressure normally rises with age, so the picture is not so clear-cut for people over 60.

No underlying cause can be found in the vast majority of cases but often there is a family history of raised blood pressure. Hypertension due to an underlying disorder (usually kidney disease), is responsible for the remaining cases. In pregnancy a severe form of hypertension can develop (eclampsia). Steroids and 'the pill' can be associated with hypertension; blood pressure returns to normal when the drugs are discontinued.

Prolonged high blood pressure can give rise to sickness and death. Hypertensive patients are prone to stroke, heart attack and heart failure.

Treatment of mild hypertension is often simple: giving up smoking and reducing weight if obese, together with restricting salt intake, are sufficient measures. If hypertension is severe, medication may be required; diuretics, beta-blockers and calcium antagonists can all be used. People with very severe, life-threatening hypertension often have papilloedema (qv) as an accompanying symptom. Treatment for essential hypertension is usually lifelong.

SEE ALSO *Sphygmomanometer*

HYPERTHYROIDISM

A syndrome associated with thyroid hormone over-secretion. It is more common in Caucasians than in other races, in women, and in early middle

H

age. Overstimulation of the thyroid, possibly by an autoimmune reaction, is the cause in the majority of cases (Graves' disease). Other causes include single thyroid tumours (toxic adenoma), which produce excessive hormone, thyroid hormone over-dosage, and hormone production by a non-thyroid tumour.

Thyroid hormones have a stimulating effect on metabolism which produces many clinical features. These include goitre, although the degree of enlargement does not correlate with the severity of the disease; increased appetite (common), although there is weight loss too because the increase does not compensate for increased energy expenditure; anxiety, tremor, insomnia and emotional instability (all common); muscle weakness; diarrhoea and menstrual irregularities (both common); tachycardia, palpitations, cardiac arrhythmias and heart failure (particularly in the elderly); abnormal eye movements and protruding eye(s).

The diagnosis is confirmed by measuring thyroid hormones. Other tests are required to establish the cause. Beta-blocking drugs may be used to relieve symptoms, but three main methods of specific treatment are used: antithyroid drugs, surgery and oral radioactive iodine. Antithyroid drugs to regulate the secretion of thyroid hormone are used in adults of reproductive age and in children. Treatment is continued for approximately 18 months. A relapse after treatment is less frequent with longer courses. Surgery is used in patients in whom drug therapy is ineffective or who suffer a relapse, and in patients with large goitres. Relapse and hypothyroidism (qv) may follow surgery. Oral radioactive iodine is used mainly in elderly patients. It is taken up by the thyroid and destroys cellular production. Relapse is rare, but the dose of radiation is difficult to judge and hypothyroidism is a relatively frequent consequence.

HYPERTROPHY

An increase in the size of a cell. This differs from hyperplasia (qv), although both may be associated with organ enlargement and may co-exist in some organs. The differentiation between the two processes is important because certain cells (for example, heart muscle) cannot multiply in order to respond to increased workload but can only increase in size, ie hypertrophy. This process of myocardial hypertrophy is the commonest form of pure hypertrophy; it is seen in conditions such as hypertension, where it affects the left ventricle (one of the two lower chambers of the heart), and chronic lung disease, where it affects the right ventricle. Valvular disease of the heart will also increase workload and may affect either ventricle. The process of hypertrophy has its limits and continued increasing workload may lead to heart failure. The enlarging cells may also outstrip the available blood supply and cause scarring cause (fibrosis).

HYPERURICAEMIA

A high concentration of uric acid in the plasma (the fluid component of blood). It carries a high risk of gout and this risk increases as uric acid levels rise. Uric acid is derived within the body from DNA breakdown in cells and outside the body from dietary sources.

Primary hyperuricaemia occurs in certain races (such as Maoris) that are genetically predisposed to high levels. Secondary hyperuricaemia can result from either over-production or underexcretion of uric acid. Over-production of uric acid is found in many conditions which cause cellular proliferation (for example, polycythaemia, leukaemia, myeloma and other malignant conditions), especially after treatment which causes cellular breakdown. Under-excretion of the acid by the kidney is found in kidney failure, alcohol poisoning, diuretic therapy, low-dose salicylate (aspirin) treatment, starvation and ketoacidosis.

Treatment is discussed under *Gout*.

HYPERVENTILATION

An increased respiratory rate. This may be a response to hypoxia (inadequate oxygen in the blood) or metabolic acidosis (increased acidity of the blood), when the treatment is that of the underlying cause, but the term is most frequently used to describe its occurrence as a reaction to stress or anxiety. Hyperventilation in anxiety produces abnormal sensations (par-aesthesiae) of the hands and around the neck, light-headedness, dizziness and palpitations. The person is obvi-ously apprehensive and sweating. In extreme cases involuntary spasm of the muscles (tetany) may occur. Pro-vided other causes of rapid respiration (such as lung disease) can be excluded, calm reassurance is all that is required for the respiration to return to normal. Breathing into and out of a paper bag may be helpful for people who are subject to recurrent bouts of hyperventilation.

HYPNOTISM

A technique used to induce a condition of altered consciousness in which a person is relaxed and yet in a height-ened state of suggestibility. An hypnotic trance is usually induced by the verbal suggestion of the hypnotist, who in a slow monotonous voice gives the subject a series of graded instructions. The subject remains fully aware of his or her surroundings but does not respond to them in the usual way. The hypnotic state is often accompanied by a failure of memory, a degree of analgesia (insensibility to pain), regression to behaviour appro-priate to a younger person and vivid imagery.

Therapeutically hypnotism may be used as an aid to relaxation, to implant suggestions of improvement (for example, to give up smoking or other addictions), or as an aid to psychotherapy by bringing about the recall of repressed memories. Hypnotism is used less today than in the past and there is insufficient evidence of its benefit in cases of psychiatric disorder.

HYPOCALCAEMIA

Inadequate levels of calcium in the circulation. There are no symptoms in mild cases, but when the condition is more marked there will be muscle cramps and spasms. Cardiac arrest may occur in severe cases.

The commonest cause of hypo-calcaemia is hyperventilation, which, by changing the acidity of the blood, reduces the proportion of calcium that is able to interact with muscle cells. Muscle function returns to normal once any such underlying cause is treated. Hypocalcaemia also results from several rare inherited conditions in which the level of activity of parathyroid hormone is low (see *Hypo-parathyroidism*), if the parathyroid glands have been affected by autoim-mune disease, or if all these glands have been inadvertently removed at thyroidectomy (qv). Even a low calcium content in the poorest diets is

H

unlikely to cause hypocalcaemia, but the condition may occur in severe osteomalacia (rickets in children) where vitamin D deficiency prevents the absorption of dietary calcium. Some patients with kidney failure or severe pancreatitis also develop hypocalcaemia. Treatment is then of the underlying cause. In cases where the parathyroid glands are absent or non-functional, highdose vitamin D or similar drugs are usually effective as treatment.

HYPOGLYCAEMIA

Low levels of glucose in the blood. Hypoglycaemia usually occurs in patients with diabetes mellitus and very rarely otherwise. By far the commonest cause is in patients with diabetes mellitus who have taken too little food, too much exercise or too much insulin (or tablet) treatment. Non-diabetic patients who have hypoglycaemia may have an insulin-secreting tumour, Addison's disease, hypopituitarism, liver disease, or an inborn error of metabolism. Hypoglycaemia may also be an exaggerated response to high levels of glucose in the blood, as seen in infants of diabetic mothers, or it can result from the stomach being rapidly emptied as a consequence of excessive alcohol ingestion or previous gastrectomy.

The symptoms of hypoglycaemia often depend on the rate at which the blood glucose has fallen. Anxiety, hunger, restlessness, palpitations, flushing and sweating are common. Abnormal behaviour may develop and progress to loss of consciousness and convulsions.

Treatment with oral or intravenous glucose rapidly brings about a cure. Preventative measures and education are important for diabetic patients.

HYPOGONADISM

Inadequate function of the gonads (testes in the male, ovaries in the female), which are hormonepro-ducing glands within the endocrine system. Hypogonadism causes infertility in females and impotence in males; the so-called 'secondary sexual characteristics' will be under-developed or absent in both sexes. Hypogonadism may be caused by a chromosomal disorder (for example, Turner's syndrome, Klinefelter's syndrome), or disease of the pituitary gland or of the gonads themselves (such as is caused by alcoholism). Diagnosis may require detailed investigation of the gonads. If the cause is chromosomal, fertility cannot be restored. Sex hormone treatment, which will generally need to be life-long, can usually achieve normal sexual appearance whatever the cause. In some patients with an endocrine cause this treatment can also restore fertility.

HYPOKALAEMIA

A low concentration of potassium in the plasma (the fluid component of blood). It occurs with reduced dietary intake (rare), loss from gastro-intestinal secretion (for example, vomiting, diarrhoea or fistula), and loss in the urine. Urinary loss may be subdivided into conditions where cellular mechanisms are faulty (such as ketoacidosis or starvation), conditions of increased kidney excretion (an excess of corticosteroids or alkalosis), and kidney disease itself (chronic pyelonephritis, for example).

The symptoms of hypokalaemia are general and non-specific, often making diagnosis difficult. They include tiredness and malaise, poor concentration and drowsiness, muscle weakness, ileus (failure of intestinal movement), thirst and excess production of urine (polyuria). Treatment consists of slowly replenishing potassium stores orally or intravenously. The underlying condition is also treated.

HYPONATRAEMIA

A low concentration of sodium in the plasma (the fluid component of blood). The symptoms are muscular weakness and thirst.

Sodium depletion is associated with water depletion and is found in patients who are unable to excrete water properly, such as those suffering with heart failure or the liver diseases cirrhosis and nephrotic syndrome. Hyponatraemia is particularly likely in these circumstances because patients are on a low-salt diet combined with high-dose diuretic therapy. Vigorous and prolonged exercise, profuse sweating, vomiting, diarrhoea, Addison's disease and burns may also bring about hyponatraemia. In these cases the condition is usually quickly corrected by the giving of sodium either orally or intravenously.

HYPOPARA-THYROIDISM

A condition caused by underactivity of the parathyroid glands, which produce the parathyroid hormone necessary for the absorption of calcium. Most commonly hypoparathyroidism is a temporary problem that occurs as a result of an operation on the thyroid with inadvertent damage to or accidental removal of one or more parathyroid gland. Other cases are probably of an autoimmune nature with circulating antibodies being produced against parathyroid hormone.

Hypoparathyroidism causes hypokalaemia (qv) and tetany (qv). Emotional instability and other psychiatric disturbances may also be associated, even at times when blood calcium is normal (so that diagnosis may then be difficult). Epilepsy, cataracts, various skin abnormalities and fungal infections may be present.

Diagnosis is made by laboratory analysis of calcium and parathyroid hormone samples taken from the patient. Treatment is to replace the lost calcium; parathyroid hormone cannot be used as it is antigenic and if given would cause the development of antibodies which would cancel out its effect. Vitamin D may also be given.

HYPOPITUITARISM

Under-production of one or more pituitary hormones, normally caused by a pituitary tumour; local surgery, radiation and vascular diseases of the blood vessels of the pituitary gland at the base of the brain are also relatively common causes. The features of the condition depend upon which hormones are deficient. Growth hormone (GH), adrenocorticotrophic hormone (ACTH), thyroid-stimulating hormone (TSH) and gonadotrophins (FSH and LH) may all be lacking.

Hypopituitarism usually sets in slowly with loss of energy, apathy and amenorrhoea. The skin becomes pale and pubic hair is lost. Blood pressure may be low. Impaired vision may also be a symptom if the cause is a pituitary tumour. Features due to lack of ACTH and TSH resemble Addison's disease (qv) and hypothyroidism (qv). Advanced cases are usually obvious as the symptoms are then striking, but in the early stages when symptoms may be mild and relatively non-specific hypopituitarism

H

may resemble other diseases. Appropriate endocrine tests (see *Endocrinology*) to measure hormonal production at rest and under biochemical stress will usually confirm the diagnosis.

The underlying cause will usually require treatment, but all patients with this condition are improved by appropriate hormone replacement. SEE ALSO *illustration on page 144*

HYPOSPADIAS

The commonest congenital malformation of the male urethra (the tube which drains the bladder): about 1 male in 350 is affected. There are five degrees of deformity:

- In glandular hypospadias, the most frequent variety, the opening is on the undersurface of the glans or tip of the penis. No treatment is generally required.

  If the opening is too small an operation called a meatotomy is performed to enlarge it.

- In coronal hypospadias the urethra is situated at the junction of the undersurface of the glans and the

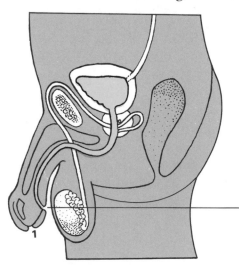

In males the urethra normally opens at the tip of the penis **(1)**. In hypospadias the opening is on the underside **(2)** or in the area between the thighs (the perineum).

body of the penis.

- In penile hypospadias the urethra opens on the undersurface of the penis.
- In penile scrotal hypospadias the urethra is situated at the junction of the penis and scrotum.
- In perineal hypospadias the scrotum is split and the urethra opens between its two halves.

These last four types require plastic surgery to attempt to correct the deformity.

Boys with hypospadias should not be circumcised as the redundant skin is useful for reconstruction during surgery.

HYPOTENSION

Low blood pressure. Low blood pressure itself is not a problem and when present naturally, rather than as a result of disease or drug treatment, it is associated with above-average life expectancy. Only when the blood pressure is too low to achieve adequate oxygen and nutrient supply to the tissues (particularly brain, heart and kidneys) is treatment required. Postural hypotension, in which the normal drop in blood pressure on standing up is not rapidly counteracted and so leads to a feeling of faintness, is common in the elderly and the previously bed-bound. It may also occur in healthy adults on getting out of a hot bath. Standing up slowly reduces the risk of this type of hypotension. Overtreatment of hypertension (high blood pressure) may also cause the condition; this is remedied by a reduction in drug dosage.

Hypotension otherwise occurs only in seriously ill patients, as a component of clinical shock; it is particularly common in severe injury, especially when there has been bleeding, in septicaemia, in peritonitis, and in severe acute heart failure (cardiogenic shock). Urgent hospital treatment with intravenous blood or fluid to correct the hypotension is required in such cases.

HYPOTHERMIA

A condition in which the body temperature is seriously below normal (usually defined as below 35°C or 95°F). Hypothermia is unusual in the young and healthy, except as a result of exposure to extreme conditions (such as immersion in cold sea water), but is relatively common in frail elderly people. In the young, a reduction in the ambient temperature activates mechanisms to conserve heart (thermoregulation); for example, blood vessels to the peripheries constrict so less blood flows through the limbs and less heat is lost through the skin. By contrast, thermoregulation in the elderly is less efficient and loss of body heat cannot be controlled. Hypothermia may also occur, and may be severe, in those debilitated by underlying disease, particularly hypothyroidism, advanced malignancy, anorexia nervosa and alcoholism. (It is not commonly appreciated that alcohol dilates blood vessels and so consumption in cold weather may lead to increased loss of body heat.) In all but the mildest cases and especially when there is an underlying debility, hypothermia has a poor outlook because it is frequently associated with septicaemia, or complicated by disturbances in heart rhythm or by metabolic problems.

Prevention is important and adequate winter heating and thick clothes are vital for those at risk. Treatment requires hospital admission (often to the intensive care unit) and very gradual rewarming; careful heart monitoring and frequent blood tests are combined with specific therapy for any underlying condition.

HYPOTHYROIDISM

A clinical condition in which the thyroid gland, the principal regulator of the rate of metabolism, is underactive and does not secrete enough thyroid hormone. The causes of hypothyroidism include defects in the pituitary gland and destruction or removal of the thyroid gland by surgery, prior administration of radio-active iodine, or radiation. Iodine is essential for normal thyroid function, being an essential component of thyroxine, the principal thyroid hormone; iodine deficiency can impair its production.

Hypothyroidism which is present at birth, due to a defect in the pituitary gland, may lead to permanent brain damage (cretinism); screening has been introduced for this condition. In adults hypothyroidism is associated with nonspecific symptoms: lethargy, constipation, cold intolerance and heavy menstruation. As the condition progresses, mental faculties become impaired and weight increases. There may be changes in the hair and voice, which become coarser and deeper respectively. In its most severe form, there is myxoedema, in which an accumulation of mucopolysaccharides (a type of carbohydrate) occurs in the skin and other tissues, leading to thickening and a characteristic expressionless face with coarse features. The heart may be enlarged with surrounding fluid. Regular bowel movement may slow down tremendously, giving rise to distension. Myxoedema coma can follow, in which there is almost always associated hypothermia. It is often fatal.

In its early stages hypothyroidism is difficult to detect clinically, particularly in the elderly, and blood tests which measure the concentration of thyroid hormone and of the thyroid stimulating hormone (TSH) secreted by the pituitary gland are necessary to diagnose the condition.

Hypothyroidism with enlargement of the thyroid gland (goitre, qv) is caused by inadequate thyroxine secretion in the blood with overstimulation of the thyroid gland by TSH to try to compensate for this defect. Causes include hereditary defects in thyroid hormone biochemistry, iodine deficiency, drugs and chronic inflammation of the thyroid (Hashimoto's disease).

Treatment is with the hormone thyroxine.

HYPOXIA

Inadequate oxygen in the blood. Hypoxia is caused by severe forms of any chest disease and by many types of heart disease. If unremedied, the condition causes permanent brain damage. Perhaps surprisingly, it causes few symptoms until very low oxygen levels are reached, at which point the patient becomes confused and may lose consciousness. Most of the breathlessness (dyspnoea) that these patients typically experience is in fact the result of carbon dioxide accumulation rather than lack of oxygen.

Treatment of hypoxia is with oxygen, and by attention to the underlying cause: for example, antibiotics for pneumonia or diuretics for heart failure. Oxygen has to be given carefully, since patients with longstanding chronic bronchitis cannot tolerate high concentrations — indeed, excess oxygen may stop their breathing completely. In these patients, oxygen is given at a concentration only slightly greater than the 21 per cent present in ordinary air.

HYSTERECTOMY

Removal of the uterus (womb). The operation is performed in severe cases of menorrhagia (heavy periods), fibroids, endometriosis, and infection, and for malignant disease of the uterus, cervix or ovaries. Surgical approach may be via the abdomen (abdominal hysterectomy) or the vagina (vaginal hysterectomy). Hysterectomy may be total, in which case the uterine body and the uterine cervix (neck of the womb) are removed, or subtotal, leaving the cervix intact. Pan-hysterectomy is the term used to describe a total hysterectomy plus removal of the ovaries and Fallopian tubes. A radical hysterectomy is usually performed for malignant disease of the cervix and involves removal of the supporting ligaments, parametria (tissues on either side of the uterus and cervix) and upper third of the vagina in addition to the uterus and cervix; the pelvic lymph glands are often removed too.

HYSTERIA

The term hysteria may be used to describe a psychiatric disorder, a particular mental mechanism (known as dissociation), or a personality type. It is as a description of dissociation that the term is most widely used in medical circles. Dissociation is an alteration of the state of consciousness whereby an individual views certain aspects of his own thought or behaviour as alien and buries them in the subconscious mind. Examples of states which may result from dissociation include amnesias, fugues, paralysis and loss of voice (aphonia). A number of conditions viewed as hysterical in the past, such as torticollis and writer's cramp, are now thought usually to have a physical basis. In the United States hysteria has been regarded by some doctors as a psychiatric disorder (Briquet's syndrome) affecting mainly women, in which a sufferer over a period of years repeatedly attends doctors with physical complaints for which no cause can be found, but this concept is not generally accepted in the United Kingdom where the term hypochondria is usually preferred in identifying such cases. As a description of personality, hysteria refers to a person with shallow, unstable emotions who is flirtatious, manipulative and unable to maintain a satisfactory sexual relationship.

IATROGENIC

A term used to describe the complications of medical management which can arise as a result of diagnostic procedures, drug therapy, administration of biologic products (whole blood transfusions, for example), mechanical therapeutic procedures (such as dialysis), surgical treatment and ionizing irradiation. The term does not imply that the condition has been caused by medical negligence. Every effort is made to reduce the incidence and severity of iatrogenic diseases. However, they cannot be eliminated altogether because they are not usually predictable.

ICHTHYOSIS

Excessive dryness of the skin, accompanied by scaliness; the word comes from the Greek, meaning 'fish-scale'. Ichthyosis is commonly seen in the elderly, especially when they are hospitalized, since the combination of a heated environment and frequent bathing dries out their already rather dry skin. Various forms of inherited ichthyosis exist, which range from a very minor dryness of the skin to a severe scaly skin disease which may be very difficult to control and is socially distressing. Excessive dryness of the skin may also be seen in association with a variety of other skin disorders, such as atopic dermatitis.

Treatment is with oily skin preparations (emollients) to rehydrate the skin. In addition to applying emollients directly to the skin, sufferers are often advised to add bath oil to their bath water and to use a modified emollient as a soap substitute to help prevent the removal of natural oils when washing.

IDIOSYNCRASY

An inherently abnormal and unpredictable response to a common drug or drugs, usually due to a genetic abnormality. The condition known as porphyria (qv) is an example and so is haemolytic anaemia (qv) due to glucose-6 phosphate dehydrogenase (G6PD) deficiency.

In individuals affected by porphyria there are abnormalities of specific enzymes involved in the synthesis of haemoglobin, which is involved in the carrying of oxygen by red blood cells. There are several different types of porphyria but in most cases sufferers develop an attack after taking one of many different common drugs (such as general anaesthetics, barbiturates, the contraceptive pill and some antibiotics); alcohol may also bring on an attack.

G6PD deficiency is a disease which affects males from Africa, the Mediterranean, and the Middle and Far East.

It is caused by a deficiency of an enzyme found in the red blood cells and results in haemolysis (qv) if certain drugs, particularly antimalarial treatments, are taken.

ILEITIS

Inflammation of the ileum, the lower small bowel. It is usually caused by Crohn's disease (qv), but may be due to a rare bacterial infection with *Yersinia enterocolita*. The inflammation may produce symptoms very similar to appendicitis, with pain in the lower right side of the abdomen and fever, or it may produce more longstanding symptoms of diarrhoea, abdominal pain, weight loss, fever or bowel obstruction. Ileitis caused by infective agents requires treatment with appropriate antibiotics. If the condition is due to Crohn's disease it can be treated either with the drug prednisolone or by surgical removal of the affected part of the bowel.

ILEOSTOMY

Surgical opening of the small bowel on to the abdominal wall to prevent the flow of faeces into the large bowel (colon). It may be a temporary measure, taken when the underlying condition is reversible with treatment, or it may be permanent (end-ileostomy) and performed after the removal of the large bowel. (The reason for removal of the large bowel may be ulcerative colitis, Crohn's disease, multiple polyps or tumours.) As a result of ileostomy, a specially designed plastic bag, which is attached to the skin by adhesive, takes the place of the large bowel and collects the faecal fluid. Modern designs of these bags neither leak nor smell, and a patient with an ileostomy can lead a full and normal life.

ILEUS

Failure of intestinal movement. As a result the abdomen becomes distended, the bowels do not open, no wind is passed and vomiting occurs. An X-ray of the abdomen will show a dilated intestine with large amounts of air and fluid. Ileus commonly occurs after abdominal operations, recovery usually taking place spontaneously over a few days; during this time the stomach is kept empty and fluids are given intravenously.

In a minority of cases ileus may be prolonged and severe; this occurs when the abdominal cavity has been contaminated by the contents of the gastro-intestinal tract (for example, in appendicitis with perforation, or after perforation of a peptic ulcer or diverticular disease of the colon), and especially if infection ensues (peritonitis). Rarely ileus can result from a neurological disorder, when nerves supplying the intestinal muscles degenerate.

Meconium ileus is common in newborn babies suffering from cystic fibrosis. In this condition bowels become blocked by thick mucus and normal intestinal movement is prevented. An operation is often required to remove the meconium.

IMMUNITY

Resistance to infections. There are two types of immunity: humoral and cell-mediated. Humoral immunity is the production of antibodies, and is the response of white cells called B lymphocytes; this is the immunity which results from vaccination (for example, diphtheria, whooping cough and tetanus, the DPT vaccination). Cell-mediated immunity is the response of white cells called T lymphocytes. It is decreased in conditions like lymphoma and may result in unusual infections such as herpes zoster or shingles.

Some children are born without humoral immunity and cannot form antibodies; this is hypogammaglobulinaemia, and results in frequent infections. Treatment involves the transfusion of antibodies. Abnormal cellular immunity mainly occurs in association with lymphocytic leukaemia or tumours of lymphoid tissue. The acquired immune deficiency syndrome (AIDS) results in a deficiency of humoral and cell-mediated immunity. As a consequence, opportunistic infections occur.

IMMUNIZATION

see *Vaccination*

IMMUNO-SUPPRESSION

A state in which the body's natural immune responses are suppressed. Immunosuppression may occur naturally, or after therapy. It is found temporarily in pregnancy, where half of the antigenic makeup of the baby is from the father and is comparable to an allograft (qv). Medical conditions caused by an over-production of antibodies (such as thyroid under-activity) rarely develop in pregnancy. Therapy to induce immunosuppression is given after organ transplantation and involves the drugs cyclosporin and azathioprine.

There are a variety of medical conditions which result from the production of antibodies against various organs, the so-called autoimmune diseases. Drugs such as steroids and cyclophosphamide are used in the treatment of these conditions because they induce immunosuppression. Steroids, for example, are very effective treatments in autoimmune haemolytic anaemia and thrombocytopenia (a low number of platelets), which result from antibody destruction of red cells and platelets, respectively.

IMPETIGO

A skin infection caused by the bacterium *Staphylococcus aureus*; it used to be very common but is less so now. It occurs mainly in children, though any age group may be affected. The typical lesion is an inflamed, weepy, rather raw area (usually just one), a few centimetres in diameter, on the surface of which the discharge forms a goldcoloured crust. Lesions are contagious and treatment with systemic antibiotics is usually necessary. The infection usually clears up within a few days after treatment.

IMPOTENCE

A common sexual dysfunction of men in which they are unable to sustain an erection adequate for penetration when attempting intercourse. The term is also sometimes used to describe the inability to ejaculate (ejaculatory impotence), which is a rarer dysfunction than erectile impotence. Erectile impotence becomes commoner with increasing age, the prevalence rising from 1 per cent in men under 35 years to 25 per cent in men at 70 years. The cause may be psychological or physical in origin. Psychological factors (anxiety, depression, sometimes latent homosexuality) are likely to be the major cause of impotence in younger men, in whom onset is often sudden and yet an interest in sex may be maintained. A range of physical factors may cause impotence, particularly in older men — these factors include physical illness such as liver disease, heart disease or diabetes mellitus, medications such as antidepressants, diuretics or antihypertensives (drugs for high blood pressure); alcoholism and drug abuse; and neurological and psychiatric disorders.

Where physical factors are causing impotence, treatment will address these. Where psychological factors are important, a behaviour therapy approach is often adopted; its aims include reducing anxiety about sexual performance with the help of joint counselling and reducing the sexual demands of the partner. It is estimated that around 75 per cent of this latter group of sufferers improve with this approach.

INBORN ERRORS OF METABOLISM

A group of inherited disorders involving a biochemical pathway. A biochemical pathway consists of a series of steps, each controlled by a particular enzyme which in turn is coded for by a specific gene. The genetic mutation responsible for an inborn error of metabolism results in a deficiency or defect of a specific enzyme. Almost 200 inborn errors of metabolism are known, the majority being inherited in an autosomal recessive pattern, some in a sex-linked manner and a few as an autosomal dominant trait.

The clinical effects may be caused by an accumulation of substances normally metabolized via the enzyme, or by a deficiency of the product of the pathway. For example, in phenylketonuria a deficiency of the enzyme called phenylalanine hydroxylase leads to a build-up of phenylalanine and a deficiency of tyrosine; these produce the clinical features of mental retardation and fair hair. If phenylketonuria is detected at birth, then a diet low in phenylalanine can be prescribed and mental retardation avoided. Newborns are screened for phenylketonuria with the Guthrie blood test; in this a drop of blood obtained by pricking the heel of the baby is tested for the presence of phenylalanine. Other examples of inborn errors of metabolism include congenital hypothyroidism (cretinism, qv) congenital adrenal hyperplasia (qv), Tay-Sachs' disease (a progressive brain disease in infants), Wilson's disease (qv), hypercholesterolaemia (increased blood cholesterol levels) and albinism (qv).

Antenatal diagnosis is available for many inborn errors of metabolism for which the enzyme abnormality has been identified, either by biochemical analysis of cells taken by amniocentesis, or by DNA analysis from specimens taken by chorionic villus biopsy. In groups of people where many are carriers for inborn errors of metabolism inherited in autosomal recessive fashion (for example, Ashkenazi Jews), it may be possible to screen potential parents to identify couples who are carriers and would benefit from antenatal diagnosis.

INCONTINENCE (URINARY)

The inability to control the bladder. Most women suffer from urinary incontinence at some time, usually during pregnancy. The commonest cause of incontinence in men is brain damage as a result of a stroke. There are several types of urinary incontinence.

Stress incontinence refers to the involuntary loss of urine during coughing, sneezing, laughing, running, jumping and so on, and is caused by weak pelvic floor muscles. It is a very common problem in pregnancy and may persist after the birth of the baby. Postnatal exercises are done to tone up the pelvic floor muscles after childbirth, preventing the development of stress incontinence and often curing it if it is a problem. Urge incontinence occurs when the bladder muscle is irritated or if there is laxity of the front wall of the bladder with partial prolapse (cystocoele); this type occurs only in women. Bed wetting is another type of incontinence, but the cause is usually in part psychological.

When simple measures, such as pelvic floor exercises, fail to cure the problem, women with urinary incontinence are usually referred to a gynaecologist. Special investigations will be done, which may include urodynamic studies (tests to measure the pressure within the bladder), cystoscopy and special X-rays of the kidneys and bladder. Depending on the underlying cause, a variety of treatments can be recommended. The patient may be referred to a physiotherapist for supervised pelvic floor exercises, drugs may be prescribed, or surgery may be considered. Incontinence is more common in elderly patients, especially in dementia in both sexes, and is much more difficult to manage; no treatment is given.

INDUCTION OF LABOUR

The initiation of labour either before (pre-term, 38–41 weeks) or after (post-term, 42 weeks or more) the normal 42 weeks' of pregnancy. The principal reasons for induction are high blood pressure in the mother (pre-eclampsia of pregnancy) and post-maturity of the fetus, which will be in jeopardy if it remains in the uterus. The method adopted will depend on the duration of the preg-

nancy, urgency for delivery and the degree of dilatation of the cervix (neck of the womb). Drugs used to induce labour are prostaglandins (which may be administered either intravenously or as vaginal pessaries) or the hormone oxytocin (which is given as an intravenous infusion); both types of drug induce contractions of the uterus. Artificial rupture of the membranes to release the 'waters' (amniotic fluid) may also be necessary to assist the process. This is carried out without anaesthesia, although some sedation may be given: a small hole is made in the amniotic membrane with a special hooked instrument, and the fluid comes out. Over 90 per cent of patients induced will deliver within 24 hours.

INFANT FEEDING

The essential role of infant feeding is to provide sufficient nutrients for normal growth over the first year of life. This is the period of most rapid growth in childhood, when birth weight is trebled. The best food for a term baby from birth is breast milk. This contains the correct amounts of water, protein, carbohydrate, fat, vitamins and minerals to ensure normal growth for the first 6 months. Ordinary cow's milk does not contain enough iron or vitamin D for infants, and a modified formula is now advised throughout the first year. If artificial feeding is planned, a modified cow's milk formula feed, which mimics the composition of breast milk, is used. Care must be taken to reconstitute powdered milk correctly, following manufacturer's instructions, and to sterilize water and utensils.

In the early weeks of life, a baby establishes a feeding pattern which is more or less repetitive from day to day. Demand feeding is best for normal term babies, who will feed

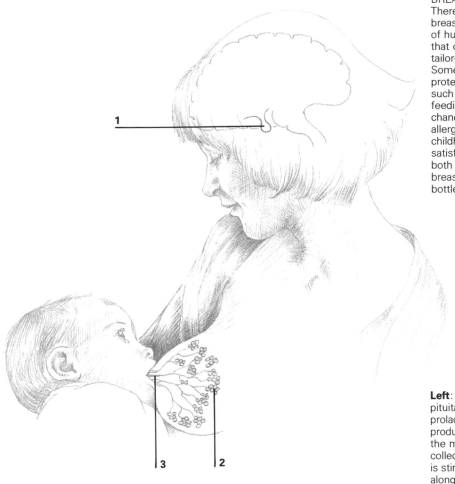

BREAST FEEDING
There are many advantages to breast feeding. The composition of human milk is different from that of other species and is tailor-made for the human baby. Some proteins in breast milk protect the infant from infection, such as gastro-enteritis. Breast feeding may reduce the chances of the baby developing allergies later in infancy and childhood. It also gives satisfaction psychologically to both mother and baby. Lastly, breast feeding is cheaper than bottle feeding.

Left: Lactation is initiated by a pituitary **(1)** hormone called prolactin. Breast milk is produced by excretions from the mammary gland which collect in the alveoli **(2)**. The milk is stimulated by suckling to flow along the milk ducts **(3)** to the nipple.

when hungry (which may be every two hours to begin with) and soon settle into a routine. Breast and modified cow's milk appear equally satisfactory for growth, which normally proceeds at about 25 g (1 oz) per day.

By the age of 4 months, most babies begin to be less satisfied by milk alone, and semi-solid food is introduced (weaning). This needs to be done gradually by trial and error. By 6 months the baby is able to chew, and may manage a rusk or biscuit. Progressively lumpier foods can be given in the latter half of the first year. By 1 year of age, the baby will take his or her meals with the rest of the family.

Milk remains an important source of nutrition in the second 6 months.

INFARCTION

The process of tissue death which is produced by the sudden deprivation of blood supply due to embolism or thrombosis. Infarction occurs in organs that have no alternative source of blood supply. The area which undergoes such a death is called an infarct. The most common organs where infarctions occur are the heart, lung and brain. The dead tissue is partially or wholly absorbed and is surrounded or replaced by fibrosis (scarring).

INFECTIOUS MONONUCLEOSIS

see *Glandular fever*

INFECTIVE ENDOCARDITIS

Infection of the endocardium (the inner surface of the heart), particularly involving the heart valves. Acute infective endocarditis is much rarer since the introduction of antibiotics for the treatment of acute infections. It occurs as a complication of infection in the bloodstream when bacteria such as staphylococci, streptococci or pneumococci may be deposited and grow on heart valves. Fever and sweating occur, together with symptoms arising from small infected emboli breaking off from the heart valves and becoming deposited in other tissues. If the heart valves are significantly damaged this may lead to impairment of heart function and heart failure.

Subacute infective endocarditis (of fairly sudden onset) mainly affects heart valves which have previously been damaged as a consequence of rheumatic fever or congenital heart disease. It is usually due to infection with a form of streptococci found in infected gums and teeth. If these bacteria enter the bloodstream — often after routine dental procedures — they may lodge in damaged heart valves. The symptoms include malaise (a general feeling of being unwell), weight loss, persistent fever, joint pains, small skin haemorrhages, anaemia and symptoms from emboli.

The diagnosis can usually be made by growing the bacteria from blood samples in the laboratory on an appropriate culture medium. The condition usually responds to appro-

priate antibiotics which may need to be taken for several weeks. The outlook depends on the duration of the condition and any cardiac damage.

INFERTILITY

The inability of a couple to achieve a pregnancy after a year of regular unprotected intercourse. Infertility affects around 10 per cent of couples. In 30 per cent of cases of infertility the cause lies with the woman, in 30 per cent with the man, and in the remainder with both. In the search for a cause of infertility both partners have to be seen

Common causes of infertility in women are failure to ovulate (produce eggs), blockage of the Fallopian tubes preventing the eggs and sperms meeting, and mucus in the cervix which kills the partner's sperm (cervical hostility). Investigations are aimed at detecting these problems. The ability to produce eggs can be shown by blood tests, ultrasound scanning or, less reliably, by keeping a daily temperature chart (most women show a transient slight rise in body temperature at the time of ovulation). Subsequent treatment is with fertility drugs. Blockage of the Fallopian tubes is often due to previous infections. This can be detected by laparoscopy (qv) or with special X-rays. If a blockage is shown, surgery may be of help, but in cases where damage is extensive the only option is invitro fertilization (IVF or a test tube baby, qv). Cervical hostility can be detected by means of a postcoital test. Mucus from the cervix is examined a few hours after intercourse to see if the sperms are managing to swim forward in it. If all the sperms are stationary, or dead, then cervical hostility can be suspected. The only effective treatment available is GIFT (see below).

The male partner should produce at least 2 ml of semen, containing between 20 and 150 million sperms per ml, at least half of which should be of normal appearance and actively swimming forward. Smaller numbers or poorer quality will result in a decreasing chance of achieving a pregnancy. Various problems such as mumps and venereal infection can lead to a poor sperm count, but in the majority of cases the cause is unknown. On the whole treatments are disappointing, although simple measures may help, such as keeping the testicles cool by wearing boxer shorts and avoiding long periods of sitting. Patience may lead to a pregnancy, but in some cases the use of donor sperm may be the only option.

If all tests are normal the problem becomes one of unexplained infertility. Here possible treatments include IVF, and gamete intra-Fallopian transfer (GIFT) where the eggs and sperm are placed together in the Fallopian tubes to allow fertilization to occur in a natural environment. SEE ALSO *Artificial insemination*

INFLAMMATION

The process by which tissue responds to injury. Acute inflammation is a result of physical, chemical or bacterial injury and consists of swelling, redness, increased local heat, pain and loss of function of the affected part (see *Whitlow* or *Stye*). In chronic inflammation there is a continuation of the acute phase, which is often followed in turn by tissue destruction, fibrosis with scarring and deformity leading to permanent loss of function (see *Rheumatoid arthritis*).

When the inflammation is viewed with a microscope, infiltration of the area by many specialized white blood cells in an inflammatory discharge is seen. These cells have different roles: some destroy or neutralize the agent causing the inflammation, while others remove dead or damaged cells and other debris. The inflammation usually subsides when the cause is removed, but occasionally the process can become self-perpetuating even if the initiating agent is eliminated.

As a general rule, treatment depends on the cause of the inflammation, but a large number of drugs (such as aspirin, paracetamol or steroids) have an anti-inflammatory effect.

INFLUENZA

The word comes from the Italian 'influenza' (meaning 'influence') as it was believed that epidemics of this acute infectious disease were due to the influence of the stars. They are now known to be caused by the influenza virus, of which there are three types: A, B and C.

The infection is highly contagious, generally occurs in the winter and may cause epidemics. Influenza is usually transmitted by droplet inhalation from sneezing and coughing. After an incubation period of 1—3 days, the onset is abrupt, with high fever, shivering, headache, sore throat and dry cough. The symptoms usually ease after 3—4 days, some tiredness and depression remaining for a few days longer. Complications may occur in the elderly and those with chronic lung or heart disease; they include pneumonia, coma, heart failure and sudden death. General measures such as bed rest, fluids and aspirin are usually sufficient. Antibiotics may occasionally be necessary when there is secondary bacterial infection (as in pneumonia).

Immunization against influenza is recommended in the elderly and those with lung or heart disease.

INSECT BITE

Most insect bites are harmless or cause a typical minor itchy sore and are usually easily treated with soothing antiseptic lotions or creams applied locally. The major hazard of insect bites comes from the transmission of infective organisms. Malaria (qv) is the most important of these world-wide, and with more extensive and rapid air travel the disease is again being seen in areas which are themselves malaria-free. Similar infections include yellow fever (qv) and filariasis (qv). AIDS does not appear to be transmitted in this way.

INSECT STING

An injury caused by the injection of toxin by an insect. The ensuing skin reaction is usually trivial, the pain, swelling and redness lasting 1–2 days unless the area becomes infected. More severe reactions lasting several days occur as a result of allergy in susceptible atopic and even in some non-atopic individuals. The incidence of allergic reaction to stings is greatest in young people under 20 years. Any reaction other than at the sting site is as a rule abnormal and an indication of severe susceptibility.

The majority of these responses are mild, consisting of itching and a rash (urticaria), but a few individuals have a severe, sometimes fatal, reaction (anaphylaxis). The shorter the period between the sting and the onset of symptoms, the more serious the reaction. Three distinct types of reaction are recognized: generalized urticaria, respiratory difficulties with bronchospasm and shock with low blood pressure. All may occur together. For the last two, immediate medical treatment is required with adrenaline and steroids. Desensitization (qv) can be tried in those with previous anaphylatic reactions to bee and wasp stings.

INSOMNIA

The inability to fall asleep or maintain adequate sleep. Insomnia is common in people of all ages, although it seems to become commoner with increasing age. Indeed, the need for sleep decreases with increasing age, and some people mistake this phenomenon for insomnia. Young people often complain of difficulty in falling asleep and older people of waking during the night. Women are particularly affected. The amount of sleep lost by sufferers is estimated to be far less than that reported by them. There are many causes of insomnia. For example, depression causes an insomnia where a person wakes early in the morning and cannot get back to sleep; alcohol dependence may cause early morning waking; anxiety may result in a delay in falling asleep on going to bed; and pain or illnesses such as emphysema, anorexia nervosa and dementia may prevent sleep.

Sleeping tablets may be of temporary benefit in treating insomnia but the disadvantages of tolerance, dependence and sedation usually far outweigh any short-term gain. In most cases of insomnia there is no underlying clinical cause and the problem may be helped by adopting practical measures, such as establishing a regular daily sleeping pattern, taking daily exercise, reducing intake of caffeine-containing drinks and alcohol especially in the evenings, having a firm mattress, or perhaps trying relaxation techniques.

INSULIN

A hormone produced by the islets of

Langerhans in the pancreas, primarily in response to high blood glucose levels (hyperglycaemia). It lowers blood glucose by stimulating the entry of glucose into the cells of fatty (adipose) tissue. In diabetes mellitus this hormone is produced in insufficient amounts, and may need to be injected to prevent hyperglycaemia and ketoacidosis (increased blood acidity characterized by an increase in ketones). Excessive insulin levels lead to hypoglycaemia (low blood glucose levels).

The effects of insulin are counteracted by other hormones such as glucagon, growth hormone (see *Acromegaly*), corticosteroids and adrenaline.

INTRA-UTERINE CONTRACEPTIVE DEVICE

see *Contraception*

INTUSSUSCEPTION

A term used to describe an abnormal process by which one part of the in-

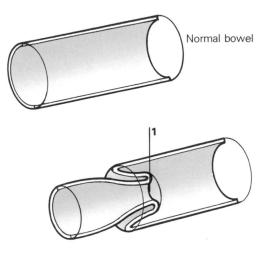

In the vast majority of cases of intussception the upper part of the bowel is pushed into the lower part **(1)**; in around 75 per cent of these cases the ileum intusscepts into the colon.

testine is pushed back into itself so that it becomes ensheathed. Typically, intussusception occurs in infants (usually males) aged between 6 and 9 months, and often without an obvious cause being found.

In adults a precipitating cause (such as a polyp or tumour) is more likely. The symptoms of intussusception are paroxysms of abdominal pain and vomiting; infants will draw up their legs and have screaming attacks. This is followed at a later stage by the passage of blood and mucus from the rectum, classically likened to redcurrant jelly.

Treatment is surgical, with manipulation of the bowel into its normal state and occasionally the removal of a gangrenous segment. Mortality is low if intussusception is diagnosed and treated within 24 hours, but rises progressively if gangrene and peritonitis develop as a result of the condition being left untreated and the intestine becoming blocked.

IN-VITRO FERTILIZATION

see *Test tube baby*

INVOLUTION

A return to a previous state or a retrograde change in a tissue or organ. A typical example of involution occurs in a woman after the birth of her child. The uterus (womb), cervix (neck of the womb) and vagina have all been stretched during pregnancy and delivery, but after the birth these tissues return to their normal size, shape and position, the process of involution taking around six weeks. The menopause is another form of involution, the female reproductive organs slowly shrinking in size due to decreased levels of hormones.

IRITIS

An inflammatory condition of the iris (the coloured part of the eye); also known as anterior uveitis and iridocyclitis. Iritis may be acute or chronic. In acute iritis the affected eye is painful, red and tender. Bright light worsens the pain and vision may be blurred. The condition can be distinguished from other causes of a painful red eye, such as conjunctivitis or acute glaucoma, by a physical examination. The cause of iritis is thought to be an autoimmune disease but in many cases it remains unknown. The condition itself is sometimes a feature of other autoimmune diseases; for example, ankylosing spondylitis, Reiter's syndrome or sarcoidosis. Except in rare cases caused by infection, when an appropriate antibiotic is given, corticosteroids (as eye drops) are the usual treatment. Drugs such as atropine can relieve spasm of the iris and alleviate pain.

In chronic iritis, pain and redness are often minimal and may be absent. The causes include juvenile rheumatoid arthritis (Still's disease), leprosy and tuberculosis, but in most cases the cause is unknown. Treatment is the same as for acute iritis.

IRON

Iron is an essential constituent of haem, part of the haemoglobin molecule (haemoglobin is the red pigment in blood). Iron is contained in food, particularly meat, and is absorbed from the small intestine and used by the bone marrow to make red cells. It is stored in the body as ferritin. A shortage of iron may result from a poor diet (this commonly occurs in babies and the elderly), increased requirements (in pregnancy), poor absorption (for example, in coeliac disease), or excessive loss (due to chronic bleeding). Ultimately iron deficiency causes anaemia with associated depression, hair loss, brittle nails and itchy skin.

Iron deficiency readily responds to therapy with ferrous sulphate. The speed of response is the same whether iron is taken by mouth or injected into the muscles or veins. It is dangerous to give iron intravenously, because severe allergic reactions can occur.

Excessive deposition of iron in bodily tissues occurs in haemochromatosis; excessive lead deposition due to severe or chronic bleeding and subsequent absorption of the blood, leaving iron deposits behind, is called haemosiderosis.

IRREGULAR PERIODS

see *Menarche, Ovulation*

IRRITABLE BOWEL SYNDROME

A syndrome of bowel disturbance and abdominal pain thought to be due to the abnormal function of the small or large bowel. It is very common, especially in women between the ages of 15 and 40, and probably one-third of adults in developed countries have occasional symptoms of it. The symptoms vary but include colicky abdominal pain (often relieved by bowel action or the passage of wind), a sensation of bloating, alternating diarrhoea and constipation, and the passage of mucus. The symptoms may be worse at times of stress. The cause of the syndrome is unknown, but the symptoms may be explained by abnormal smooth muscle activity in the colon and introspection and anxiety about bowel function. There is no association between the syndrome and cancer or colitis (inflammation of the colon).

Treatment involves a high-fibre diet and some people may benefit from taking a drug to relax the smooth muscle. The symptoms often resolve with time. In other cases patients are clearly depressed and the symptoms may resolve with anti-depressant medication.

ISCHAEMIA

Tissue damage (often transient) due to reduced blood supply, as distinct from infarction (death of tissue) due to loss of blood supply. Ischaemia may be caused by general circulatory failure (which sometimes occurs after cardiac arrest or arrhythmia), or may be due to local narrowing of blood vessels (for example, as a result of thrombosis). In some circumstances a combination of factors may be involved.

The symptoms of ischaemia depend upon the organ affected. For example, the narrowing of blood vessels to the heart muscle (coronary arteries) will result in ischaemia when the heart is required to do more work during exercise. This may cause pain, known as angina pectoris. Ischaemia and pain may be reversed when exercise is stopped. If permanent blockage (occlusion) of coronary vessels takes place with thrombosis, then ischaemia will lead to injury and death of the cells of the heart muscle (myocardial infarction).

ISHIHARA'S CHARTS

A series of coloured plates used to detect colour blindness. The plates consist of numbers or symbols presented against several different backgrounds. Both symbols and backgrounds are made up of different coloured spots. The hue, brightness and depth of the colour on each plate differ only slightly so that the symbols cannot be distinguished from the background by people with defective colour vision.

ISOTOPES

Gamma ray-emitting radioactive particles are used in medicine mainly as a diagnostic tool. By attaching an isotope to an inert compound tolerated by the body, nearly every organ in the body can be imaged and either anatomical or functional information generated. After administration, usually by intravenous injection, the compound (radio-pharmaceutical) is taken up by the target organ and the gamma rays emitted collected by a gamma camera linked to a computer. The resultant information can be processed and recorded onto film. Computerized tomography has replaced the use of isotopes in some regions of the body, notably the central nervous system (see *Brain scanning*). Areas where the technique remains valuable and provides unique information are:

- Bone: isotope scans are used to detect bone disease such as osteomyelitis (qv) and metastatic deposits and are often positive long before there is visible change on a radiograph.
- Renal scanning generates both anatomical and functional information. It is particularly useful in assessing kidney function after transplant operations.
- Lung scanning has a unique role in the detection of pulmonary embolism.
- Thyroid: isotopes are used for imaging the gland and may also be administered in high dose to the overactive thyroid; the concentrated radioactivity is taken up by

and destroys the overactive tissue. This method is usually only used when surgery and drugs do not control thyrotoxicosis (qv).

- Cardiology: used to detect myocardial ischaemia and damage.
- Infection: isotopes can be attached to white blood cells to detect abscesses and other infections.

IUCD/IUD

see *Contraception*

IVF

see *Test-tube baby*

JAUNDICE

Yellow pigmentation of the skin due to an accumulation of the pigment bilirubin in the blood. Normally the red pigment in the blood, haemoglobin, is broken down by the liver to form bile. This is yellow; it is excreted into the bile ducts and then into the bowel, where it gives the stool its characteristic brown colour. Any disturbance of this process leads to an increase of bile in the blood. The yellow bile, as it accumulates in the skin and particularly in the whites of the eyes, imparts a yellow tinge. This progresses to a deep yellow-brown colour like a very deep sun tan.

Jaundice is a symptom of this disturbance. Early diagnosis and treatment are needed to prevent kidney failure and spontaneous bleeding developing. Jaundice can be divided into three types: prehepatic, hepatic and post-hepatic.

Pre-hepatic jaundice occurs when there is excessive pigment released into the blood from the breakdown of the blood cells (haemolysis, as in haemolytic anaemia), and the stools remain brown.

Hepatic jaundice occurs when the liver is unable to make the bile; this can be due to infection (viral hepatitis A and B and non-A, non-B, leptospirosis), poisons (carbon tetrachloride, alcohol), some drugs (chlorpromazine, halothane or the contraceptive pill), or to cirrhosis. In this type of jaundice the liver is enlarged and the stools may become pale. Blood tests help to distinguish the underlying cause in the hepatic and pre-hepatic types.

Post-hepatic jaundice, also known as obstructive jaundice, is due to blockage of the bile duct, often as a result of stones in the common bile duct or damage to the bile duct resulting from a stone or cholangitis (qv) causing a stricture. Occasionally it is due to pressure from outside the duct caused by a growth in the pancreas or gallbladder. In post-hepatic jaundice the liver is working and the urine becomes dark with bile. The stools are pale. Techniques used in the investigation and treatment of post-hepatic jaundice include ultrasound, which may show dilated bile ducts in the liver and a stone or mass blocking the duct, and endoscopic retrograde cholangic pancreatography (ERCP), which can outline the duct from below the blockage (using X-rays) and even remove the stone. Using this method, a fine tube can be passed into the dilated ducts to drain bile and improve the condition of the patient prior to surgery.

Mild jaundice (normal or physiological pre-hepatic jaundice) not infrequently develops a few days after birth, as the fetal red cells are haemolysed. Only in cases of rhesus incompatibility (see *Haemolytic disease of the newborn, Kernicterus*) is treatment necessary.

In all types of jaundice, treatment depends on the underlying cause.

J

KAPOSI'S SARCOMA

A skin cancer. Kaposi's sarcoma is a common sign of AIDS in male homosexuals who are infected with the human immunodeficiency virus (HIV). It is virtually never seen in people infected with HIV for other reasons — for example, haemophiliacs and drug addicts. The first lesion may appear anywhere on the skin as a red 'strawberry-like' mark; it may later multiply. It commonly occurs on the face, particularly the nose, but can also be found in the gut and lungs, where bleeding results. The cause is unknown, but it has been suggested that it could result from an infection by a virus which stimulates the uncontrolled multiplication of cells lining blood vessels in the skin. Before the advent of AIDS, Kaposi's sarcoma was mainly seen in elderly Jewish men in northern Europe.

Treatment of the condition is very unsatisfactory and includes make-up, local X-ray therapy and the drug interferon.

KELOID

The cellular overgrowth of fibrous tissue in a scar at the site of a skin injury. Keloid is often seen in black races and in pregnant women of all races. True keloid in white races is rare and the only common site is over the sternum or breast-bone. It is important to distinguish between true keloid and the far commoner hypertrophic scar, which is often wrongly referred to as keloid. The hypertrophic scar appears as a thick red scar which gets no worse after six months and generally fades. (Compression treatment (perhaps with elastic appliances) is particularly useful in flattening and maturing this type.) True keloid continues to get worse and may progress for many years. Treatment is difficult. If the keloid is cut out and the area sewn up, recurrence is certain. Radiotherapy has been attempted with mixed results. Local steroid injections may help.

KERATITIS

Inflammation of the cornea (the transparent layer of tissue at the front of the eye). The commonest causes are infection and injury, but nutritional deficiency and hypersensitivity reactions may also be associated with this condition. Damage can occur in neurological conditions where sensitivity of the cornea is lost, and also in lacrimal disorders where the normal flow of tears is interrupted or impaired through disease of the lacrimal glands. Keratitis is characterized by burning or smarting, blurring of vision and sensitivity to light.

It can be treated by an opthalmologist with eye drops. Scarring may occur, forming a localized grey opacity, and if central can result in loss of vision with a blind spot in the centre of the visual field. Treatment of this complication is by replacement with a graft from another cornea, taken from a person who has just died (see *Corneal grafting*).

KERNICTERUS

A neurological complication which sometimes results from jaundice in haemolytic disease of the newborn (qv). Maternal antibodies cross the placenta and react with antigens on the red blood cells of the baby, resulting in destruction of the baby's red cells. Bilirubin, a breakdown product of the pigment haemoglobin contained in the red cells, then increases in the bloodstream of the baby to produce kernicterus. The baby may appear normal at birth, but soon develops severe jaundice and looks yellow. Kernicterus may cause the death of the baby, or lead to permanent brain damage, with spasticity, mental deficiency and deafness.

Treatment is by exchange transfusion of the baby's blood (when all the blood is exchanged); the blood that is transfused is crossmatched with the mother's. Phototherapy is an additional treatment: this involves exposing the baby to intense blue light, which destroys bilirubin in the baby's circulation.

KETOACIDOSIS

Acidosis (increased acidity of the blood) characterized by an increase in ketones, which are produced when fat stores are used for energy. An excessive breakdown of fat for energy occurs in prolonged fasting and leads to excessive ketone formation and acidosis; ketones are used in this situation as an energy source at a time when glucose levels in the cells are low. The usual cause of ketoacidosis is uncontrolled diabetes mellitus, when insulin deficiency leads to high blood glucose but low glucose in the cells so that again there is excessive fat breakdown. Diabetic ketoacidosis, which gives a typical sweet smell to the breath, may also occur at times of increased insulin requirement in a known diabetic patient, when the insulin dosage has not been appropriately adjusted (during infections or surgical procedures, for example).

KIDNEY

The kidneys are paired organs which lie on the rear wall of the abdomen, behind the peritoneum (abdominal cavity) and beside the spinal column.

Each kidney is about 12 cm (5 inches) long, weighs about 150 g (5 oz) and has about one million glomeruli. Such a large reserve of glomeruli means that a person can live quite normally with only one kidney.

Structure of the kidney: **1** cortex; **2** pyramid (containing glomeruli); **3** medulla; **4** pelvis; **5** ureter.

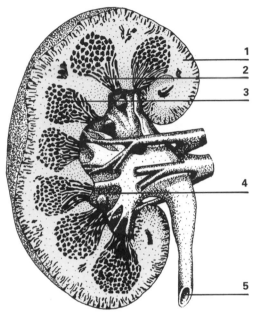

The principal function of the kidneys is the elimination of toxic waste-products of the body's metabolism, as well as the maintenance of stable fluid and electrolyte levels. Blood reaching the kidneys through the renal arteries is filtered by a network of tiny capillaries (glomerulus) housed in a capsule (Bowman's capsule). Plasma (the fluid component of blood) filtered from the blood enters Bowman's capsule before passing down the tubules, where useful substances (such as glucose) are reabsorbed. The vast majority of water passing into the tubules is reabsorbed too, under the influence of antidiuretic hormone secreted by the pituitary gland at the base of the brain; only a small proportion of it is excreted as urine. The ingestion of large quantities of fluid will suppress release of the

K

hormone, resulting in increased urinary volume to maintain a stable total body water level. Alcohol also depresses hormonal secretion.

KIDNEY FAILURE

Failure of the kidneys, renal failure, means that they no longer remove soluble waste products (including urea and excess acid) from the body. It is conveniently divided between acute and chronic forms. Renal failure is best diagnosed from blood tests, but urine examination and kidney biopsy are often required to establish the cause. There are no specific symptoms.

Acute renal failure occurs when kidney function is suddenly impaired, usually with little urine production (oliguria). The cause may be severe untreated hypotension (low blood pressure) or dehydration, in which blood flow to the kidneys is inadequate; renal disease, such as glomerulonephritis; or complete obstruction to urine flow, which occasionally happens with stones in the ureter as a result of urolithiasis or an enlarged prostate.

The prompt hospital treatment required for acute kidney failure may include short-term dialysis; this is often sufficient to prevent the development of chronic renal failure, and the patient eventually returns to full health.

Chronic renal failure may follow severe acute renal failure but more often develops insidiously as a result of progressive renal disease (glomerulonephritis, nephrotic syndrome, pyelonephritis, longterm use of nephrotoxic drugs); it is commoner in diabetics. Daily urine volume may be increased (polyuria) and is rarely low, either because damaged glomeruli allow excessive amounts of fluid to pass or because reabsorption by the tubules is impaired; sometimes both factors coincide. In mild cases no treatment is required, although the patient may be advised to drink plenty of fluid. In severe cases — termed end-stage chronic renal failure — the patient will die within weeks unless some form of dialysis is commenced or a kidney transplant is performed.

KIDNEY STONES

see *Nephrolithiasis*

KLINEFELTER'S SYNDROME

A sex chromosome disorder occurring in 1 in 1,000 males. Affected males have two X and one Y chromosomes (XXY), instead of the normal male pattern (XY). Infertility is the rule, the testicles are small, secondary sexual characteristics (such as pubic hair) are poorly developed, and gynaecomastia (breast enlargement) occurs in about 40 per cent of cases. The limbs are elongated and about 20 per cent of sufferers are mildly mentally retarded. Treatment with testosterone, a male sex hormone, may improve secondary sexual characteristics but not infertility. For parents of a child with Klinefelter's syndrome the risk of having a further child with the same disorder is higher than that of the general population. Neither parent has a chromosomal abnormality and the reason for the risk is at present unknown.

KNOCK KNEES/BOW LEGS

These are known medically as genu valgum (knock knees) and genu varum (bow legs). In knock knees, the knees touch and the ankles are wide apart; in bow legs, the knees are wide apart when the ankles are together.

Both conditions occur in children around 2 years old. They cause great concern to parents, but at around 6 years the deformities disappear. Usually they require no treatment. Very rarely there is underlying rickets, or damage to one side of the growing plate of the bone (due to a fracture through the growth plate), and for these cases osteotomy (qv) may be required. 'Genu recurvartum' refers to overstraightening of the knee, which rarely requires treatment; when surgical treatment is necessary, it is usually for recurrent dislocation of the kneecap.

KWASHIORKOR

A form of malnutrition in which the diet contains near-adequate amounts of energy but is deficient in protein. It is most commonly found in Third World countries in infants aged between 9 and 24 months who have been weaned on a diet deficient in milk and other protein-rich foods. The imbalance in the diet leads to acute biochemical disturbances. Growth fails and there is muscle-wasting in the limbs, although the baby often looks chubby either because of oedema (excess fluid beneath the skin) or excess fat (caused by the diet's high carbohydrate content relative to protein intake). The child is apathetic and irritable. The skin may be abnormally pigmented and ulcerated. The hair is fine and sparse and in black children may lose its curl and become red in colour. Diarrhoea and vomiting are common, and the child is more prone to infection. The disease may be complicated by other illnesses endemic in the Third World, such as malaria, dysentery and in-ternal parasites which result in malabsorption (qv).

Adding more protein to the diet will prevent the condition recurring, once the acute biochemical disturbances and infections are treated with intravenous fluid and/or antibiotics as appropriate. Severe cases may lead to death.

KYPHOSIS

Excessive forward curvature of the spine. It may be localized to one segment of the spine, as occurs after injury or destruction of the vertebra by tumour or tuberculosis, or generalized, as in adolescent kyphosis.

In adolescent kyphosis parts of the vertebrae fail to grow properly and become wedge-shaped; this results in a round-shouldered stance. Pain is unusual and treatment is rarely necessary. Occasionally a period in a plaster cast around the chest to take the weight off the spine may be advisable during the phase of rapid growth (about 8—14 years in girls and 9—16 years in boys).

Kyphosis may be associated with a lateral curve of the spine, when it is referred to as a kypho-scoliosis (see *Scoliosis*).

LABOUR

Labour, or parturition, often popularly spoken of as the confinement, is the process by which babies are expelled from the uterus (womb) via the birth canal.

The signs that labour is beginning are:
- Regular contractions of the uterine muscle. These become progressively stronger and more frequent
- Expulsion of the mucus plug from the cervix (neck of the womb)
- The waters breaking. The mem-

branes containing the amniotic fluid around the baby, break, producing either a sudden gush or a slow trickle.

Labour contractions can be painful and the mother usually requires some pain relief. This can be given in the form of an epidural block, a special type of local anaesthetic (see *Epidural anaesthesia*); an injection, usually of pethidine (called demerol in the USA); or in a mixture of oxygen and nitrous oxide which is breathed through a mask.

When labour is started artificially, this is called an induction (qv). Labour may be induced if there is any risk to the baby's or mother's health.

It is sometimes necessary to use obstetric equipment such as a ventouse (qv) or forceps to aid delivery. Their purpose is to speed up delivery if there is severe fetal distress, in cases of unusual presentation, or to shorten a prolonged second stage. Forceps assist the delivery of the baby by gentle traction and/or rotation of the fetal head. A ventouse works by suction. Some form of painkiller is usually given to allow correct use of these instruments.
SEE ALSO *Ventouse*

In late pregnancy the head of the fetus settles into the brim of the pelvis (1). The cervix gradually opens (2) as the fetal head presses down. The membranes break when the head broaches the ring of the vulva (3) and the baby is pushed down the birth canal. The birth is aided by the obstetrician who first applies downward and backward traction (4) and then lifts the head gently upwards (5) to minimize damage to the mother's perineum.

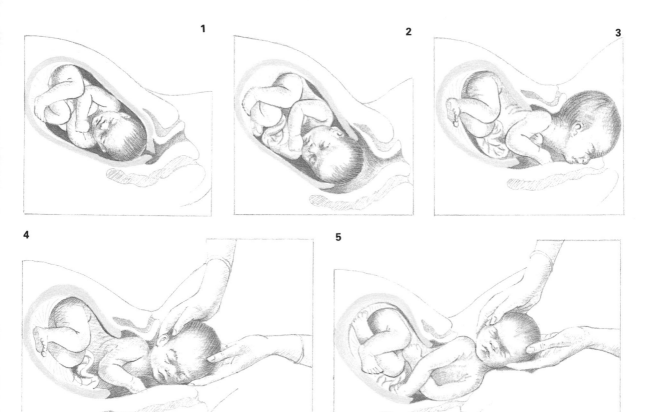

LABYRINTHITIS

Inflammation of the labyrinth, the part of the inner ear which controls balance. The labyrinth lies behind the cochlea and consists of a series of membranous sacs and ducts within the bony vestibule of the petrous bone of the skull. Three semicircular canals in planes at right angles to each other each contain a receptor organ that is stimulated by movement of the endolymphatic fluid contained within.

Inflammation may result from infection spreading from the outer ear (as in chronic or acute otitis); via the bloodstream; or from the meninges (the membranes covering the brain and spinal cord), as a result of meningitis. Many other infections may also affect the labyrinth, such as syphilis, scarlet fever, typhoid fever, typhus, and viral infections such as influenza, measles, mumps and herpes zoster.

The inflammation causes irritation of the vestibule so that the receptors are falsely stimulated to send impulses to the brain suggesting movement is occurring. The false perception of movement that this produces leads to dizziness (vertigo). Labyrinthitis clears up as the cause of the inflammation is treated, equilibrium is restored and the dizziness subsides, but function is not usually restored to the labyrinth itself. The brain simply adjusts to the lack of signals coming from the receptors. Hearing, if lost, does not usually return.

LAMINECTOMY

Strictly, laminectomy means a surgical approach to the spinal canal by removing the laminae (plates of bone at the back of the vertebrae) of one or more vertebrae together with their intervening ligaments. The procedure may be carried out on one side only (laterally) so that only half the lamina is removed, or bilaterally, in which case the bony projections at the back of the vertebrae (called the spinous processes) and ligaments are also removed. Laminectomy allows access to the spinal canal and spinal cord, for the removal of spinal tumours, for example.

The removal of a slipped disc is often called a laminectomy. This is an incorrect use of the term; strictly it should be called a laminotomy of fenestration. In this operation an opening in the ligamentum flavum (a ligament in the spinal cord) is made and lamina above and below are nibbled away to allow the disc to be removed.

LAPAROSCOPY

An investigative technique that can be used to assess the extent of any disease process but is mainly employed to check the Fallopian tubes in cases of infertility. Laparoscopy may also be used in the treatment of infertility (for example, to remove an ovum from the ovary for subsequent in-vitro fertilization — see *Test tube baby*) and as an operative procedure (in female sterilization, for example). As a diagnostic tool, it is especially appropriate for investigations of chronic pelvic pain, suspected ectopic pregnancy or small ovarian cysts.

In laparoscopy a small incision is made below the umbilicus and into the abdominal cavity, which is then filled with carbon dioxide gas by means of a special needle. This gives the surgeon a clear view of the pelvis and other abdominal structures. The laparoscope — a rigid instrument with a diameter of 6–10 mm ($\frac{1}{4}$–$\frac{1}{3}$ in) — is then inserted through the incision. The procedure is usually performed under a general anaesthetic.

LAPAROTOMY

A general term applied to any operation in which the abdominal cavity is opened. The exact diagnosis, extent of disease and operative procedure are usually uncertain until the time of the operation.

The abdomen is opened through one of various possible approaches, such as an upper midline scar or a transverse (Pfannenstiel or 'bikini') scar. All the structures are then inspected, a diagnosis is made and surgery undertaken as indicated.

Occasionally the disease process is so advanced that the surgical treatment is not possible, such as in advanced cases of certain cancers. A piece of affected tissue (biopsy) is taken so that definitive diagnosis can be made by the pathologist, and appropriate treatment (such as chemotherapy) instituted.

LARYNGITIS

Acute simple laryngitis is a superficial inflammation of the mucous membrane of the larynx (voicebox) and is usually due to infection. This may be either part of a generalized upper respiratory infection or a sudden localized laryngitis. The cause in both cases is usually a virus. Injury due to over-use of the voice and irritation from inhaled fumes, especially tobacco smoke, may also cause laryngitis.

Treatment is by voice rest and steam inhalations with menthol to help loosen viscous secretions. Alcohol and tobacco should be avoided. Antibiotics are prescribed if the infection is caused by bacteria.

The inflammation usually subsides in a few days but hoarseness may persist for up to two weeks.

Chronic laryngitis occurs when laryngeal inflammation has healed with fibrosis and scarring. The tissues are dry, causing a cough and hoarseness. An otorhinolaryngologist should perform a laryngoscopy to exclude other conditions which can mimic laryngitis, such as cancer, polyps and vocal cord nodules; these require surgery.

LARYNGOSCOPY

A technique for viewing the larynx (voice-box), performed by an otorhinolaryngologist (ear, nose and throat specialist). There are two techniques: indirect and direct laryngoscopy.

Indirect laryngoscopy is performed without an anaesthetic, the patient sitting upright. A mirror is placed obiquely at the back of the mouth and illuminated by light reflected from a mirror worn on the laryngologist's forehead. This technique requires the tongue to be held and co-operation from the patient. The vocal cords can be seen to move when the patient sings a note.

Direct laryngoscopy, as its name suggests, involves looking directly at the vocal cords through a straight illuminated tube passed through the mouth and pharynx under general anaesthesia. Operative procedures, such as the removal of polyps, can be undertaken with this technique.

LAVAGE

Washing out or irrigating an organ or cavity. The two most common types of lavage are gastric lavage and peritoneal lavage.

Gastric lavage, commonly known as stomach-pumping, is used to treat patients who have taken a drug overdose or ingested other irritant poisons such as paraquat or the leaves, roots, berries or resins of many plants.

It involves passing a tube (large bore if the poisoning agent is tablets or other large matter) into the stomach and washing out the remains of the substance with a warmed fluid.

Peritoneal lavage is a continuous infusion of saline into the peritoneal cavity of the abdomen combined with an outflow for removing the waste products of metabolism, such as urea. It is used in cases of kidney failure when haemodialysis is either not available or inappropriate. The peritoneum functions as a semi-permeable membrane (see *Dialysis*).

Lavage of the peritoneal cavity may also be performed using an antibiotic solution in order to remove infected material. This procedure is carried out after many abdominal operations, particularly if sepsis is a risk (for example, as a result of an operation for peritonitis or bowel removal).

LAXATIVE

A substance that increases bowel action, used particularly to relieve constipation. Common stimulant laxatives include senna, cascara, phenolphthalein and bisacodyl. Bulk laxatives include bran, ispaghula husk, and a sugar that cannot be ingested — lactulose. The long-term use of stimulant laxatives should be avoided, as these substances may deplete the body of certain minerals, affect organs such as the kidney, or alter the delicate balance of bowel function. Certain foods with a high dietary fibre content may enhance bowel action and have a laxative effect — for example, bran cereals or fruit.

LEAD POISONING

Lead poisoning most commonly occurs in those involved in the production of lead (especially white lead) or who use lead or its salts in the course of their work; for example, lead smelters, pottery workers, painters and dyers. It has occurred as a result of children chewing toys or cot-sides painted with lead-based paint, and in individuals who have accidentally ingested lead, but such instances are rare. The symptoms of lead ingestion are variable. Anaemia is usually one; other features may include severe colicky abdominal pain due to intestinal spasm, constipation, and a blue line on the gums (due to a deposit of lead sulphide). The peripheral nerves (outside the brain and spinal column) may be affected and produce muscle weakness, particularly at the wrists and fingers. The effects of lead on the central nervous system may include agitation, restlessness, mental changes and epileptic seizures. A raised level of lead in the blood will confirm the diagnosis.

Treatment is by administration of a chelating agent, which binds lead in the body and facilitates its excretion by the kidneys.

LEGIONNAIRES' DISEASE

This disease was first recognized after a large outbreak of fever and pneumonia among war veterans (Legionnaires) who attended a convention in Philadelphia in 1976. It is caused by a bacterium called *Legionella pneumophilia* which is found commonly in water. The illness can occur as an isolated case or in outbreaks.

It is contracted by inhaling fine water droplets from the contaminated cooling towers of airconditioning systems and shower heads. Although healthy people can become infected, the risk of both infection and death is higher in older patients and in those with chronic disease of the lungs, heart and kidney, and cancer.

After an incubation period of 2–10 days the illness gradually begins with fever, a dry cough, headache, confusion, abdominal discomfort and diarrhoea. The infection does not respond to the usual antibiotics. The diagnosis is generally confirmed by blood tests and examination of the patient's phlegm. The best treatment is a long course of the antibiotic erythromycin.

LEISHMANIASIS

A group of tropical diseases caused by infection with the Leishmania parasite. People become infected by the bite of certain types of sandfly. The most serious type of leishmaniasis is called 'kala-azar', which is prevalent in India, China, Africa, Eastern Europe and the Mediterranean and mainly affects children and young adults. It causes fever, anaemia and enlargement of the liver, spleen and lymph glands. Diagnosis is made by bone marrow and blood tests.

'Oriental sore' is another form of leishmaniasis; this occurs in Asia. A crusting papule develops at the site of the sandfly bite and heals slowly. Another type of leishmaniasis, called espundia, is found in South America. This form may involve the nose and lead to destruction of the nasal cartilage.

Effective drugs exist to combat leishmaniasis, but treatment depends on which form the disease takes.

LEPROSY

A chronic disease of low infectivity (that is, few people exposed actually develop the condition) caused by the *Mycobacterium leprae* bacterium. Worldwide there are more than 10 million people with leprosy, nearly all of them in Asia, Africa and Latin America. The cases found in developed countries are in immigrants from these areas. The disease can only be acquired after prolonged and close contact with an infected person. The incubation period is between 3 and 5 years.

Leprosy mainly affects the skin, nose and nerves and gives rise to whiteish skin patches where sensation is lost, nodule formation with ulceration and cord-like thickening of the nerves. The loss of sensation leads to injury, ulceration and ultimately the dropping off of toes, fingers and sometimes other parts of the limbs. Diagnosis can be made by skin biopsy. Leprosy can be treated with drugs such as dapsone and rifampicin.

LEPTOSPIROSIS

A disease caused by a spirochaete bacterium called *Leptospira*; it occurs worldwide. People become infected as a result of skin contact with water contaminated by the infected urine of animals such as rats, pigs and dogs. Infection is more common in people who work in sewers, rivers, wet fields and farms, but may also be contracted by swimming in contaminated water. Those whose occupations put them at risk of developing the disease should wear protective clothing.

Most infections lead to a relatively mild febrile illness similar to influenza. Sometimes a more serious form called Weil's disease may occur, leading to fever, jaundice, bleeding and occasionally liver and kidney failure; this type is transmitted to people via the urine of rats. A less serious form of leptospirosis, called canicola fever, is transmitted by dogs and pigs and usually causes mild meningitis in people.

The infection usually responds to antibiotics.

LEUCOCYTOSIS

A temporary condition in which the white cells in the blood increase in number. This commonly occurs as part of the body's response to bacterial infections, and any condition of stress (such as bleeding) and shock. Steroid treatment may also result in a high white blood cell count. In contrast to leukaemia (a 'cancer' of white blood cells in which very high blood counts may occur) the white cells in leucocytosis appear normal and no abnormal forms are seen.

LEUKAEMIA

The leukaemias are a group of malignant diseases characterized by the presence of abnormal white cells in the blood. These cells grow in the bone marrow or lymphatic tissue, impairing the production of normal cells. As a result there is anaemia, neutropenia (a low number of the white cells that fight infection), and thrombocytopenia (a low number of platelets — cells which help to stop bleeding). The abnormal white cells circulate in the blood and spread to other organs; they cause enlargement and ultimately poor function of these organs. The common sites of spread are the liver, spleen, the lymph nodes, the linings of the brain (the meninges), the brain itself, the skin and the testes. Many causes for leukaemia have been established, including infection with viruses, exposure to radiation, heredity, and exposure to chemicals.

There are two main types of leukaemia; myeloid and lymphoid. In myeloid leukaemia the cells are derived from a granulocyte (a type of white cell produced in the bone marrow), and this form is most common in adults. In children, the leukaemia most commonly seen is lymphoid, where the original cell was a lymphocyte (produced in lymphatic tissue such as occurs in the spleen, lymph nodes, thymus and tonsils).

Treatment for acute leukaemia involves several courses of chemotherapy and often bone marrow transplantation. Many such cases, especially in children, can now be cured.

LEUKOPENIA

A low white blood cell count. The most important contribution to leukopenia is a reduced number of neutrophils, the cells which fight bacterial infection. There are a variety of causes of leukopenia, including drugs, infections, vitamin deficiencies of B_{12} or folic acid, leukaemia and X-ray treatment.

LEUKOPLAKIA

A white patch or raised area with sharply defined edges, present in the mouth and on the tongue. In more severe cases the affected area hardens and cracks may appear on its surface, scraped off in parts. The probable cause of the lesion is chronic irritation due to, for example, pipe smoking or illfitting dentures. Leukoplakia is precancerous in its severe form, being the commonest precancerous lesion in the oral cavity. Any ulcerative lesion of the mouth persisting for more than two weeks should be examined medically. In the early stages of oral cancer, lesions are rarely painful, unlike non-malignant ulcers which have a similar appearance.

Treatment of leukoplakia is not usually necessary. Severe cases may require surgical removal of the lesion, but this is not always feasible.

L

LICHEN PLANUS

A frequently itchy skin condition of unknown cause which can affect any area of the body, including the penis, scalp and the mucous membranes in the mouth. The pulse side of the wrist is the part most typically affected. The appearance of the condition is characterized by individual lesions consisting of 0.5 cm (1/5 inch) diameter, flat-topped, polygonal pimples on which a white lacy network is visible on the surface — the so-called Whickham's striae. When lichen planus occurs on the lower legs, lesions may be much thicker and more scaly, sometimes resembling psoriasis (qv); when the scalp is affected, baldness with some scarring may result.

In most cases the itching responds to treatment with corticosteroids applied directly to the affected part; this may also improve the appearance of the lesions. The condition usually improves spontaneously with time.

LIGATION

Tying off a structure (such as large blood vessels and other tubes) using a ligature, or cord, during a surgical operation. A variety of natural materials (such as silk, catgut, cotton or even metal), or synthetic materials (such as nylon, Dacron, and polypropylene) may be used for this purpose.

LIPOMA

A smooth, soft, discrete swelling which is mobile. Lipomas are small collections of extra fat contained in a fibrous capsule. Most commonly they lie just under the skin, but can be found anywhere in the body. They are harmless. In one variety, called Dercum's disease, the lipomas are multiple and often tender. They can be removed under local anaesthetic and sometimes are if their unsightliness or tenderness cause concern.

LISTERIOSIS

An infection caused by the bacterium *Listeria monocytogenes*, which commonly infects animals such as cattle. This organism is widely distributed in the environment (including soil) but only rarely causes disease in humans. Those particularly at risk from infection via the consumption of contaminated food (the usual method of transmission to humans) are pregnant women and patients whose immune systems are being suppressed (for example, as a result of cancer treatment with cytotoxic drugs). In most cases the symptoms of listeriosis resemble influenza. A form of meningitis may be evident in severe cases. The infection can cause meningitis in the newborn, and in pregnant women may cross the placenta and infect or even kill the fetus. The diagnosis is established by blood culture (culturing a sample of blood to see if bacteria grow).

The disease may be effectively treated with a number of antibiotics, including penicillin derivatives and co-trimoxazole. Pregnant women are advised not to eat soft, ripened cheeses such as Brie and Camembert, as the organism may be found in them. The risk of infection from poultry, meat and frozen foods can be eliminated by ensuring that they are properly cooked through before consumption.

LITHIUM

A naturally occurring salt used widely as a treatment for manic depressive psychosis and less commonly for severe recurrent depression. Once started, lithium treatment is normally continued for at least five years.

Lithium may produce toxic effects and so blood tests are taken every three months in order to monitor toxicity levels. For this reason it is not generally prescribed if kidney function is poor or during pregnancy. The toxic side-effects include tremor of the hands, thirst, weight gain in the longer term and, rarely, kidney damage.

LIVER FAILURE

Inability of the liver to perform its normal functions due to severe damage resulting from viral infection, toxins, alcohol, chemicals or drugs. The normal liver removes toxic substances produced in the bowel (ammonia, for example); produces proteins (particularly albumin and the factors involved in blood clotting); stores and processes vitamins; and excretes bile as a waste product, which also aids the digestion of fats. When the liver fails, toxic substances accumulate and irritate the brain and nervous system (hepatic encephalopathy) to cause coma. The patient bleeds easily due to the inadequate production of blood clotting factors. The pigment bilirubin accumulates to cause a yellow discoloration of the eyes and skin (jaundice). Fluid and salt are retained in the abdomen (ascites) and legs (oedema).

Treatment involves blood transfusion and giving clotting factors, cleansing the bowel to prevent the accumulation of toxic substances, vitamin and calorie supplements, and expert nursing until the liver recovers or a new liver is transplanted.

LONG SIGHT

see *Hypermetropia*

LOUSE

see *Pediculosis*

LSD

see *Drug dependence*

LUMBAR PUNCTURE

A technique for sampling the cerebrospinal fluid which surrounds the brain and spinal cord. A small amount of local anaesthetic is infiltrated into the skin and soft tissues at a point between two of the lumbar vertebrae

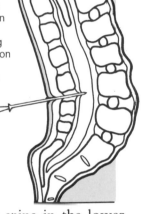

To obtain a sample of cerebrospinal fluid a fine needle is passed beween the spinal vertebrae and into the cavity containing the CSF. The patient lies on his or her side with the spine flexed as much as possible to aid the procedure.

(the bones of the spine in the lower part of the back). A fine needle is then passed between the vertebrae into the spinal cavity to where the cerebrospinal fluid lies. Cerebrospinal fluid samples can be analyzed for the presence of blood (to detect subarachnoid haemorrhage, for example), inflammatory cells, micro-organisms or malignant cells, and protein and sugar concentrations may be measured. In cases of suspected meningitis, for example, evidence of infection is looked for in the cerebrospinal fluid. Lumbar puncture is also of value in the investigation of a variety of neurological conditions (for example, multiple sclerosis).

However, it can be a dangerous procedure and for this reason is never undertaken lightly. In patients with increased intracranial pressure (when a brain tumour is present, for example), lumbar puncture can cause rupture of certain parts of the brain.

LUNG CANCER

There are two types of lung cancer: primary and secondary. Primary lung cancer is the commonest form of cancer in men, with a peak incidence between the ages of 50 and 70. Its incidence is rising in women. The main cause of primary lung cancer is cigarette smoking. Secondary lung cancer is caused by spread from other primary tumours, most commonly in the gastro-intestinal tract or breast.

Lung cancer may be of several tissue types and these determine whether it develops centrally or peripherally. The squamous type usually occurs in central sites and tends to spread locally; adenocarcinoma is typically found in peripheral sites (the glands) and is often associated with previous lung scarring as a result of asbestosis for example — this type usually spreads via the bloodstream; the undifferentiated carcinoma type indicates cancerous cells (often so-called oat cells) which form no particular pattern; bronchio-alveolar cell carcinoma starts in the small airways.

Symptoms vary and in its early stages the condition may produce none. Initial signs are the development of a cough or a change in a 'smoker's' cough, the coughing of blood, and recurrent or poorly resolving pneumonia which fails to clear up as quickly as expected with antibiotic treatment. Early detection gives a chance of cure by complete removal of the tumour and part of the lung around it. However, the cancer may only be detected when it is already too late to attempt a cure. At this stage nonspecific signs of cancer may be present, such as loss of weight and appetite and physical weakness. Areas and structures near the lung may be affected; for example, the laryngeal nerve, indicated by hoarseness; fluid may collect outside the lung in the chest cavity; the gullet (oesophagus) may be involved, causing difficulty in swallowing. The cancer may also spread to distant sites, the lymph glands, neck, brain, liver, adrenal glands and bone being the commonest. Certain systemic syndromes due to cancer, such as high blood calcium concentrations, inappropriate secretion of antidiuretic hormone or ACTH may occur. Clubbing of the nails may be found.

Investigations of cases of suspected lung cancer involve biopsy tests and evaluation of how far beyond the lung and lung cavity malignancy extends. Heart and lung function is assessed if an attempt at curative surgery is being considered. If surgery is not possible or the tumour cannot be completely removed, radiotherapy and/or chemotherapy are usually given.

LUPUS ERYTHEMATOSUS

see *Systemic lupus erythematosus*

LYMPHADENO-PATHY

Enlargement of the lymph nodes. This may be seen on the surface of the body as 'lumps' in the neck, armpits and groin. The lymph nodes situated in the centre of the chest (the mediastinum) may be seen on chest X-ray and those at the back of the abdomen (retroperitoneal lymph nodes) by CT scan. The causes of lymphadenopathy include infections, such as glandular fever, tuberculosis or HIV infection (see *AIDS*); malignant tumours, such as lymphomas (cancer of the lymph nodes), or secondary cancer from a tumour elsewhere; and inflammatory conditions such as sarcoidosis.

In children, lymphadenopathy is a very common response to infection, and disappears when the infection clears up. In all cases the underlying cause of the lymph node enlargement is established before treatment is given.

LYMPHATIC SYSTEM

The system of tiny tubules that permeate the body and drain excess tissue fluid (lymph) from the tissue spaces to the blood system. Lymph is formed when plasma (the fluid component of blood) passes out from tissue capillaries to bathe the tissues with essential substances for metabolism. Unlike capillaries, some lymphatic vessels are blind-ending in the tissue spaces but may gradually join up to form progressively larger

The main lymphatic nodes and vessels: **1** cervical nodes; **2** right lymphatic trunk; **3** axillary nodes; **4** thoracic duct; **5** cisterna chyli; **6** aortic nodes; **7** iliac nodes; **8** inguinal nodes.

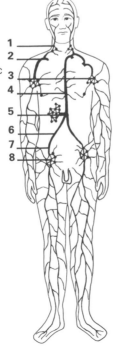

vessels. Lymphocytes, a type of white blood cell, in the nodes are responsible for the destruction of bacteria, which drain to the nodes. Lymph nodes may therefore be enlarged and tender if there is infection in the areas of the body drained by them. Tumour cells may also spread from a primary site via the lymphatic vessels to form secondary cancerous deposits in distant organs (metastases).

LYMPHOMA

The replacement of the normal lymph node with the growth of abnormal malignant cells. Lymph node enlargement in the neck, armpits and groin with palpable swellings is usually the first symptom.

Lymphomas are a group of disorders, and are divided into two main types: Hodgkin's lymphoma and nonHodgkin's lymphoma. Hodgkin's lymphoma has a recognizable cell, the Reed-Sternberg cell, which proliferates. It occurs predominantly in young men, and has a good prognosis (outlook) if treated with radiotherapy or drugs. In the many forms of nonHodgkin's lymphoma, the lymphocytes (a type of white blood cell) are abnormal and proliferate. These lymphomas do not have such a good prognosis. Treatment is also by radiotherapy and/or chemotherapy.

Burkitt's lymphoma is a very unusual type of lymphoma found in African children, and commonly causes one or more localized swellings in the jaw.

LYMPHO-GRANULOMA VENEREUM

A venereal disease caused by a member of the chlamydia group of organisms

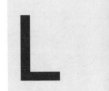

(*Chlamydia trachomatis*). The incubation period is 1–12 weeks; usually 7 to 12 days. Initial symptoms are enlarged lymph nodes in the groin and the formation of a papule or vesicle, which then forms a relatively painless ulcer. Abscesses may form at other sites of the body. Extensive scarring may occur if early treatment with antibiotics is not given. Repeat courses of antibiotics may be necessary and abscesses may need surgical drainage.

MAGNETIC RESONANCE IMAGING

Also called nuclear magnetic resonance (NMR), this is a recently developed technique of diagnostic medical imaging. Its most important advantage over existing methods, such as X-rays, is that it does not utilize ionizing radiation.

The technique is based on the physical principle that charged particles in atomic nuclei precess around their axis of spin. The proton spin axes are aligned in a strong magnetic field and are then excited by the application of an electromagnetic pulse. As the precessing nuclei return to their state of equilibrium they emit radiowaves. Gradients in the magnetic field cause the radiofrequencies to vary with the position of the emitting nuclei. This achieves spatial resolution, allowing computed images to be produced.

The technique is used mainly for investigating the central nervous system, the musculoskeletal system and malignant tumours. MRI has proved to be considerably more sensitive than CT in detecting diseases of the brain and spinal cord; multiple sclerosis in particular. It is also a good method of investigating sciatica,

because it requires neither radiation nor the introduction of dye into the spinal cord; the ability to image in any plane is used to produce longitudinal pictures of the cord and nerve roots. Similarly, the cartilages (menisci) of the knee can be investigated without the introduction of dye or an anthroscope into the joint. MRI is often the investigation method of choice in the assessment of spread of malignant tumours, because of its sensitivity to subtle changes in tissue-water content.

Scan times are relatively long and this has limited the use of MRI in the chest and abdomen, where respiratory movement degrades the images. This situation will undoubtedly change in the near future as developments lead to faster scan times.

MALABSORPTION

Failure of the body to digest and absorb food. This may result in malnutrition, anaemia, weight loss and the passing of bulky, greasy, offensive stools. Malabsorption has many causes, making diagnosis difficult and lengthy. The problem may be in the lumen or tube of the bowel (as in lack of bile or pancreatic insufficiency for example), in the wall of the bowel (as in infections, coeliac disease or sprue), or, rarely, outside the wall of the bowel (when, for example, cancerous deposits block the channels carrying nutrients from the bowel).

Investigations include blood tests to measure protein, calcium, iron, and the vitamins B_{12} and folate; X-rays (possibly including an examination to monitor the passage of barium through the small intestine); ultrasound examination or a CT scan of the pancreas and a biopsy of the mucous membranes of the small bowel.

Further investigations may be required to make an accurate diagnosis.

The treatment of malabsorption involves eliminating the underlying illness, and eliminating from the diet specific foods and food products that are not being absorbed properly, such as gluten and other wheat products (see *Coeliac disease*).

MALARIA

A disease caused by malarial parasites which enter the blood after a bite from an infected female mosquito. It mainly occurs in Africa, South America, the Indian subcontinent and South-east Asia.

The symptoms of malaria usually start with the person feeling cold and shivery, followed by high fever and physical collapse. Then the temperature falls, with profuse sweating, and the person feels better until the next attack two or three days later. This pattern continues until treatment is given; in some types of malaria death may follow quickly unless treatment is prompt.

Malaria is usually treated successfully with drugs such as quinine and chloroquine. Recently, however, resistance to antimalarial drugs has been increasing and family practitioners are regularly advised as to which antimalarials are appropriate in which parts of the world. Preventative measures, such as wearing suitable clothing and using mosquito nets and mosquito repellents, are increasingly important.

MALIGNANT

The word 'malignant' is used to describe several life-threatening medical conditions. Malignant tumours (cancer) are aggressive tumours which show a capacity to invade and destroy the surrounding tissue. Malignant hypertension is an uncommon but serious form of high blood pressure which tends to occur in younger patients; very high levels of blood pressure are reached, leading to death unless promptly treated. Malignant hyperthermia is a rare and sometimes fatal condition that tends to run in families. It is characterized by muscle rigidity and very high fever brought on by the use of certain anaesthetic drugs; other family members similarly at risk can be identified by blood tests. Malignant tertian malaria is a form of malaria which can be rapidly fatal unless it is treated promptly.
SEE ALSO *Benign*

MAMMOGRAPHY

The examination of the breasts by X-rays; in the past it has mainly been used in the investigation of a lump in the breast before biopsy.

Clinically undetectable early cancers can be discovered by mammography and can, therefore, theoretically be treated at a much earlier stage. Long-term studies of screening asymptomatic women by mammography have concluded that there would be a significant reduction in the death rate from breast cancer if such screening were established. As a result some countries are setting up national breast screening programmes. Benign lumps would also be detected, leading to a number of women with benign breast disease undergoing biopsy.

The examination is conducted using special X-ray equipment suitable for the study of soft tissues. The breast is compressed so it is as flat as possible, allowing for greater soft tissue detail. Tumour tissue is denser than breast tissue, especially in post-menopausal women, in whom glandular tissue has been replaced by

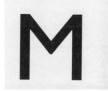

fat. Cancer of the breast may have the appearance of grains of salt, which show up fairly easily on an X-ray.

MANIA

A persistent state of euphoria out of keeping with a person's circumstances. The term is often used interchangeably, but incorrectly, with 'hypomania'. A manic person may report feeling full of energy and be observed to be always on the move, sleeping little and adopting new interests. Sometimes mania will lead to spending money excessively, becoming promiscuous, dressing in outlandish clothes or pursuing religion with great fervour. Speech will often be increased in rate and amount, in some cases becoming incoherent. Generally patients will over-estimate their abilities, viewing themselves as particularly intelligent, strong or important. These opinions may progress to grandiose delusions of having a special identity or special powers Hallucinations occur rarely.

Sufferers are usually admitted to hospital where initial treatment will often entail the use of strong tranquillizers. In the longer term many sufferers will go on to have further mood swings as part of a manic-depressive psychosis (qv).

MANIC-DEPRESSIVE PSYCHOSIS

A mental disorder in which states of euphoria (mania) and depression alternate; also known as bipolar affective disorder. This psychosis usually starts in adolescence or young adulthood. Sufferers report a history of mood disorders in around one-fifth of close relatives, suggesting an important genetic contribution. Recent work has identified specific genetic markers in some families. People who have a tendency to regular 'ups and downs' (the cyclothymic personality) are generally viewed as being at greater risk of developing manic-depressive psychosis. The course of the disorder is variable, some sufferers having one episode only but the majority going on to have further episodes. Between episodes sufferers behave normally.

Treatment includes the use of anti-depressants, electroconvulsive therapy (ECT) and strong tranquillizers. Hospital admission is necessary in severe cases. Lithium and, less commonly, the drug carbamazepine are used as long-term preventative treatment where a person has generally had three distinct episodes.

MANTOUX TEST

see *Tuberculin test*

MARFAN'S SYNDROME

An inherited disorder of connective tissue characterized by disproportionately long bones in the arms and legs. Affected individuals consequently are tall and their arm span exceeds their height. Other distinctive features are long fingers and toes, a high arched palate, hyperextensible joints ('doublejointedness'), dislocation of the lens of the eye and dilatation of the aorta (the main artery) close to where it joins the heart. The last mentioned may lead to aortic incompetence (see *Aortic regurgitation*) and rupture of the aorta. Affected individuals need ongoing medical surveillance to detect these complications at an early stage.

MASTECTOMY

Surgical removal of the breast. All

forms of mastectomy involve removal of the breast together with the nipple, but there are a number of variations. Radical mastectomy used to involve removal of the breast, a large area of skin, and a large amount of deeper tissue including part of the chest wall muscle together with all the fat and lymph nodes of the armpit. This deforming operation is no longer used in the treatment of breast cancer, as no more patients survived than those who had undergone less radical forms of treatment. Simple mastectomy involves removal of the breast, nipple and an area of skin. This operation may be combined with surgery to the armpit to remove any affected lymph nodes.

Nowadays, many early breast tumours are being treated by a wide local excision of the tumour followed by radiotherapy to the remainder of the breast. This operation clearly has many psychological and cosmetic advantages over mastectomy.

Mastectomy is performed under general anaesthesia and involves a hospital stay of 7–12 days. Post-operative physiotherapy to the shoulder is usual to prevent stiffness. When the woman is discharged, she is supplied with a temporary soft prosthesis (artificial spare part) to wear under her bra. After the wound has healed completely (four weeks) a permanent prosthesis is supplied. Some surgeons will now perform a breast recon-struction either at the same time as the mastectomy or, more usually, at a later date. Excellent cosmetic results can be obtained: however, not all cases are suitable, particularly those with advanced disease.
SEE ALSO *Breast cancer*

MASTITIS

Inflammation of the breast. The term refers to an acute infection which occurs after pregnancy when the breasts are engorged with milk and as a result of a small crack in the nipple permitting a staphylococcal infection. This results in cellulitis, fever, pain and swelling, and requires treatment with antibiotics and surgical drainage of the abscess.

The term 'mastitis' is also used incorrectly to describe a series of chronic changes in the breast which are better known as fibrocystic or fibroadenomatous disease (see *Fibroadenoma*). The cysts and fibrous areas which form give the breast a general lumpiness, and are tender prior to the monthly period. Occasionally the cysts may cause a blood-stained discharge. They require investigation, with aspiration of the cyst and a mammogram. A biopsy is usually performed because of the difficulty in distinguishing these lumps from breast cancer.

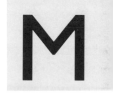

MASTOIDECTOMY

An operation which involves clearing the mastoid air cells, which lie around the ear, using an electric drill and an operating microscope. The advent of antibiotics has meant that the operation is now much less commonly performed. However, it is required when there is disease of the mastoid, usually as a result of chronic infection (for example, in meningitis or brain abscess) spreading from the middle ear, and occasionally in cases of mastoiditis (inflammation of the mastoid).

In simple mastoidectomy the operation is confined to the mastoid bone, and the middle ear cavity and external canal are left untouched. Hearing is hardly affected. When the disease is more severe and widespread, a 'window' is drilled through into the middle ear to leave a mastoid cavity which can be periodically inspected and cleaned by an otorhinolaryngologist (ear, nose and throat specialist). The eardrum and the system of sound-transmitting ossicles (tiny bones) in the middle ear may need to be reconstructed as a result. The mastoid cavity so produced is at risk of becoming infected, and in up to a quarter of cases the ear continues to discharge. The operation is therefore not undertaken lightly, but is necessary when a life-threatening infection, such as meningitis or a brain abscess, results from prolonged ear infection.

MEASLES

A highly infectious viral disease which occurs mainly in pre-school age children. The incubation period is about ten days, and spread is by droplet infection from coughs and sneezes. The first symptoms are fever, catarrh, conjunctivitis and a cough (which may progress to croup), followed by a red rash, which begins behind the ears and soon spreads to cover the body. The illness usually lasts about ten days. Minor complications, such as ear infection and pneumonia, are common and need antibiotic treatment. Encephalitis (inflammation of the brain) is a rare and serious complication. Though measles is an uncommon cause of serious illness in developed countries, the death rate is high in areas of the world where malnutrition is rife. Effective immunization is available, and vaccination should be given in the second year of life. It is very exceptional for measles to be contracted by the same person twice.

MECONIUM

A thick, dark green substance composed of mucus, intestinal cells and bile (giving the colour) which is contained in the bowels of a baby before birth. The meconium is usually discharged within the first 24 hours of life. A delay of more than 48 hours may indicate some form of intestinal obstruction. Early passage of meconium before birth stains green the amniotic fluid surrounding the baby in the womb and is associated with fetal distress. If it is inhaled before delivery (meconium aspiration) the baby suffers severe breathing difficulty at birth as the small airways become obstructed. Emergency respiratory care to suck out the meconium may then be required.

MEGACOLON

A distended segment of the large bowel (colon) of variable length. The affected segment usually lacks tone because of a defect in or damage to the intrinsic nerves that normally control muscle contraction in the bowel wall, and is nonfunctional. Megacolon is often accompanied by a partial obstruction in the bowel, with the contents being held up before the dilated segment. Megacolon is rare in infants but may be seen in the inherited Hirschsprung's disease (qv), in which the nerves that provide normal tone and function in the bowel wall are absent. In adults the cause may be unknown or may be associated with a South American parasitic disease called Chagas' disease, which damages the nervous supply to the bowel. Treatment may involve surgery or, alternatively, intensive therapy with laxatives. The syndrome of toxic magacolon is a rare feature of severe inflammatory bowel disease (ulcerative colitis or Crohn's disease qv) and requires urgent and expert management in hospital.

MELAENA

A black, sticky stool composed of partially digested blood. The bleeding is usually from a peptic ulcer in the stomach or duodenum; less commonly it is from gastritis (inflammation of the stomach lining), cancer of the stomach, oesophagitis (inflammation of the oesophagus) or oesophageal varicose veins or varices. Bleeding from sites lower down the bowel is usually red when it is passed, as it has not undergone the chemical changes of the digestion process.

Anybody with melaena needs urgent hospital admission. The patient's blood pressure and pulse rate are closely monitored, a fall in the former or an increase in the latter indicating that the lost blood volume must be replaced by transfusion. Blood may also be transfused to treat shock or acute anaemia. Patients aged over 60 years need special care until they have recovered from the haemorrhage. Thereafter accurate diagnosis of the causes of the melaena are provided by endoscopy, which may also be used to treat the bleeding site by laser beam, heater probe or injection. Some patients may require emergency surgery to control continuing haemorrhage.

MELANOMA

An extremely serious form of skin cancer, the incidence of which is rapidly increasing in the Western world. The malignant cell is the melanocyte, which is normally present in human skin and is necessary for the production of skin and hair pigment. What exactly causes normal melanocytes to turn into malignant melanomas is not known, but the relatively recent preoccupation of white races with sunbathing and also migration from temperate to sunny climates are thought to be important factors. Exposure to sunshine in short, sharp bursts (as on a summer holiday) by people not normally exposed may be more harmful than constant exposure by people used to it, such as outdoor workers. In some individuals there is a family history of melanoma and multiple moles.

A melanoma may arise from a previously existing mole or from an otherwise normal area of skin. It is, however, common to develop harmless moles during the teens and twenties and the appearance of these is not serious. Suspicious signs in a pigmented lesion suggesting a possible melanoma include asymmetry and irregularity of outline, size greater than 1.5 cm ($\frac{1}{2}$ inch), alterations in colour, increasing size and spontaneous bleeding. Individuals with suspicious-looking lesions should be referred to a dermatologist (skin specialist) for assessment.

Early recognition and surgical removal substantially improve the survival rate; the deeper into the skin a melanoma penetrates, the poorer the outlook.

MENARCHE

A girl's first period and one of the manifestations of sexual maturity or puberty in girls. In Western Europe the average age of menarche is 13 years. A doctor should be consulted if menstruation is delayed after the age of 16 years and a physical examination conducted to exclude any abnormalities, such as an imperforate hymen or other malformations of the uterus or vagina. If nothing abnormal is found, menstruation will probably start spontaneously within a year or two, such is the wide variation in its onset.

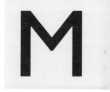

MÉNIÈRE'S DISEASE

A common disease of the part of the inner ear which controls balance (the labyrinth). Its cause is unknown although a variety of theories have been put forward and there is clearly an excess of fluid in the labyrinth. The condition is slightly more common in men, usually appears between the ages of 35 and 55 years, and is characterized by attacks of vertigo (qv), a type of dizziness, accompanied by deafness and tinnitus. These attacks occur with remissions of varying length. With each attack deafness tends to worsen. Tinnitus may be very troublesome and may be exaggerated or change in quality during an attack of vertigo. Similarly deafness may increase transiently or there may be a feeling of fullness in or behind one ear before an attack so that some patients are forewarned. Initially the symptoms of Ménière's disease may be reversible with treatment but later deafness becomes permanent; sounds are distorted so that hearing aids may not be tolerated.

Drugs which dilate the arteries and increase blood supply to the cochlea and labyrinth in the inner ear are generally ineffective, but diuretics and antihistamines seem to help in some cases. About 75 per cent of cases are partially controlled by non-surgical means. Surgery or ultrasound can be used to destroy the labyrinth to relieve the vertigo, but will not improve the deafness.

MENINGIOMA

A tumour arising from the membranes surrounding the brain and spinal cord. Meningiomas are usually slow-growing and are considered benign. Size is variable. A meningioma causes localized neurological effects due to pressure on the underlying brain, which atrophies. Symptoms of increased intracranial pressure (within the skull), such as headache, vomiting and papilloedema (congestion and swelling of the optic disc), often occur late as these tumours grow very slowly as a rule.

Treatment is by surgical removal; this may be technically difficult because some tumours obtain part of their blood supply from the underlying brain, but nevertheless removal usually results in permanent cure.

MENINGITIS

Infection of the membranes covering the brain and spinal cord (meninges). The majority of cases occur in childhood and are caused by bacteria or viruses. Tuberculous meningitis is now rare in developed countries following the general decline in tuberculous infection, but continues to be common in the Third World.

Bacterial infections are the most important cause of meningitis; they are common, potentially lethal, and yet are completely curable with early antibiotic treatment. The *Meningococcus* bacterium is usually responsible for meningitis in older children and adults. In infants, other bacteria are more common. In babies, symptoms may be nonspecific, with fever, vomiting and lethargy. There may be a bulging anterior fontanelle (soft spot — the depression on the top of the head, where the three bones of the skull meet), indicating a rise of pressure in the cerebrospinal fluid (CSF) which surrounds the brain and spinal cord. Older children and adults complain of headache and stiff neck, and dislike bright light. The diagnosis is made by lumbar puncture (removal of a small amount of CSF from the subarachnoid space around the spinal

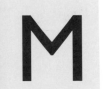

cord). Complications such as deafness and hydrocephalus are uncommon, provided antibiotic treatment is prompt.

Of the many viruses that can cause meningitis, those responsible for mumps and influenza are frequently implicated. The illness in cases resulting from viral infection is usually relatively mild (though the symptoms of headache and neck stiffness are present), and is distinguished from bacterial infection by the findings on lumbar puncture. No treatment is required, and full recovery is the rule.

MENINGOCOELE

see *Spina bifida*

MENISCUS

A piece of cartilage within the knee joint. A tear of one of the two meniscii within the knee is the commonest of all knee injuries and often occurs in playing football. The damage is caused when the knee is twisted and flexed while the body weight is on that leg. The acute swelling usually resolves within a few days and the knee sometimes unlocks spontaneously, but subsequent attacks of locking and swelling often occur either after further minor injury or, in a few cases, for no apparent reason. In some cases the original injury was thought trivial and only later locking and swelling indicated that a tear had occurred. Treatment is by meniscectomy (removal of the torn portion of the meniscus). This can now be performed endoscopically (see *Arthroscopy*).

MENOPAUSE

Literally, menopause means cessation of menstruation. It is, however, often used in a broader sense to mean the preceding months or even years of gradual reduction in the amount and frequency of menstrual loss due to irregularity in ovulation, a time medically known as the climacteric. The average age at which a woman reaches the menopause is 51 years, but this can vary. Menstruation ceases as a result of the ovaries becoming exhausted of immature eggs and therefore being unable to respond to the hormonal stimulus from the pituitary gland. Common symptoms are hot flushes, sweating and dryness of the vagina. Sexual desire is unaffected in most women.

Hormone replacement therapy (qv) may be prescribed for women in whom these symptoms are distressing.

MENORRHAGIA

Excessive bleeding with a period (menstruation), which may be either prolonged, heavy or both. It is abnormal for the menstrual cycle to be less than 21 days, or for the duration of menstruation to be more than 7 days. An excessive loss is usually reckoned to be one in excess of 80 ml (3 fl oz) of blood per cycle.

The various causes include psychosocial (chronic anxiety, for example, is thought to be relevant in some cases) and endocrine (involving hormones) problems, bleeding diseases, disorders of the uterus (such as polyps of the endometrium or lining of the womb) or complications of pregnancy, miscarriage, and delivery (retained products of conception). If, after a history and examination, uterine abnormality is suspected, a diagnostic curettage (D & C) is often necessary to identify the problem; a polyp, for example, would be removed surgically.

In patients in whom menorrhagia is a secondary symptom, treatment is directed to the underlying primary

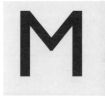

cause. Antiprostaglandin or progestogen treatment may be prescribed for cases caused by hormone malfunction. Hysterectomy is necessary in a few patients in whom medical treatment has been unsuccessful.

MENSTRUATION

see *Menarche, Ovulation*

MERALGIA PARAESTHETICA

A condition in which tingling and burning pain are felt in the skin of the outer part of the thigh as a result of pressure on a small nerve (called the lateral cutaneous nerve of the thigh); this nerve passes under the inguinal ligament in the groin and transmits sensory stimuli from the skin of the thigh. The nerve is prone to compression at this site (the fold of the groin), particularly in overweight people. A reduction in weight usually brings relief. If this fails, it is sometimes necessary to cut the inguinal ligament in order to decompress the nerve.

METABOLISM

The process by which living organisms maintain and regulate cells, tissues and organs. Metabolism involves utilizing the breakdown products of food to supply energy and essential components to keep the biochemical process in balance and to enable the body to counteract any stress that disturbs this, such as heat, cold, injuries, infection and surgery.

METASTASIS

The process by which cancer spreads to distant parts of the body, and the secondary tumours resulting from this process. Metastasis is caused by a clump of malignant cells breaking away from the main or primary tumour and travelling by blood or lymph vessels to distant sites where, if they survive, they grow and develop into tumours. Sometimes these so-called secondaries grow so rapidly as to become much larger than the primary tumour.

In most cancers the commonest form of spread is via the lymph vessels to the lymph nodes. Invasion of a vein by the tumour results in metastasis by blood. Once tumour cells enter the blood they tend to lodge in the liver, lungs, bones and brain. The capacity to spread by metastasis varies among malignant tumours. Cancers of the breast and lung, melanomas and sarcomas metastasize early.

MIGRAINE

A recurrent form of intense headache, often accompanied by visual disturbances and vomiting. The underlying cause is not known but is thought to involve the constriction and dilatation of the arteries to the brain at different stages of the headache. Stress, menstruation and certain foods are factors that may trigger these vascular changes, in which various biochemical substances, such as prostaglandins, may play a part. Migraine is a common disorder, especially in women, and occurs in most age groups; it is less common in the elderly. Typically an attack begins with the warning signs of malaise (a general feeling of being unwell) or depression, followed by visual disturbances (bright flashing lights or transient loss of part of the field of vision). There may be other signs of neurological disturbance, such as paraesthesiae and weakness, but these are less common. These early symptoms then run into the painful stage: a throbbing headache develops, often over the whole of the head, or sometimes on one side only; nausea and vomiting may also occur. An attack may last several days. Migraine may be easy or difficult to diagnose, as symptoms may vary in severity and content. It must be distinguished from psychogenic or tension headaches, and underlying vascular abnormalities of the brain.

Treatment involves avoidance of factors known to trigger an attack and the use of analgesics (painkillers) and anti-emetics (to prevent vomiting); the drug ergotamine taken in the early stages may abort an attack. If attacks are frequent, preventative treatment with betablockers, tricyclic drugs or the drug pizotifen may be necessary.

MINERALOCORTICOID

One of a group of hormones which regulate the balance of salt and water in the body. Mineralocorticoids are secreted by the cortex or outer part of the adrenal gland and exert their effects mainly on the kidney. The principal mineralocor ticoid is aldosterone. Overproduction of aldosterone results in Conn's syndrome (qv) and is also a complication of other conditions, such as heart failure and cirrhosis of the liver (secondary aldosteronism). Under-production of aldosterone is very rare; it usually occurs as part of the syndrome of Addison's disease (in which the adrenal cortex is destroyed) or hypopituitarism (deficiency of one or more pituitary hormones).

MISCARRIAGE

see *Abortion*

MITRAL INCOMPETENCE

A defect of the mitral valve, which is situated between the left atrium and the left ventricle of the heart; the atrium receives from the lungs oxygenated blood which the ventricle pumps to all parts of the body. The valve is composed of two leaflets which normally form a water-tight seal when the left ventricle contracts, preventing blood washing back to the left atrium. When the valve is incompetent this seal is broken; a murmur develops and after a while the function of the left ventricle deteriorates to produce heart failure, with increasing breathlessness and fatigue.

The commonest cause of mitral incompetence is rheumatic heart disease. Other causes include rupture of one of the papillary muscles that anchor the valve (as a result of a heart attack), infection of the valve (endocarditis), and a prolapsing mitral valve leaflet syndrome; the last-mentioned often produces a characteristic click and murmur, which can be heard on listening to the heart through a stethoscope.

The severity of incompetence is assessed by means of special X-rays of the heart chambers. Treatment consists of surgical replacement of the mitral valve.

MITRAL STENOSIS

A condition caused by narrowing (stenosis) of the mitral valve in the heart. Mitral stenosis is nearly always a consequence of damage to the valve as a result of rheumatic fever. Narrowing of the valve causes raised pressure in the left atrium and, ultimately, raised pressure in the blood vessels in the lungs. This makes the lungs stiffen

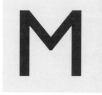

and results in shortness of breath. In more advanced cases fluid may accumulate in the small air spaces (alveoli) of the lung, in a condition known as pulmonary oedema; this results in severe breathlessness, particularly when lying flat. Mitral stenosis may be associated with rhythm abnormalities of the heart, especially atrial fibrillation (see *Arrhythmia*). Other complications include heart failure and systemic and pulmonary embolism.

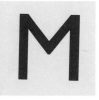

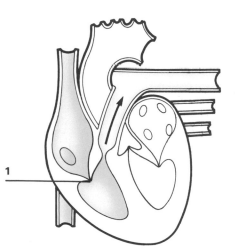

The symptoms of narrowing of the mitral valve **(1)** sometimes do not become apparent until many years after an attack of rheumatic fever.

Treatment of mild cases may involve the use of diuretics to prevent the development of pulmonary oedema and appropriate treatment of any rhythm disorder with digoxin, betablockers or calcium antagonists, depending upon the nature of the disturbance. In more severe cases surgical treatment may be necessary either to stretch the valve (valvotomy) or replace it with an artificial one.

MITTELSCHMERZ

Abdominal and pelvic pain felt during ovulation. The term comes from the German and means midcycle pain. Mittelschmerz is thought to occur as a result of irritation of the lining of the abdomen (peritoneum) by blood that escapes into the abdomen when the ovary releases an egg two weeks before a period. The pain, which is shortlived, can be relieved by simple painkillers. An alternative treatment is the oral contraceptive pill, which cures Mittelschmerz by preventing ovulation.

MOLE

see *Birth mark*

MOLLUSCUM CONTAGIOSUM

A viral infection of the skin which produces 0.3 cm (1/10 inch) domed lesions, often grouped fairly closely together; classically these lesions have a small depression on the surface from which their creamy contents can be expressed by careful squeezing. The condition is commoner in children and is highly contagious. In adults, the appearance of uncontrollable, widespread, lesions suggests immunosuppression (as in AIDS, for example).

Anything which causes the lesions to become inflamed may lead to their clearing up. The doctor may therefore apply a variety of caustic substances to them or physically remove their surface with tweezers.

MONGOLIAN BLUE SPOT

see *Birth mark*

MONGOLISM

see *Down's syndrome*

MORNING SICKNESS

Nausea and morning vomiting are

common in the early weeks of pregnancy. Some women feel sick in the mornings, some at other times, some all day long.

Morning sickness is thought to be due to hormonal changes in early pregnancy, but the causes are poorly understood. For the majority of pregnant women the nausea will settle and disappear altogether around the twelfth to fourteenth week. It is seen more often in women who are prone to travel sickness and those in their first pregnancy. Severe sickness suggests the possibility of multiple pregnancy.

Medication is avoided in the treatment of morning sickness unless vomiting is very severe. Helpful measures include eating small amounts and avoiding foods that exacerbate the nausea; tight clothing can also make the nausea worse.

MORPHINE

see *Heroin*, *Analgesic*

MOTOR NEURONE DISEASE

A progressive degeneration of the cells in the brain stem and spinal cord where the motor (or movement) nerves are situated; these supply the voluntary or skeletal muscles. The higher pathways which carry motor instructions to these cells, allowing the brain to control movement, also degenerate. Sensory cells and pathways are not affected.

Motor neurone disease (called amyotrophic lateral sclerosis, or ALS, in the United States) takes three principal forms: progressive muscular atrophy, in which there is wasting, weakness and fasciculation (twitching) of muscles — this often begins in the hands or feet, sometimes on one side only and progresses steadily (frequently over several years) until paralysis is widespread and eventually affects breathing; amyotrophic lateral sclerosis, in which spasticity of the limbs is the principal initial feature; weakness and wasting come later; and progressive bulbar palsy, in which the muscles of speech and swallowing are affected first. In general all of these symptoms finally develop. The disease ends in death, between 2 and 10 years from its onset, normally due to pneumonia or other infections.

The cause of motor neurone disease is unknown, and as yet there is no cure, although there are many forms of supportive treatment, including the provision of appliances and sometimes assisted respiration.

MULTIPLE SCLEROSIS

A degenerative disease of the nervous system in which myelin (a substance which provides an insulating sheath around the nerves) is lost, so that the nerves are no longer able to conduct impulses; it is also known as disseminated sclerosis and frequently abbreviated (MS or DS). The cause is unknown. MS characteristically affects several different parts of the body at different times (relapses), initially with near or total recovery (remissions) between episodes. Diagnosis is dependent on the occurrence of typical symptoms indicating involvement of at least two different body sites and on at least two different occasions; however great the suspicion of MS, it will not be confirmed until this stipulation is satisfied. The condition is slightly more common in women. Two thirds of cases begin between the ages of 20 and 40.

There is a bewilderingly wide range of symptoms, but among the more

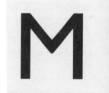

common are temporary blindness (usually only in one eye), difficulties in control of the hands (particularly for small delicate movements), and difficulty with walking and balance. A number of tests are helpful in supporting the diagnosis (and to exclude other neurological diseases). For example, in MS electrical transmission within the brain is delayed, and this can be assessed by flashing light at the eyes and recording (by means of EEG) the so-called 'visual evoked response'. A lumbar puncture often reveals abnormal proteins in the cerebrospinal fluid. CT scanning but, even better, MRI scanning (Magnetic Resonance Imaging) may show abnormal areas within the brain where myelin has been lost — so-called 'plaques'.

There is no established treatment for MS although high-dose steroids may help to reduce the duration and severity of individual relapses. The disease often runs a slow and insidious course with minimal loss of function after a relapse, but occasionally it progresses rapidly, leading to paralysis, incontinence, inability of the patient to care for himself or herself, and eventually to death, usually from respiratory complications. Intelligence and awareness are normally not impaired. The attitude of sufferers to their disease varies and while depression is common some develop a semi-euphoric outlook.

MUMPS

A viral disease of relatively low infectivity which mainly affects children between 5 and 11 years of age. The incubation period is 14—21 days. Transmission is by droplet infection from coughs and sneezes. The first symptoms are usually a headache, fever and malaise (a general feeling of being unwell), followed one or two days later by characteristic pain and swelling of the salivary glands, usually the parotids on one or both sides of the face. A high fever occurs at this stage and may persist for up to a week; it may herald one of the many possible complications, such as meningitis, orchitis (testicular inflammation) or pancreatitis.

There is no specific treatment, though painkillers may help. Prevention is by the measles, mumps and rubella (MMR) vaccine. It is very rare for mumps to be contracted by the same person twice.

MURMUR

A sound associated with turbulent blood flow. A murmur may occur when blood flows through a narrow channel into a large one, at a high rate, or when backflow occurs against the normal forward movement of blood. The loudness of the sound is not a reliable indicator of severity, and many murmurs, particularly in children or in pregnant women, may not be associated with any underlying abnormality. Murmurs may occur during the contraction phase of heart action (systole) or during the resting phase (diastole), or be continuous throughout the cardiac cycle. The duration, character and timing of the murmur, and its associated clinical features, all give pointers to the underlying cause.

MUSCULAR DYSTROPHY

A group of uncommon muscle diseases which are genetically determined and progressive in nature. Most are inherited, but some occur as new mutations in patients without a family history of the disease. The rate of progression depends on the type of abnormality. The commonest is the Duchenne type, the inheritance of which is sex-linked and so occurs only in boys. Typically the young child is slow to walk and has difficulty climbing stairs because of the weakness of his upper leg muscles. The disease progresses to involve other muscle groups so that by the age of about 10–12 years the child usually requires a wheelchair. Most patients are of normal intelligence; only a few are educationally subnormal. Some develop disease of the heart muscle. Death usually occurs in the twenties due to respiratory infection or cardiac failure.

Some forms of muscular dystrophy are inherited in autosomal dominant fashion: examples are myotonic dystrophy, which usually becomes apparent in middle age when an inability to relax muscle groups voluntarily occurs, together with cataracts and frontal baldness, and the facioscapulohumeral form which affects the face and limbs. Autosomal recessive forms of dystrophy are less common, and may come on in childhood or adult life.

No specific treatment is available. Genetic counselling is important, especially since the isolation, characterization and sequencing of the gene responsible for the Duchenne type in 1988. This discovery has led to accurate detection of female carriers of the gene and to antenatal diagnosis by chorionic villus sampling.

MUTATION

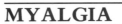

A change in genetic material. The smallest mutation possible is a change in a single DNA base (point mutation), affecting a single gene. Large mutations, such as parts of chromosomes being missing or in the wrong place, may affect many genes. A mutation occurring in a reproductive germ cell or gamete (sperm or ovum) will be inherited. Most mutations are spontaneous, but certain factors such as some chemicals (for example, mustard gas) and ionizing radiation (as in X-rays) can increase the rate of mutation. Mutations may result in the appearance of certain inherited diseases, such as haemophilia and Duchenne muscular dystrophy, in previously unaffected families.

MUTISM

A state in which a person does not speak and makes no attempt to communicate verbally despite an adequate level of consciousness. It is a central feature of stupor (qv). Mutism also occurs in a number of psychiatric conditions, including depression and schizophrenia. It may also be the result of brain disease such as dementia, of multiple sclerosis and tumours, as well as of general metabolic disorders such as hypothyroidism and hypoglycaemia.

MYALGIA

Aching of muscles. A non-specific symptom which can be associated with many acute illnesses, particularly viral infections such as influenza. Myalgia may be due to underlying muscle disease such as myositis, infections of the muscle or polymyalgia rheumatica. Treatment is of the underlying cause.

MYASTHENIA GRAVIS

A rare muscle disease characterized by excessive fatiguability (weakness increases as the affected muscle is used), leading to an inability to sustain

M

muscular activity. Myasthenia gravis is an autoimmune disease in which there is a failure of transmission of nerve impulses to the muscle. Transmission of the impulses from nerve to muscle depends upon the release of a substance called acetylcholine from nerve endings and its combining with specific receptors on the surface of the muscle fibre. In this condition, antibodies against the acetylcholine receptor, produced in the thymus gland, are present in the circulating blood. The disease may be mild or severe and its course variable. It is twice as common in women as men and usually starts between 20 and 50 years of age. The muscles most frequently involved are the eyelids, external eye muscles, muscles for chewing, swallowing and speech, and respiratory muscles. The most common symptoms are drooping eyelids (ptosis), double vision, slurred speech and difficulty in swallowing. Muscle weakness may be minimal at the start of the day, but increases with use. Weakness of the respiratory muscles can be so severe that the patient requires temporary artificial ventilation.

Drugs such as pyridostigmine or neostigmine can restore neuromuscular transmission and dramatically improve weakness, at least temporarily. In more severe cases, corticosteroids, azathioprine (an immunosuppressive drug), plasmapheresis (the replacement of plasma with plasma protein to eliminate circulating antibodies) or thymectomy (surgical removal of the thymus gland) may be tried.

MYELOGRAPHY

see *Radiculography*

MYELOMA

Uncontrolled growth of plasma cells in the bone marrow. Plasma cells are cells which produce antibodies in response to infection. In myeloma an abnormal type of protein or antibody, called a paraprotein, is produced by the growth of a group or 'clone' of plasma cells. This growth can be measured in the blood as plasma cells have a very characteristic appearance under the microscope, with the nucleus situated at one end of an oval-shaped cell. Myeloma causes anaemia. In some cases there is dissolution of bone which may be seen on X-ray as 'holes'; fractures may occur as a result. The abnormal protein or paraprotein is excreted in the kidneys, and blockage of the tubes in the kidney by deposits of this protein can result in kidney failure.

Myeloma is treated with drugs (chemotherapy) and, to help relieve pain in the bones, radiotherapy. Myeloma is predominantly a disease of the elderly.

MYOCARDITIS

Inflammation of the heart muscle (myocardium) Myocarditis usually occurs after infection with viruses such as Coxsackie B, influenza and echovirus, diphtheria, acute rheumatic fever and toxoplasmosis. Radiation, drugs and chemicals may also cause myocarditis. Symptoms are those of the disease which is causing the inflammation (fever in viral infections, for example), together with breathlessness, chest pain and an irregular heart beat. Treatment is of the underlying cause. Complications such as heart failure and cardiac arrhythmias (abnormalities of cardiac rhythm including heart block) may also require treatment; see individual entries. The outlook is generally good, but is dependent on the cause and severity of any complications.

MYOCLONUS

Irregular or rhythmical muscle jerking movements with brief muscle contractions resembling an electric shock. These cannot be controlled by willpower and commonly occur in association with anxiety or on going to sleep. Myoclonus may also be familial, be found in association with metabolic disorders such as liver or kidney failure, or occur with structural brain disease. Certain types of myoclonus may respond well to drug therapy.

MYOPATHY

A general term for any disease of muscle. Causes include inherited disorders such as the muscular dystrophies, inflammatory diseases such as polymyositis, hormoneinduced myopathies due to thyrotoxicosis or corticosteroid therapy, and metabolic myopathies from alcohol, vitamin D deficiency or drugs. The principal symptom of a myopathy is weakness, the precise pattern of which will depend on the cause. Muscle pain, cramps and wasting may be features. Investigations for a suspected myopathy include clinical examination, biochemical tests, electromyography (EMG) and muscle biopsy.

MYOPIA

Short-sightedness. In this condition the parallel light rays entering the eye do not focus clearly on the retina but at a point in front of it. As a result, images falling on the retina are out of focus and appear blurred.

Correction is achieved by means of glasses with concave lenses which decrease the refraction of light and bring the point of focus further back. A similar effect can also be achieved with the use of contact lenses. More

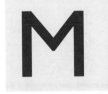

In myopia the parallel light rays entering the eye focus at a point in front of the retina (**above**). The problem is corrected (**below**) by means of a concave lens which reduces the refraction of light and brings the point of focus futher back.

recently, surgery to alter the shape of the cornea has been introduced. This technique is still being developed but even so has proved strikingly successful in many cases.

SEE ALSO *Astigmatism*, *Hypermetropia*

MYOSITIS

Inflammation of muscle. This may be due to a variety of causes, including infection or the side-effects of drug therapy. Myositis may also be due to an immunological disorder, in which case the condition is termed polymyositis. Polymyositis usually occurs in middle age; it is characterized by weakness, particularly in the muscles around the hips and shoulders, and may be associated with a rash (dermatomyositis). In some people the condition may be found in association with underlying malignant tumours.

Treatment is of the underlying cause; most cases of polymyositis respond to steroid or immunosuppressive treatment.

MYOTONIA

An inability of muscles to relax normally after contraction. There are two types of myotonia: dystrophia myotonica and myotonia congenita.

M

Dystrophia myotonica is a rare hereditary disorder which has its onset between the ages of 15 and 40 years. Affected individuals are of characteristic appearance with frontal baldness, ptosis (drooping of the upper eyelids) and wasting of the facial, shoulder and pelvic muscles. Mental abnormalities and cataracts are also common. Myotonia congenita is also inherited but, in contrast to dystrophia myotonica, is first noted at birth or in early childhood. There is no muscle wasting and no long-term ill effects but the muscles are stiff and slow to relax, especially in cold weather. Myotonia is readily recognized in the electromyogram (EMG) and can be relieved by drugs such as phenytoin, but the dystrophic features in dystrophia myotonica are uninfluenced by treatment.

NAEVUS

The medical term for a mole. Naevi are entirely benign skin lesions which appear throughout childhood and early adult life and are of no medical consequence. They consist of localized collections of cells in the skin which produce melanin (the normal skin pigment), resulting in the characteristic appearance of domed, smoothly symmetrical, slightly pigmented or darker brown lesions on any body site. Moles may become darker in pregnancy; this is usually of no significance. If a mole changes in character a doctor should be consulted as the change may indicate melanoma (qv). The tendency to develop many moles may run in families, but most people have at least a few.

Various other types of cellular collections in the skin may also have the suffix 'naevus' as part of their name, but these are all much rarer than common moles.

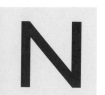

NARCOLEPSY

Falling asleep in the absence of fatigue and in inappropriate circumstances. True narcolepsy is rare. The cause is largely unknown but up to 40 per cent of patients have a family history of the condition. It may be an autoimmune disorder (see *Auto-immune disease*). Sufferers can be roused from an attack as from normal sleep. Night-time sleep is often disturbed. Tricyclic antidepressants, less often amphetamines, may be used in treatment as they stimulate 'waking centres' in the brain.

NARCOTIC

A strong hypnotic and analgesic drug; the term is often used as a synonym for narcotic analgesic. Narcotics such as morphine and pethidine are widely employed in medicine to control severe pain, and are commonly used after operations, for the treatment of renal or biliary colic, and in the care of the terminally ill. Their use is accompanied by side-effects such as nausea, vomiting and constipation. Narcotics can also produce a state of euphoria.

NAUSEA

A feeling of sickness that may precede vomiting and is often accompanied by an excess of saliva. Nausea, like vomiting, may be triggered by strong, unpleasant smells, horrific scenes or severe pain. It commonly occurs in early pregnancy, when it is a prominent feature of morning sickness (qv). Most severe illnesses produce nausea, which is also a common side-effect of some drugs and antibiotics.

Nausea may be relieved by some antihistamine and related drugs.

NECROSIS

The death of cells in tissues or organs as a result of any type of injury — for example, burns, electric shock; lack of blood supply or lack of oxygen. Necrosis disrupts the cell structure and produces inflammation in the area around the injury. The cells causing the inflammation also have a role in removing the dead material and in the process of healing. Massive necrosis of a vital organ usually leads to death — for example, massive heart attack.

NEPHRECTOMY

An operation to remove one or both kidneys; the terms unilateral nephrectomy and bilateral nephrectomy are used to describe the respective operations. Common reasons for unilateral nephrectomy include live donor kidney transplantation, malignant disease, renal injury with uncontrolled bleeding, a non-functioning, persistently infected kidney or a nonfunctioning kidney causing severe hypertension (very high blood pressure).

Bilateral nephrectomy is usually performed in patients who are in renal failure and receiving dialysis, or who have already had a successful transplant replacing one kidney and now require removal of the other, non-functioning kidney, or in patients whose own kidneys are causing severe hypertension, are a persistent source of infection or are very enlarged as a result of polycystic kidney disease (qv).

Usually nephrectomy involves a hospital stay of one week and a recuperation period of about 6—8 weeks.

NEPHROBLASTOMA

see *Wilm's tumour*

NEPHROLITHIASIS

The presence of stones (calculi) in the upper urinary tract. The symptoms, causes, investigation and treatment of nephrolithiasis are similar to those for stones in other parts of the urinary tract (see *Urolithiasis*).

The treatment of nephrolithiasis has changed dramatically in recent years. Percutaneous operations, in which the stone is approached via a small tract made from the skin into the kidney, are replacing more traumatic open operations. The stone is located and then broken up by instruments or ultrasonic probes passed down the tract. The technique called extra-corporeal shock wave lithotripsy, in which the stones are broken up by ultrasonic shock waves, is even less disturbing to the patient because it does not require any form of invasive surgery. However, not all stones are suitable for this treatment and the apparatus is extremely expensive. As with urolithiasis, the identification and treatment of underlying metabolic abnormalities is important if stones are not to recur.

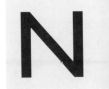

NEPHROTIC SYNDROME

The group of symptoms which coincide in this disorder are proteinuria, hypoalbuminaemia and oedema. Often a sign of glomerulonephritis (qv), nephrotic syndrome develops when extremely high levels of protein in the urine (proteinuria) lead to reduced levels of a protein called albumin (hypoalbuminaemia) in the blood, which in turn causes oedema of the legs (and face in children) and often ascites. Blood cholesterol levels are increased (hypercholesterolaemia) and in chronic cases premature coronary heart disease may develop.

A renal biopsy is usually performed to determine the type of glomerulonephritis. Minimal change glomerulonephritis accounts for 28 per cent of cases (and is the most frequent cause of nephrotic syndrome in children), membranous glomerulonephritis 25 per cent, and focal glomerulonephritis 15 per cent, with a large number of other rarer types making up the balance.

General treatment consists of a reduced-salt, normal protein diet and diuretics to control the oedema and ascites. In both adults and children corticosteroid therapy has proved most successful in treating minimal change glomerulonephritis and preventing the development of kidney failure. It may also be tried in other types of glomerulonephritis, although the response rate is much poorer. The reason for this failure is not known. Treatment in these cases is therefore complicated and may involve immunosuppressive drugs and steroids.

NEPHROTOXIN

An agent (for example, a drug, chemical, or antibody) which damages the kidney. Nephrotoxins may produce a variety of kidney diseases ranging from proteinuria (excessive protein in the urine) and mildly impaired function of the renal tubules to acute and chronic kidney failure. Drugs are an important cause of kidney damage, mainly as a result of individual hypersensitivity to them, although there have been dose-related cases. Examples of drugs that can cause renal damage are: NSAIDs (causing acute and chronic renal failure), aminoglycoside antibiotics, such as gentamicin (acute renal failure), outdated tetracycline antibiotics (acute renal failure), penicillamine (nephrotic syndrome) and ladiographic contrast material (acute renal failure). Chemicals poisonous to the kidney include some metals (arsenic, gold, lead, lithium), organic compounds (carbon tetrachloride, ethylene glycol) and the weedkiller paraquat; however, cases of kidney damage resulting from exposure to such agents are rare.

SEE ALSO *Anaphylaxis*, *Iatrogenic disease*

NERVOUS BREAKDOWN

A common lay term used to describe an episode of psychiatric illness that causes a complete disruption of a person's work and social life. Often the illness will lead to hospital admission. A number of different psychiatric disorders may result in a nervous breakdown; for example, affective disorders such as depression and mania, schizophrenia and severe neuroses. Recovery is often complete.

NEUROFIBRO-MATOSIS

A dominantly inherited disease characterized by spots of increased skin pigmentation and many benign tumours of the sheaths surrounding the nerves, particularly on the trunk. These can be small or several centimetres in diameter. Depending on their position (in the spinal canal or within the skull, or in one or both acoustic nerves, for example), they can give rise to serious pressure effects and need surgical removal. There may be associated overgrowth of fibroblast cells (which produce collagen, the main component of connective tissue), giving rise to grotesque deformities. About 30 per cent of patients have neurological disturbances. There is no cure for the underlying cause.

NEUROPATHY

In its broadest sense this term refers to any disease or lesion of one or more nerves. In practice, however, it is often used to refer to disease which affects the functioning of the peripheral nerves (or cerebrospinal nerves) passing from the spinal cord to the muscles. Such a disorder is often first evident through malfunction of that part of the nerves at the furthest point from the neurone cell body in the spinal cord (where the nucleus is located) so that sensation and reflexes are diminished. A distinction is usually made between neuropathy affecting single nerves (mononeuropathy) and that involving many (polyneuropathy). Single nerves may be affected as a result of injury or pressure (as in carpal tunnel syndrome, for example). Many nerves may be affected by metabolic disorders (for example, diabetes mellitus) or autoimmune diseases (for example, rheumatoid arthritis).

Treatment depends upon the cause. Corticosteroid treatment may help in some autoimmune cases.

NEUROSIS

One of a group of psychiatric disturbances that are often viewed as being of psychological and not physical origin (ie, of a psychogenic nature). The members of this group include anxiety neuroses, phobias, obsessional neuroses, hysteria and hypochondriasis. Most patients with a neurosis have a mixture of symptoms (anxiety — a prominent symptom of all neuroses — depression, irritability and obsessional thoughts). Such non-specific neuroses are the most common psychiatric disorders; specific neuroses such as a phobic anxiety state, for example, are less common. They occur more often in women and are for the most part transient or fluctuating, most episodes passing in the course of a year. Generally, neurotic patients do not confuse their experiences with reality, unlike psychotics who commonly have delusions or hallucinations.

Treatment approaches include psychodynamic psychotherapy, behaviour therapy, antidepressant tranquillizers and beta-blockers.

NICOTINIC ACID

Part of the B complex of vitamins and essential for many complex biochemical reactions within the body; also known as niacin or vitamin B_3.

The main dietary sources of nicotinic acid are meat (especially liver), peanuts, fish, wholemeal cereals (refined cereals contain reduced amounts of nicotinic acid because bran is removed during the refining process) and pulses.

Deficiency results in a condition called pellagra, which is characterized by dermatitis, diarrhoea and demetia. The skin changes initially resemble sunburn but later ulceration and secondary infection may occur. In chronic cases the skin thickens, becomes dry and scaly and has a brown pigment.

NOCTURIA

Excessive or excessively frequent urination at night. This occurs when the volume of urine produced during sleep exceeds the capacity of the bladder or when the bladder is incompletely emptied each time so that the urge to urinate is more frequent.

Nocturia is found in a number of illnesses. For example, in most kidney disorders inability to concentrate

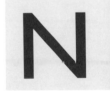

urine leads to increased amounts of dilute urine; and in diabetes mellitus very high sugar levels in urine promote excessive urination. Nocturia also occurs if bladder capacity is reduced by infection, tumours, stones or compression during pregnancy. Prostatic disease or enlargement is also a common cause of nocturia because of incomplete emptying.

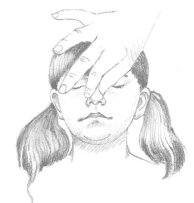

A nosebleed can be stopped by pinching the fleshy part of the nose with the fingers. This works by compressing the vessels on the septum between the nostrils. Serious nosebleeds may require the doctor to apply further pressure by packing the nose with gauze or an inflatable catheter.

NON-SPECIFIC URETHRITIS (NSU)

An inflammatory condition of the urethra, the tube that drains the bladder. Certain types of micro-organism cause this very common sexually transmitted disease; *Chlamydia trachomatis* is responsible for most cases. Both men and women are affected. In women the pelvis is also inflamed, which can lead to pain and (usually temporary) sterility. Most cases respond well to antibiotics. Couples should abstain from sexual intercourse until the cure is complete.

Children born to infected mothers may have their eyes infected during passage through the birth canal, producing the condition known as ophthalmia neonatorum. This can be successfully treated with an antibiotic eye ointment.

NOSEBLEED

Nosebleed (known medically as epistaxis) can be the result of local causes, such as injury to the nose, rhinitis (inflammation of the membrane of the nose), or, rarely, malignancy; of a specific disease of the blood such as leukaemia or thrombocytopenia (a deficiency of blood platelets which hinders clotting); or of a more general disorder, such as hypertension (high blood pressure). Frequently, however, no specific cause is found and the bleeding occurs spontaneously from the vessels at the front of the nasal septum (the partition between the nostrils). This may be initiated by slight injury (often from nose picking) or by atmospheric drying of the nasal mucus leading to crusting; when the crust is dislodged by blowing the nose or picking, bleeding may occur. Nosebleeds are more likely to occur if the blood vessels in the nose are prominent or telangiectasia (qv) is present.

The amount of bleeding can vary from the trivial to lethal. Blood may flow back into the pharynx and often appears in the opposite nostril. Sometimes the bleeding may be entirely into the pharynx. Such blood is occasionally inhaled or swallowed, to be coughed up later as a suspected haemoptysis or haematemesis.

NSAID

Non-steroidal anti-inflammatory drug, a class of medication that includes an extensive range of different compounds such as aspirin, indomethacin, naproxen and ibuprofen. The precise way in which these drugs act is not clear although they have effects on a variety of biological processes involved in inflammation. NSAIDs are therefore predominantly used in the treatment of conditions that have inflammation as a central feature — for example, rheumatoid arthritis and ankylosing spondylitis, in which they may markedly improve functional activity.

NSAIDs may cause a variety of side-effects including rashes, gastro-intestinal disturbance and ulceration of the stomach. Patients display a marked variation in response to different NSAIDs and for this reason these drugs require careful prescribing and subsequent monitoring of their effects.

NYSTAGMUS

Involuntary rhythmic movement of the eyes (usually in unison) in either a horizontal or vertical direction. There are two types: jerk or phasic nystagmus, and oscillating or pendular nystagmus. In the first type, the commoner of the two, the eyes move rapidly in one direction (the quick phase) and then recoil more slowly (the slow phase). Both phases may be repeated several times or may continue for as long as the gaze remains in one direction. Jerk nystagmus is seen in disease of the labyrinth of the inner ear (labyrinthitis), in drug intoxication (as with barbiturates) and in problems involving the brain-stem and cerebellum (as, for example, in multiple sclerosis). The symptoms which may be produced by these underlying causes include nausea, vomiting and vertigo (an illusion of rotation or of the world rotating around one).

Oscillating or pendular nystagmus is seen in patients in whom central vision is lost, usually due to disease of the retina (the light-sensitive lining at the back of the eye). Miner's nystagmus is also of the pendular type and is caused by years of working in poor light.

OBESITY

Obesity may be defined as an increase of more than 20 per cent over the ideal weight for age, height and sex. It is common in countries where carbohydrate foods (sugars and starches) form a major part of the diet.

In the majority of cases of obesity there is no underlying medical cause. Any age group may be affected: for example, infants fed on modified cow's milk, schoolchildren brought up on an unrestricted carbohydrate diet of sweets and cakes, and adults with a lifelong indulgence in high-carbohydrate foods and a sedentary occupation, or in whom alcohol intake is excessive or pregnancy frequent. The common factor in all these cases is consumption of carbohydrates exceeding the energy requirements of the individual.

The incidence of heart disease, high blood pressure diabetes mellitus (in the middle aged), gallstones, hiatus hernia and osteoarthritis is much higher in the obese than in the rest of the population.

An underlying hormonal abnormality is the most likely cause of obesity that is not due to overeating; hypothyroidism and Cushing's syndrome are examples. Other less common causes are the side-effects of some drugs, head injury with damage to the hypothalmus, brain tumours and disorders of the ovaries.

Tests are usually done to rule out any of the underlying causes of obesity outlined above. In cases of obesity due to overeating, treatment is difficult since its success largely depends on the willingness of the individual to break a lifelong habit.

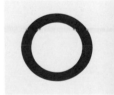

OBSESSION

A recurrent idea, thought, image or

impulse which cannot be suppressed; also known as obsessional neurosis. The term may be used to describe either a common personality trait (such as precision, thoroughness and tidiness) or a particular neurosis. It is when the obsessions become so intense as to dominate the individual's waking life to the exclusion of other activity that a true obsessional neurosis exists. Obsessional neurosis is rare and usually develops in young adulthood. Some of the thoughts which come into the sufferer's mind may be of a violent or sexual nature. The sufferer recognizes the thoughts as his own and often regards them as absurd. Often these thoughts will be accompanied by rituals or acts; for example, a person with obsessional thoughts about being dirty will repeatedly wash his hands.

Treatment is often psychological, using behaviour therapy.

OCCLUSION

A technique that shuts things in or out. For example, in tubal occlusion the Fallopian tubes are either tied or clipped, so preventing sperm from fertilizing ova. Occlusion can also be applied to other structures. For example, an occlusive dressing on a wound is one which is sealed to shut out infection. The term is also used in dentistry, to describe the quality of the 'bite' (that is, the juxtaposition of the upper and lower teeth – see *Orthodontics*).

The term can also mean blockage or obstruction.

OEDEMA

Excess fluid beneath the skin or in one or more of the cavities of the body. Oedema only becomes clinically evident once several litres have accumulated and there is an increase in weight. It is found in several medical conditions and may be localized or widespread. Its distribution in the body is an important clue as to its cause. Localized oedema is due to inflammation or local blockage of blood or lymph vessels. Heart, kidney, liver and gut disease are the major causes of more widespread oedema. Fluid may accumulate in one of several ways: because a rise in pressure in the capillaries (tiny blood vessels) forces fluid out of them and into surrounding tissues (as in heart failure); because of damage to the capillaries (as in inflammation); or lack of sufficient protein concentration in the blood to keep fluid in the circulation. The last-mentioned occurs in kidney disease, either as a result of protein being lost (in nephrotic syndrome, for example) or insufficient amounts of protein being manufactured (as in cirrhosis of the liver).

Treatment depends upon the cause.

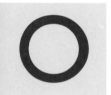

OESTROGEN

A steroid hormone produced mainly by the ovaries, although smaller amounts are produced by the adrenal glands and by fatty tissue sited all over the body. Oestrogen is responsible for the development of female sexual characteristics and the maintenance of these characteristics throughout the reproductive phase. Production of oestrogen by the ovaries increases at puberty and then fluctuates in a regular cyclical pattern until the menopause, when production of oestrogen falls to very low levels.

Oestrogen is the major component of the combined oral contraceptive pill and of hormone replacement therapy (qv).

OOPHORECTOMY

The surgical removal of an ovary. The ovaries are the source of the majority of the female sex hormones (oestrogens and progesterones) and removal of them both renders the patient menopausal as well as infertile. Oophorectomy involving both glands is only performed before the menopause if they are seriously diseased.

The operation is performed for malignant disease of the ovary (both ovaries are usually removed) and occasionally for benign cysts when it is impossible to preserve any functional ovarian tissue. Other conditions for which oophorectomy may be required are cancer of the uterus or cervix (womb or neck of the womb), or destruction of the ovary as a result of sepsis or endometriosis.

It is usual practice to remove the uterus (hysterectomy) as well when the ovaries have to be removed.

OPHTHALMOPLEGIA

Paralysis of the muscles that control the eyeballs. One or both eyeballs may be affected in this type of ocular muscle palsy, which prevents their movement in one or more directions. Ophthalmoplegia has many causes. One of the most common is disease of the small arteries that supply the nerves of the muscles; this often occurs as a complication of diabetes mellitus. Ophthalmoplegia may also be caused by pressure on the nerves, such as by aneurysm (dilatation of an artery) or a tumour close to where the nerves pass inside the skull, by diseases of the muscles (myasthenia gravis, for example) and finally by disease of the cells in the brain stem from which the nerves supplying the muscles of the eye arise (as in multiple sclerosis).

Treatment depends upon the cause.

OPPORTUNISTIC INFECTION

An infection which occurs when the immune defences of the body are low. This commonly happens after treatment with cytotoxic drugs used in the treatment of cancer which kill the normal cells present in the bone marrow. Opportunistic infections also occur in individuals infected with the human immunodeficiency virus (HIV) and their presence is an important factor in a diagnosis of AIDS (qv). These infections are unusual, and often stem from organisms which normally cause infections in animals. Common opportunistic infections are Pneumocystis pneumoniae, cytomegalovirus, herpes zoster (shingles), doxoplasmosis, and variants of tuberculosis.

Treatment is difficult because of the poor immunity of the affected individual but involves antibiotics and/or antiviral agents.

OPTIC ATROPHY

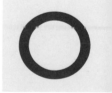

The progressive loss of nerve cells in the optic nerve. These cells transmit visual information from the retina (the light-sensitive lining at the back of the eye) to the midbrain, and thence by another set of nerve cells to the occipital cortex at the back of the brain. The loss of optic nerve cells leads to a reduction in the sharpness of vision, especially in the centre of the field of vision, and in some cases to 'holes' in the visual field (scotoma). Eventually blindness results.

Causes include diseases of the optic nerves, nutritional factors which pick out this group of nerve cells, and compression of the optic nerves. The disease group includes general diseases of the brain such as multiple sclerosis, which frequently affects the optic nerves, and a group of hereditary brain disorders which also affect movement, the ataxias. Optic atrophy is also a feature of certain inherited diseases of the eye, such as retinitis pigmentosa. It has also been found in beriberi (thiamine deficiency) and pellagra (niacin deficiency). Nutritional (B vitamin) deficiency is the probable cause of so-called tobacco/alcohol amblyopia which, in severe cases, can progress to optic atrophy. Compression of the optic nerves may be due to a tumour, injury or inflammation in the eye socket. Tumours of the pituitary gland often compress the optic chiasm, where the two optic nerves meet to 'swap' fibres. If the cause of compression is found, or if a vitamin deficiency is identified very early, it may be possible to remedy the condition; otherwise optic atrophy cannot be treated.

ORCHIDECTOMY

Surgical removal of the testis. Orchidectomy is performed in cases of suspected testicular malignancy, in undescended testis left untreated since childhood, in cancer of the prostate and, very rarely, when a testicular abscess has severely damaged the organ. The operation is performed through an incision in the groin; the testis is delivered to this point, where it is inspected and, if necessary, removed. If malignancy is suspected, during the operation the spermatic cord is clamped at the level of the inguinal canal in order to prevent the spread of tumour cells while the testis is manipulated.

Orchidectomy as a late treatment for undescended testis is usually advised to eliminate the risk of malignant change; 1 in 10 testicular cancers is associated with testicular

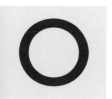

maldescent. In cases of cancer of the prostate, bilateral orchidectomy may help the condition to regress, by cutting the supply of many male hormones to the carcinoma, which is hormone-dependent.

ORCHITIS

An acute infection of the testis which causes fever, swelling and severe pain. It occurs after puberty, and is caused by mumps or other viruses. Occasionally orchitis is due to bacteria carried from elsewhere in the body, or rarely from sexually acquired infections. These and tuberculosis also infect the epididymis, the thick structure on the side of the testis which is the collecting system for sperm.

Treatment consists of relieving the pain and, if bacteria are responsible, taking antibiotics. Orchitis often clears up but the result may be a useless and atrophied testis. Occasionally surgical examination of the testis is required to exclude other causes; an abscess in the testis, for example, is treated like any other abscess but if the organ is severely damaged removal (orchidectomy) may be necessary.

ORTHOPNOEA

Difficulty in breathing (dyspnoea) when lying down. Affected individuals often sleep propped up on several pillows or, in extreme cases, in a chair. Orthopnoea is usually associated with heart failure, especially of the left side of the heart. This leads to congestion of the lungs with blood and subsequently leakage of fluid into the air spaces (pulmonary oedema). Orthopnoea may also occur in emphysema and in acute asthmatic attacks. Treatment is of the underlying cause.

OSSIFICATION

The process by which bone is formed. Specialized cells called osteoblasts are responsible for bone formation. Ossification starts with the laying down of collagen fibres (collagen is a protein, and the main component of connective tissue such as skin, tendon, ligament and bone), followed by the deposition of a cementing protein and impregnation by calcium crystals. Calcium, vitamin D, phosphorus, proteins and some hormones are necessary for normal ossification.

OSTEOARTHRITIS/ OSTEOARTHROSIS

A common age-related condition characterized by degenerative changes in the joints; half of all people over the age of 60 have some signs of osteoarthritis. The changes consist of a gradual wearing away of the cartilage overlying the ends of the bones and the formation of cysts in the bone beneath. Osteoarthritis may occur for no known reason or may be secondary to other conditions; these include previous injury, inflammatory joint disease and metabolic diseases. In some individuals there is a strong family history of osteoarthritis.

Pain is the main symptom of osteoarthritis. This is exacerbated by usage of the joint, tends to be worse at the end of the day and is generally relieved by rest. Joints commonly involved include the hip, knee and those at the base of the big toe and thumb and at the tips of the fingers. Joints of the spine may also be involved (spondylosis).

No specific treatment can reverse the disease process. Treatment is therefore aimed at reducing symptoms, particularly by means of painkilling drugs. In some patients, particularly those with advanced hip and knee disease, joint replacement surgery may be necessary. Occupational therapy or physiotherapy may be required in some cases to help patients adapt to their condition.

The condition is distinct from rheumatoid arthritis (qv), one of the most crippling of all rheumatic diseases.

OSTEOGENESIS IMPERFECTA

A group of rare inherited disorders characterized by fragile bones. The cause is not known but is thought to involve an abnormality of collagen, which forms the intercellular fibres of connective tissue. In the most severe form of osteogenesis imperfecta, fractures of bones may occur either before or during birth; these babies usually die in the newborn period. The main feature in children less severely affected is a tendency for bones to fracture in response to only minor stress (brittle bone disease). The condition may be accompanied by skeletal deformities with increased spinal curvature and shortness of stature, discoloured and abnormally shaped teeth, joint hypermobility ('double-jointedness'), thin skin, and blue sclera (in which the 'whites' of the eyes appear blue).

There is no known effective treatment for this condition.

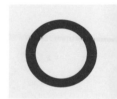

OSTEOMALACIA

A disease, also known in children as rickets, in which the bones become softened as a result of a deficiency of the vitamin (D) that is required for calcification of bone. Deficiency can occur in a number of ways: through insufficiency in the diet (fatty fish, such as mackerel and herring, is the richest source of vitamin D); lack of exposure to sunlight (vitamin D is produced in the skin on exposure); as a result of diseases of the liver or kidneys interferring with the processing of vitamin D and its absorption from the gut; and through drugs such as anticonvulsants upsetting liver metabolism. Vitamin D deficiency is found particularly in the elderly and Asian immigrants who are vegetarian, have a diet containing very little of the vitamin, and are rarely exposed to sunlight.

Symptoms associated with osteomalacia include non-specific aches and pains around the shoulders, chest, back and thighs. Areas over the bones may feel tender, and bone fractures may develop in the elderly. Weakness of the muscles, particularly around the shoulders and hips, may be noticed. Blood tests and X-rays may be used to help establish a diagnosis of osteomalacia. Treatment of any underlying cause and medication with calcium and vitamin D may be required.

OSTEOMYELITIS

Infection of bone, usually due to bacteria but sometimes due to other types of micro-organism such as viruses and fungi. Micro-organisms may reach bone via the bloodstream, from other sites of infection or as a result of injury. The infection often causes severe pain in the affected bones; onset may be either insidious and gradually worsen, or sudden (as is often the case in children). Fever and nausea may accompany the infection; if osteomyelitis comes on gradually there may be malaise (a general feeling of being unwell) and weight loss.

Treatment of acute osteomyelitis requires bed rest and therapy with appropriate antibiotics. In some circumstances surgery to release pus from bone and to promote healing is required. Some cases, especially those not vigorously treated, can become chronic and difficult to eradicate.

OSTEOPETROSIS

'Marble bone' or Albers-Schönberg disease, a group of rare diseases which is found in its severest form in children. It is inherited as an autosomal recessive trait (see *Recessive pattern of inheritance*) and may cause blindness due to pressure on the optic nerve as well as suppression of bone marrow function and early death in infancy. In its less severe forms, usually dominantly inherited (see *Dominant pattern of inheritance*), there are multiple fractures. The defect is due to a disturbance in function of cells called osteoclasts which are involved in the normal constant remodelling of bone. As a result, bone structure is haphazard and lacks its usual strength. There is no known cure for the condition. Bone marrow transplantation may help.

OSTEOPOROSIS

Loss of bone substance; this results in the bones becoming more fragile and liable to fracture. Some degree of osteoporosis is part of the normal ageing process and is symptomless. A severe form of osteoporosis may be seen in postmenopausal women and in the elderly of both sexes (senile osteoporosis). The cause is unknown. The female sex hormone oestrogen may have a significant role to play in post-menopausal osteoporosis and there is evidence that hormone replacement therapy is of value in retarding bone loss in this group of women. The most common symptom of osteoporosis is severe back pain, accompanied by loss of height and a characteristic stooped posture because the weight of the torso causes wedge-shaped compression fractures of the vertebrae in the spine. Pain is only felt at the time of a fracture and goes away as the fracture heals. Minimal injury results in fractures of other bones, particularly the hip and the wrist. Senile osteoporosis resulting in hip fracture is a major cause of death and disability in the elderly. Ten to fifteen per cent of patients die within three months of such fractures and a significant majority of the remainder are left immobile. Osteoporosis may also occur in patients who have been immobile for a long period and is often seen in cases of fractured limb (disuse osteoporosis); maintenance of bone health and retention of calcium depend upon muscular contraction during movement. It may also occur in Cushing's syndrome, long-term steroid therapy, hyperthyroidism and alcoholism; in all of these conditions the body loses calcium, which is withdrawn from the bones.

OSTEOTOMY

A special operation which involves dividing a bone, re-aligning it and then fixing it in its new position. Holding it in the new position is achieved by means of plaster of Paris or plates (fixation). An osteotomy is performed to correct the bony deformities that may result from congenital disorders (for example, congenital dislocation of the hip or knock knees/ bow legs), disease (such as rickets), tuberculosis (or Paget's disease of bone) or badly united fractures (particularly of the elbow or shinbone). It can also be used to relieve the pain of osteoarthritis by improving the affected joint's range of movement (especially the hip and the knee).

OTITIS

Inflammation of the external auditory canal (otitis externa) or the middle ear space (otitis media).

Most cases of otitis externa are caused by infection resulting from injury; the remainder are reactive, caused by eczema. The condition is very painful because fluid produced by the infection swells the tightly bound skin of the external canal. Treatment is with topical antibiotics. Otitis externa never causes deafness.

Otitis media usually begins as an acute infection after a common cold. Many cases are caused by a virus and so antibiotics are sometimes of little value, but nevertheless should be given in case the infection is bacterial. Children frequently suffer from it because of poor resistance and adenoids. The infection produces redness and swelling of the eardrum, and fever. As with otitis externa, the build up of pus causes great pain. The eardrum will eventually perforate unless the pressure is relieved, causing a slight discharge. Healing usually occurs naturally. Recurrent attacks, especially if associated with failure of the eardrum to heal, can lead to chronic otitis media with persistent discharge, known as otorrhoea. The vast majority of cases of otitis media resolve with no residual hearing impairment, but occasionally deafness in one ear may result.

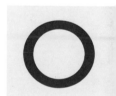

OTOSCLEROSIS

A disease which causes slowly progressive conductive deafness as the chain of ossicles (small bones) transmitting sound from the eardrum to the cochlea is stiffened by bony overgrowth and those bones which are normally immobile fuse together. The cause of otosclerosis is unknown.

Two-thirds of cases begin between the ages of 11 and 30 and tend to run in families. The deafness starts in one ear but in 90 per cent of cases progresses to the other. Typically it reaches a peak in the twenties, after which there is little further deterioration.

Apart from deafness most patients have occasional tinnitus; in about a quarter of sufferers this is a serious problem. Dizziness is also common but usually momentary, accompanying a change in posture.

Other causes of conductive weakness have to be excluded before the diagnosis can be made; these include a break in the chain of ossicles after injury or infection, and Paget's disease (qv).

The deafness can be corrected by the use of a hearing aid or by an operation called stapedectomy (qv).

OVARIAN CYST

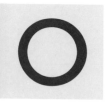

Cysts which form in the ovaries can either be simple (benign) or cancerous (malignant). Benign cysts are more common and often arise in young women. However, malignant cysts are a major cause of death from cancer in women.

Cysts often occur in both ovaries at the same time. Usually they remain painless until their weight and the distension caused by their increasing size cause abdominal swelling and discomfort. Benign cysts generally are not larger than 6–8 cm ($2\frac{1}{2}$–3 in), although this is by no means the rule and many very large cysts are benign too. Complications that may arise include bleeding into the cyst and, rarely, infection. Ultrasound is very helpful in diagnosing and determining the size of ovarian cysts.

All cases of ovarian cyst are treated surgically (see *Oophorectomy*). If the cyst is benign, removal of it alone may be possible. Otherwise the ovary is removed together with the cyst. For malignant cysts, an extensive operation is often required.

For dermoid cyst, see *Teratoma*.

OVULATION

The production and discharge of eggs (ova) from the ovary. The ovary contains thousands of immature follicles, each one containing a potential egg or ovum. During a woman's reproductive years these follicles are stimulated to develop by a hormone called follicular stimulating hormone (FSH) secreted by the pituitary gland. Only one follicle usually reaches full maturity during each menstrual cycle, although occasionally more than one ovulation will occur (this can lead to multiple pregnancies). The process of ovulation usually occurs two weeks prior to menstruation.

At ovulation an egg (ovum) escapes (**left**) from a mature follicle and finds its way down the corresponding Fallopian tube (**middle**) into the womb. If the egg is not fertilized and implanted in the womb, it is shed at the time of the menstrual period (**right**).

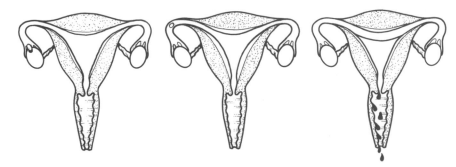

At the time of ovulation the ovary starts to produce a special hormone called progesterone in addition to oestrogen. These hormones prepare the womb lining (endometrium) for a fertilized egg. If a fertilized egg does not implant in the womb, the lining is shed at the time of the menstrual period.

Ovulation usually starts at puberty and continues through to the menopause, although at the extremes of reproductive life it may occur rather irregularly. Ovulation can be suppressed by the use of the contraceptive pill and stimulated by certain fertility drugs. Use of the latter increases the likelihood of multiple pregnancies.

PACEMAKER

A device which takes the place of the heart's natural pacemaker, the sinuatrial node, and transmits an electrical impulse to the heart muscle. Pacemakers are often fitted permanently in patients who have a slow heartbeat (bradycardia) and in whom attacks of unconsciousness (Stokes-Adams attacks) occur. They may also be fitted temporarily; after a heart attack, for example.

The lithium batteries used in permanent pacemakers may last up to ten years before they need replacing. In sophisticated pacemakers the electrical impulse is sent to more than one chamber of the heart so that the natural heart muscle contraction is accurately reproduced. Some of these advanced dual-chamber pacemakers can increase the number of impulses sent to the heart muscle when exercise is taken, thus increasing the output of the heart as in a normal individual.

Most pacemakers are used to regulate a slow heart rate, but there are types which are employed to detect and stop life-threatening tachycardias (rapid heartbeats) in cases where drug therapy has failed.

Fitting a pacemaker involves passing one end of a wire into the heart **(1)** via a large vein and attaching the other end to a box housing a lithium or mercury battery and impulse generator **(2)**. If the pacemaker is temporary, this control unit is attached to the chest wall. A permanent pacemaker is implanted beneath the skin.

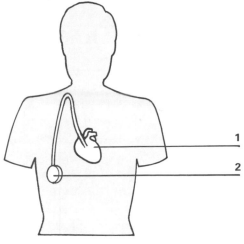

PAGET'S DISEASE OF BONE

A disease of the elderly in which bones may become enlarged, softened and deformed. The cause of the condition is unknown but there appears to be an imbalance in the normal processes of bone renewal which leads to the rate of renewal being greatly increased. The new bone formed has an abnormal structure and is therefore weak.

Most people who have the disease have no symptoms, and it is only discovered accidentally after an X-ray or blood test for another condition. When they are present, symptoms will depend on which bones are affected and to what extent. Pain may be felt, particularly if the weight-bearing bones in the lower spine and pelvis are involved. The long bones of the limbs may become warm and enlarged, and fracture. Involvement of bones in the skull or spine may cause pressure on nerves.

P

Treatment is only required in people who have symptoms; pain relief may include the use of simple painkillers or non-steroidal anti-inflammatory drugs. For severe cases, other forms of treatment — for example, the drugs calcitonin, etidronate or mithramycin — may be required.

PAGET'S DISEASE OF THE NIPPLE

In this condition the nipple of a middle-aged or elderly woman develops eczema, which appears as a fine scaly rash with slight redness and itching; it gradually progresses to soreness, bleeding and ulceration with eventual erosion of the nipple. The eczematous rash is an early sign of a cancerous growth of the breast which is initially confined to one of the milk ducts. Early treatment by mastectomy often cures the condition.

Paget's disease of the nipple is not related to Paget's disease of bone.

PALLIATIVE THERAPY

Treatment that makes someone feel better but is not curative. Palliative therapy is often used in the context of treatment for cancer. For example, when cancer of the pancreas blocks the common bile duct and the drainage of bile into the gut, a palliative operation is performed to bypass the blockage, but the cancer remains. Similarly, palliative radiotherapy shrinks a mass of tumour, but eventually the tumour will return.

PALPITATION

A change in heart rhythm or an increase in the force of the beat of which the affected individual is acutely aware. Palpitations are a common symptom of anxiety. They may also be a symptom of anaemia, overactive thyroid gland, tumours of the adrenal glands, abnormal heart rhythm, or a sideeffect of drugs such as caffeine. Persistent abnormalities in heart rhythm do not usually give rise to palpitations, whereas recent, transient and episodic changes do.

PANCREAS

An organ situated in the upper abdomen which produces the enzymes for digestion, bicarbonate to neutralize the acid coming into the small intestine from the stomach, and also some gut hormones (most importantly insulin to control sugar and fat metabolism). The production of alkalis and enzymes for food digestion is referred to as the pancreatic exocrine function: products are secreted into a duct system, in the form of pancreatic juice, which flows into the upper small bowel. The hormones are secreted into the bloodstream as a part of a process called the pancreatic endocrine function which is carried out by specialized cells grouped together in the islets of Langerhans within the pancreas. Malabsorption of vitamins, fats and other essential nutrients occurs if the exocrine pancreas does not function properly. Diabetes mellitus will occur if the endocrine pancreas fails. Both functions may be disrupted if the pancreas is either removed surgically or severely damaged by disease.

PANCREATITIS

Inflammation of the pancreas. It is characterized by pain in the upper abdomen which is often severe, spreading through to the back, and may be associated with vomiting. Fever, shock and generalized symptoms may also

P

be present in acute pancreatitis, which can be a life-threatening acute illness. In acute pancreatitis the pancreas is digested by its own enzymes. The commonest cause of acute pancreatitis is either a gallstone lodged at the end of the common bile duct or alcoholism. Rarer causes include drugs (steroids and the oral contraceptive pill), injury, high blood calcium or high blood fats.

Patients with chronic pancreatitis have recurrent bouts of abdominal pain, and ultimately the ability for the organ to produce the enzymes for food digestion may be impaired, leading to malabsorption. Diabetes mellitus may develop if the diseased gland cannot produce enough insulin. Chronic pancreatitis is mostly due to excess alcohol ingestion.

Treatment of acute pancreatitis requires hospital admission for resuscitation with intravenous fluids and possible surgery. Treatment of chronic pancreatitis includes powerful pain-relieving agents, a low-fat diet and the replacement of enzymes to aid digestion. Ultimately, surgical removal of the pancreas may be necessary if the pain is very severe.

PAPILLOEDEMA

An abnormal swelling of the optic disc, at the site where the optic nerve leaves the retina (the lightsensitive lining at the back of the eye). Papilloedema is usually a sign of increased pressure inside the skull (intracranial pressure) caused by a lesion such as a brain tumour, although there are other, less ominous causes such as very high blood pressure and abnormalities of the system of veins draining the retina. Symptoms are usually those of the underlying disease, and include headaches and vomiting from increased intracranial pressure. Vision may well be normal. Eventually, a prolonged increase in intracranial pressure may compress the optic nerve and thus produce optic atrophy (qv). Very rarely severe papilloedema exerts such pressure upon the artery supplying blood to the retina that there is a risk of the tissues of the retina infarcting, or dying, resulting in sudden and permanent blindness.

Papilloedema is detected by examining the retina with an instrument called an ophthalmoscope. A CT scan generally identifies the cause. Treatment depends upon the underlying cause.

PAPILLOMA

A benign collection of cells, within any epithelial surface such as the skin, leading to a small nodule or other lesion of some kind. (Epithelium is the cell tissue of the outer surface of the body, and also of its closed cavities.) The commonest example is the basal cell papilloma (also known as a seborrheic wart), a very common skin lesion in the elderly, which is of unknown cause and is harmless. These rather warty brown lesions frequently appear on the trunk, and increase in incidence with advancing age. The term 'papilloma' may also be used to describe benign growths in other epithelial tissues such as the bladder and the bowel.

PAPULE

A solid, raised lesion on the skin which generally measures less than 1 cm ($\frac{1}{2}$ inch) across and has clearly defined edges. Papules may be flat, pointed or blunt, and are formed by the thickening of one or more layers of the skin. Papules occur as the result of viral infections (for example,

P

warts), bacterial infections (such as syphilis) and in drug-induced rashes. The deposition of cholesterol, a fat, in the skin gives rise to yellowish papule formation.

PARAESTHESIA

An abnormal sensation in part of the body due to interference with the sensory nerves serving that region. Common sensations of this type include tingling, prickling, pain, tightness and the feeling of a band around a limb or the trunk.

The abnormality causing the sensation may lie in the nerves around the spinal cord, the spinal cord itself or in the brain. A common example of paraesthesia is the sensation of pain running down the leg when a nerve root is compressed by a slipped disc.

PARACENTESIS

The drawing off of fluid (ascites) from the abdominal (peritoneal) cavity. This is performed either to aid diagnosis, when the cause of the ascites is unknown or infection is suspected, or as a form of treatment, when the volume of fluid that has accumulated is sufficient to cause distressing distension of the abdomen and even impairment of breathing.

To draw off the fluid, a small tube is inserted through the skin of the front of the abdomen, under a local anaesthetic.

PARALYSIS

Permanent or temporary loss of voluntary movement of all or part of the body. The affected limb(s) may be stiff (spastic) or flaccid, depending on the site and nature of the paralysis.

Paralysis may be less than complete (paresis), may affect all or part of one side of the body (hemiparesis), or all the limbs (quadriplegia (qv), or the trunk and legs (paraplegia, qv). In the paresis or hemiparesis caused by a stroke, the paralysis is spastic, the reflexes very brisk and sensation may be reduced. Spastic weakness also occurs in cases of paralysis caused by injury to the upper spinal cord. In a very low spinal injury, in which only nerve roots below the spinal cord are damaged, the paralysis will be flaccid. Bladder control is retained in most cases of hemiparesis, in contrast to those of complete spinal paralysis in which control is lost of the bladder and the bowels. Some forms of spinal paralysis are temporary — for example, in the rare Guillain-Barré syndrome (qv). Temporary paralysis is also found after epileptic seizures and in a rare condition (called familial periodic paralysis) in which recurrent attacks of flaccid paralysis occur in association with very high or very low potassium concentrations in the blood. Flaccid paralysis can also be caused by pharmaceutical derivatives of the plant extract curare, such as tubocurarine.

PARALYSIS AGITANS

see *Parkinson's disease*

PARANOIA

Paranoia is when a person has beliefs or ideas about himself or herself, usually concerned with persecution but also with jealousy or love. It occurs in various degrees of severity. The person with a paranoid personality will often feel criticized, suspicious and unwilling to trust others and have no insight into his or her condition. More severe problems occur in people with paranoia syndromes who hold a fixed, rigid system of beliefs which they believe others oppose only for malicious motives. Such people may engage in frequent litigation, quarrel often with neighbours, and will sometimes be driven to violence. A common paranoid syndrome, and possibly a sign of schizophrenia, is morbid jealousy in which a person believes his or her partner to be unfaithful; this is also known as the Othello syndrome. More common than these syndromes of paranoia is paranoid schizophrenia, where a person may have delusions of persecution — for example, that the neighbours are plotting to murder him or her. The paranoid personality is not influenced by treatment but paranoid schizophrenia is treated like other schizophrenic illnesses (see *Schizophrenia*).

PARAPHIMOSIS

An uncommon complication which occurs when a tight foreskin is pulled back over the glans (tip) of the penis and then cannot be returned. In paraphimosis the foreskin forms a tight collar in the groove between the shaft and glans which prevents the return of blood from the glans. As a result, the glans becomes painful and swollen. Once swelling has started, it becomes progressively more difficult to pull the foreskin forward into its normal position. This may not be possible even under an anaesthetic in an established case, and surgical release of the constricting band of foreskin is then needed. Circumcision is advisable to prevent recurrence.

PARAPLEGIA

Spinal paralysis involving the trunk and lower limbs. In paraplegia the arms function normally, in contrast to spinal paralysis at a high level in which only a few shoulder movements and breathing are possible (quadriplegia). If the level of the spinal cord damage is low (below the level of the ribs), then the person affected can usually walk with leg braces but is likely to be partially dependent on a wheelchair. In general the higher the level of spinal cord damage the more help the person needs.

Control of the bladder and bowel is initially lost after paraplegia develops; with training some patients can regain bladder control, which is important because residual urine in the bladder predisposes to infection, stone formation and obstruction of the kidneys. Immobile patients in whom sensation is reduced or absent require frequent turning and attention to their skin to prevent the development of sores. Constipation is a frequent problem.

PARATHYROID GLAND

One of several small glands (usually four but variable in number) situated behind the thyroid gland near the base of the neck. They secrete a hormone called parathormone, which is responsible for controlling the distribution of calcium and phosphate in the body. Secretion of the hormone is stimulated by a fall in blood calcium or an increase in phosphate levels. Overactivity of the parathyroid glands (hyperparathyroidism) produces increased calcium levels in the blood (hypercalcaemia) and bone disease (softening and cyst formation in the bone) and occurs in kidney failure and with benign tumours (adenomas) of a single gland. Treatment is by removal of the adenoma, or of all the glands in patients with renal failure (total parathyroidectomy). Underactivity of the parathyroid glands (hypoparathyroidism) may result from pa-

P

rathyroidectomy or occur as an autoimmune disease; symptoms that arise from low blood calcium include sensations of pins and needles in the extremities and muscle spasms. These symptoms respond to calcium supplements and vitamin D derivatives.
SEE ALSO *illustration page 144*

PARATYPHOID FEVER

An illness which occurs as a result of infection by the bacterium *Salmonella paratyphi*; it resembles typhoid but is generally milder. The disease is endemic in many parts of Asia, the Middle East, Africa and Latin America, and in some Mediterranean countries.

People usually become infected by eating contaminated food. Water polluted by infected faeces and urine in turn contaminates fruit, vegetables and seafood. Infection can be spread by contaminated hands and by flies. Diagnosis is made by culturing the bacteria from blood, faeces or urine.

The infection responds to treatment with antibiotics. Vaccines are ineffective.

PARESIS

see *Paralysis*

PARITY

This term refers to the number of children to whom a woman has given birth and includes all live births, and stillbirths after 28 weeks of pregnancy (viability). A woman who has borne a child capable of independent life, or viable, is called parous.

A nullipara is a woman who has never reached 28 weeks in a previous pregnancy, although she may have been pregnant more than once (multigravida).

PARKINSON'S DISEASE

A disease of the nervous system characterized by an involuntary tremor, rigidity and slowness of movement. Facial expression is absent in the affected person. Also evident are stooped posture, monotonous voice, and limited limb movements (walking, for example, involves small quick steps in a shuffling gait). Tremor, often most noticeable in the hands at rest, is of lower frequency than the shaking that typically affects a person when he or she is suffering from an attack of nerves. Voluntary movement will usually reduce or abolish this tremor.

Parkinsonism is predominantly a disease of the middle-aged and elderly. It arises spontaneously and occasionally runs in families. Apparently a degenerative disease of the midbrain, Parkinsonism causes the depletion of a chemical neurotransmitter called dopamine, which is essential to the proper regulation of movement and posture. The disease can be debilitating in its later stages. A form of Parkinsonism (post-encephalitic Parkinsonism) has occurred as a common sequel of encephalitis lethargica, an epidemic disease which was widespread in Europe just after the First World War. Parkinson's disease may also arise as a complication in patients who are receiving phenothiazine tranquillizers; these are used in the treatment of schizophrenia and other psychotic states.

The principal drug used in the treatment of Parkinson's disease is levodopa. The dosage of this drug is often limited by side-effects, but modern adjuvant preparations and newer drugs called dopamine agonists, such as bromocriptine, have been developed to reduce these.

PARONYCHIA

Inflammation of the skin around the nails. This disorder is commonly seen in people who habitually have their hands immersed in water for prolonged periods; housewives with young children, bar staff, nurses and hairdressers are typical examples. The normally tight bond between the nail and the surrounding skin becomes loose and the resulting penetration of fluid predisposes to inflammation and infection from organisms, usually candida (qv), though other types are also frequently found.

Paronychia is managed by keeping the hands as dry as possible for several weeks, the sufferer wearing cotton gloves (to absorb perspiration) within rubber globes whenever his or her hands are immersed in water. The application of skin creams alone is never successful, so physical protection is vital. If unprotected immersion cannot be avoided, an emollient (oily skin preparation) should be applied immediately before and after. Antibiotics and an anticandidal cream or lotion as treatment in addition to the measures mentioned above may be required. The condition is slow to clear up and relapses may occur swiftly if the hands are not diligently protected.

PAROTITIS

Inflammation of the parotid glands. The parotids are salivary glands situated in the tissues of the cheeks. Saliva produced in the glands passes along a tube (Stensen's duct) which opens on the inside of the cheek, near the back teeth. Inflammation may be caused by a virus or bacterium, or be part of a generalized disease. The commonest cause is mumps. Bacterial infection may occur in newborn babies and in debilitated patients (for instance, after a stroke or chronic kidney failure), and requires antibiotic treatment. Inflammation of parotid and other salivary glands may occur in some rheumatoid and malignant diseases. Recurrent attacks of parotitis may be associated with an abnormal drainage system for saliva (sialectasis) and with stones in the duct. Occasionally an abscess forms, and is treated surgically.

PEDICULOSIS

Infestation with lice. These insects feed upon the dead outer layers of human skin and find ideal conditions in the clothing of the homeless and neglected. The skin rash that lice can cause may resemble dermatitis (qv) or, alternatively, may look like multiple reactions to insect bites. The diagnosis is established by examining the clothing of the affected individual, especially the seams where lice tend to gather. Washing and steam ironing the clothing is usually sufficient to eradicate the infestation.

Pediculosis capitis is the head louse (often called 'nits') and is seen especially in children. It is treated with a special medicated shampoo that kills both the lice and its eggs.

PELVIMETRY

Measurement of the size and shape of the pelvis. This is necessary during pregnancy to assess whether the pelvis is small or distorted and therefore more likely to cause problems during delivery.

Major abnormalities of pelvic size or shape can be detected by means of an internal (vaginal) examination, which is performed by an obstetrician. More exact information can be obtained from a pelvic X-ray, which

P

is done in unusual cases only (such as a breech presentation) and not until the last month of pregnancy. The amount of radiation used is very small and does not harm the fetus.

PEMPHIGUS

A serious skin disorder characterized by blisters. It usually appears between the ages of 40 and 60. The cause is unknown. The basic disorder is an autoimmune attack upon the epidermis (outer layer of the skin) which is directed against the protein that bonds the individual epidermal cells together. This attack leads to a separation of the epidermal cells from each other, with consequent blister formation within the normally compact epidermis. The blisters are easily ruptured and frequently the doctor will find just the eroded remains, often scattered widely over the body. Erosions often also appear in the mouth; in fact, these changes may precede the skin findings by many months.

Treatment is with systemic cortico-steroids. Complications are frequent, and result either from widespread skin erosions (such as septicaemia) or directly from steroid therapy.
SEE ALSO *Impetigo*

PEMPHIGUS NEONATURUM

see *Impetigo*

PEPTIC ULCER

A disease characterized by recurrent ulceration of the upper part of the small bowel (duodenal ulcer) and the lower part of the stomach (gastric ulcer). Approximately 10–20 per cent of people have a peptic ulcer at some stage in their lives. The precise causes of peptic ulcer disease remain unknown but two factors are thought to play a central role. The first is the amount of acid that the stomach produces (patients with duodenal ulceration secrete more acid) and the second is infection of the stomach with a bacterium called *Campylobacter pylori*. Other important factors include smoking, taking aspirin-like drugs and family history. Contrary to popular belief, stress does not seem important.

Symptoms include pain in the abdomen overlying the stomach, sometimes going through to the back; this pain is especially felt just prior to meals or late at night when acidity in the stomach is highest.

Complications such as severe bleeding, narrowing of the stomach outflow by scar tissue (pyloric stenosis), or perforation of the ulcer may require surgery.

Treatment is with acid-lowering drugs such as ranitidine or cimetidine. If infection in the form of *Campylobacter pylori* is present, the patient may receive a short course of antibiotics and bismuth (a heavy metal). Peptic ulceration is a chronic disease and successful treatment does not mean that the patient will be trouble-free; patients may either require repeated short courses of treatment or small doses of ranitidine or cimetidine to hold the condition in remission.

PERFUSION

The flow of blood through the small blood vessels, supplying blood to organs and tissue. If perfusion is poor, the oxygen supply is affected and there is a build-up of waste products. Perfusion is dependent on a good blood pressure and the potency (or 'openness') of small blood vessels. A sign of poor perfusion is coldness of the nose, fingers and toes.

PERICARDITIS

Inflammation of the pericardium, the fibrous membrane that surrounds and protects the outer surface of the heart. Acute pericarditis has many causes, most often viral infections, such as Coxsackie B, and heart attack; other causes include acute rheumatic fever, tuberculosis, systemic lupus erythematosus and kidney failure.

Symptoms are of the underlying disease, together with central chest pain and breathlessness. The condition may be detected by an ECG tracing (see *Electrocardiography*). NSAIDs are given to suppress inflammation and relieve pain. The outlook is generally good but depends on the underlying cause. Complications include pericardial effusion, in which fluid accumulates in the space between the pericardium and the heart. This interferes with the normal filling of the heart and when severe can cause cardiac arrest and death if the fluid is not drained.

Constrictive pericarditis may follow acute pericarditis, particularly when tuberculosis is the cause of the inflammation. The pericardium becomes thickened, rigid and calcified, and the heart is unable to fill properly. Symptoms are similar to those of heart failure, with fluid and swelling (oedema and ascites) in the abdomen and limbs, but the patient may not feel particularly breathless as there is less oedema in the lungs. Aspiration of the fluid effusions may produce temporary improvement, but in many cases surgical removal of part of the pericardium will be required.

PERIOD PROBLEMS

see *Amenorrhoea*, *Dysmenorrhoea*, *Menorrhagia*, *Mittelschmerz*, *Premenstrual tension*

PERITONITIS

Inflammation of the lining of the abdominal cavity (peritoneum) as a result of an accumulation of blood or bowel contents within the cavity. There are many causes of peritonitis but usually it is due to the perforation of a gastric or duodenal ulcer, of an infected appendix, or of the large bowel, either as a result of obstruction or diverticulitis (qv). The symptoms are severe abdominal pain, with fever and collapse of the circulation.

Initial treatment aims to relieve the pain and correct the low blood pressure (resulting from shock), and is followed immediately by surgery. Despite receiving such prompt treatment, peritonitis is still responsible for an appreciable number of deaths. It is particularly serious in the very young and the elderly.

PERSEVERATION

A term used to describe the senseless repetition of words or deeds by those suffering from organic brain disease. A person thus affected may respond appropriately to a question or command and then continue to give that same reply or perform that same action when a range of different answers or responses is required. For example, a patient may correctly touch his nose with his index finger when asked to do so but will then continue to touch the nose when asked to touch the left shoulder.

PES CAVUS

A foot with an abnormally high arch and therefore an unusually high instep; also known as claw foot. The clawing of toes usually accompanies pes cavus. In many cases the cause of the condition is unknown, but it

P

occurs in some neurological diseases (such as Friedreich's ataxia), and spinal dysraphism (maldevelopment of the lower spinal cord associated with spina bifida) or previous poliomyelitis may be responsible. Pes cavus is sometimes found in spondylolisthesis (congenital malalignment of the vertebrae in the lower part of the spine).

Treatment is generally unsatisfactory; special shoes may be helpful and in severe cases surgical tendon transfers, joint fusion or excision may help to improve the deformity or function of the foot.

PESSARY

These are either instruments designed to support a displaced or prolapsed uterus (womb), or suitably shaped bodies that are inserted into the vagina to deliver drug treatment.

A prolapsed uterus is often treated with surgery, but in some circumstances, perhaps if the patient is medically unfit or pregnant, a non-irritating polythene plastic pessary can be used instead to support the vagina and uterus. The pessary can cause infection or ulcers of the vagina, so patients are seen every 3—6 months for assessment.

Pessaries used to deliver drugs to the vagina are solid round or oval bodies. The pessary melts in the vagina, releasing whatever drug it contains. The drugs may be as varied as spermicides (for contraception), antibiotics (for infection) or prostaglandins (for inducing labour).

PETECHIA

A small area of bleeding from small blood vessels under the skin. Petechiae appear as small red dots. They commonly occur when there is an ab-

normality of the blood platelets, either because the number of platelets is low (for example, in thrombocytopenia) or because there is an abnormality of function (for example, in leukaemia).

PHAEOCHROMO-CYTOMA

A rare tumour, usually of the medulla or inner layer of the adrenal gland, although it can arise elsewhere. It is usually benign and some patients with the condition have tumours called chromaffonomas in other organs. The tumour secretes the hormones adrenaline and noradrenaline, which cause extremely high blood pressure (severe hypertension) together with an unduly rapid heartbeat (tachycardia). Occasionally the hormone secretion is intermittent, resulting in typical attacks; these consist of pallor, palpitations, headaches, sweating and nausea as well as very high blood pressure. If untreated the complications of hypertension (such as brain haemorrhage or kidney damage) can occur. Surgical removal of the tumour is the treatment of choice, but if this is not possible drug therapy is used.

PHARYNGITIS

Inflammation of the pharynx; this cavity lies behind the nose and mouth and provides the passage of communication to the larynx (voice-box) and oesophagus.

Inflammation is usually caused by both viruses and bacteria. Pharyngitis is more common in cold, damp weather and when resistance is low. It may occur in epidemic form in closed communities. Other causes are swallowing hot fluids or corrosives (for example, acids or strong alkalis, such as caustic soda), injury resulting from surgery, or abrasion or grazing.

Pharyngitis is sometimes an early stage of measles, scarlet fever, glandular fever or influenza.

The symptoms are sore throat, especially on swallowing, swollen glands in the neck (lymphadenopathy), fever and sometimes earache due to referred pain. Rest, fluids and aspirin usually ensure recovery within a few days. However, aspirin must be avoided in children because there is evidence that in rare cases it can cause a disease called Reye's syndrome.

PHENYLKETONURIA

see *Inborn errors of metabolism*

PHIMOSIS

Narrowing of the opening of the prepuce of the penis so that the foreskin cannot be readily retracted over the glans. Phimosis is usually congenital but may be acquired as a result of inflammatory fibrosis. Usually it is first noticed as a ballooning of the foreskin on urination or as an infection of the foreskin and glans or tip (balanitis). In its severe form the preputial orifice may be reduced to a mere pinhole. The treatment is circumcision.

PHLEBITIS

see *Thrombophlebitis*

PHLEBOGRAPHY

An X-ray examination of the veins; also called venography. Phlebography is usually used to investigate the veins of the calf and the leg in cases of suspected thrombosis, although virtually any vein in the body may be examined in this way. It is still regarded as the most accurate method of detecting deepvein thrombosis.

Veins are not distinguishable on ordinary X-rays, so it is necessary to make them opaque by injecting a non-toxic dye or contrast agent into one of the veins in the foot. Tourniquets are applied above the ankle and knee in order to contain the contrast agent in the region to be examined.

More sophisticated phlebographic techniques include the insertion of fine tubes (catheters) into the venous system; a contrast agent can be introduced through the tube to highlight individual veins deep within the body. It is also possible to take blood samples through the catheter; this technique is used in the search for very small hormone-secreting tumours.

PHOBIA

A neurosis in which the sufferer experiences anxiety when he or she is in particular situations. The anxiety is out of proportion to the demands of the situation, cannot be reasoned away and generally leads to an avoidance of the situation. Most phobias are commoner in women. The most common severe phobia is agarophobia. A social phobia is one in which a person feels anxiety in the presence of others, sometimes with a fear that he or she will fail to perform or will behave in a humiliating way. Examples include fear of writing, speaking, eating or urinating in the presence of others. Simple phobias are those which involve a single, often distressing fear − for example, of animals, heights, illness, dying, flying and so on. Animal phobias are particularly common in children.

In many phobias avoidance of the feared situation is thought to maintain the problem and so treatment usually entails exposure to it. Behaviour therapy is often used. Systematic desensitization is a technique often employed in conjunction with relaxation training to gradual expose the sufferer to the feared situation. Flooding, on the other hand, entails sudden exposure and appears to be at least as effective as other treatments. Medication, such as antidepressants and beta-blockers, is sometimes of benefit.

PHOTOPHOBIA

Abnormal sensitivity of the eyes to light. This may occur in an attack of migraine and also in any illness associated with fever. If the sensitivity is severe, meningitis may be indicated; in this case, marked drowsiness and severe neck stiffness may also be present. Detailed examination of the eyes should be sought if the symptoms are pronounced.

PHOTOSENSITIVITY

Excessive sensitivity of the skin to the effects of sunlight. The commonest cause is the ingestion of photosensitizing drugs, such as certain common diuretics, tranquillizers and antibiotics, to which some individuals are idiosyncratically sensitive. The skin becomes inflamed in those areas subjected to greatest exposure (usually the face, back of the neck and backs of the hands). In some cases, even the protection offered by clothing is insufficient and only areas additionally covered by underclothing are spared. The photosensitizing agent is sometimes difficult to track down, especially in those who habitually indulge in self-medication (over-the-counter laxatives, herbal remedies and so on).

Systemic diseases such as systemic lupus erythematosus and porphyria may also induce photosensitivity.

Other causes, such as xeroderma pigmentosum, are exceedingly rare. Treatment is directed at the underlying cause, such as identifying and discontinuing the offending drug.

PILES

see *Haemorrhoids*

PILL, THE

Oral hormone contraceptive preparations. These are among the most reliable methods of contraception available and are widely used, especially in industrialized countries. There are two main varieties of pill: combined preparations (containing the hormones oestrogen and progestogen) and progestogen-only preparations.

Combined preparations are used by a majority of women who choose oral contraception. They are very effective and work by stopping the release of an egg each month from the ovaries. The most serious side-effect of this pill is blood clotting (thrombosis). Other adverse effects include headache, dizziness, nausea, water retention, weight gain, tiredness, depression and a decrease in sexual drive. Women unsuited to combined preparations include those who smoke, who have a history of vascular disease or have high blood pressure. The risk of developing heart and blood vessel disease increases with age and other factors, such as lifestyle. Women who are on the pill are therefore advised to periodically review their method of contraception with a doctor or family planning clinic. Some women experience a delay of several weeks in returning to normal fertility after they have stopped taking the pill.

Progestogen-only preparations (the mini-pill), which are used by a minority of women, are slightly less effective than combined preparations. They work by thickening the cervical mucous and making the womb lining unwelcoming to fertilized eggs. The mini-pill has to be taken every day; there is no pattern of 21 days-on, 7-days off. The commonest side-effect is irregularity of periods, with spotting and bleeding between periods. Unlike the oestrogen-containing pill, the mini-pill does not raise blood pressure and is therefore suitable for women with high blood pressure. It is also useful if the woman is breast-feeding, since milk yield is unaffected, and for women in whom oestrogen side-effects are troublesome or expected.

The 'morning after' pill may be used if unprotected intercourse has taken place. These preparations have to be used within 72 hours for them to be effective. They are designed as an emergency method only.

Studies have failed to prove conclusively any link with the pill and breast or cervical cancer.
SEE ALSO *Contraception*

PITYRIASIS

A term which is used to describe any scaly skin condition. The two commonest skin conditions of this type are pityriasis versicolor and pityriasis rosea. All other such conditions bearing the prefix 'pityriasis' are rare.

Pityriasis versicolor is a minor infection of the skin which produces multiple, slightly scaly patches of increased or, more often, decreased pigmentation, about 1−2 cm (½−1 in) in diameter, scattered widely over the trunk. The condition is often first noticed when the affected areas fail to tan after prolonged exposure to sun. Treatment is directed against the infection and is in the form of a lotion.

Pityriasis rosea is a condition of unknown cause which often begins as

a single red scaly patch followed after a day or two by the wide-spread eruption of 1−2 cm (½−1 in) similar lesions. The condition produces no symptoms and clears up spontaneously after 6−8 weeks. If itching is a problem, then a mild steroid may be helpful.

PLACEBO

A 'pretend' or 'dummy' treatment. In order to establish whether a particular form of treatment works, it is important to compare the results with no treatment. Thus, one group of patients is given the treatment under test and another group receives the 'placebo'. In most trials this is 'double-blind': neither the patient nor the doctor knows which treatment is being given. Such trials are usually necessary in order to determine the efficacy of a new drug, especially in order to compensate for the substantial psychological benefit which any new treatment, even if subsequently shown to be of no benefit, may produce (the 'placebo' effect).

PLACENTA

The placenta, or afterbirth, is the organ through which the fetus obtains nourishment before birth. It develops from the fertilized egg and is connected to the fetus by the umbilical cord.

The placenta is expelled from the

P

The placenta acts as the lungs, liver and kidneys of the fetus. Oxygen for the energy needs of the fetus is transferred from the mother's circulation (1), where it is carried on red blood cells, to the blood of the fetus. Carbon dioxide and other waste products are transferred from the fetus to the mother's blood.

uterus (womb) shortly after the birth of the baby, during the third and final stage of labour. Most women are given an injection of the drug syntometrine during or immediately after the birth of the baby. This makes the uterus contract and expel the placenta quickly, which in turn prevents excessive blood loss. The midwife usually examines the placenta to ensure that it is whole. Otherwise infection or bleeding may result.

PLACENTA PRAEVIA

A condition in which the placenta or afterbirth is positioned low in the uterus (womb), covering the cervix (neck of the womb) and blocking the baby's passage to the vagina. It is a very dangerous condition and is usually associated with recurring episodes of vaginal bleeding in the last two months of pregnancy. The baby is invariably born by Caesarean section

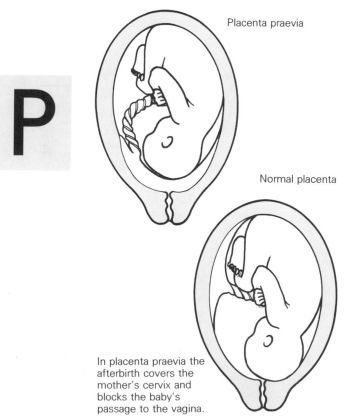

Placenta praevia

Normal placenta

In placenta praevia the afterbirth covers the mother's cervix and blocks the baby's passage to the vagina.

because the placenta blocks the birth canal. If the first episode of bleeding is very heavy, an emergency Caesarean section may be done. If the first bleed is light, the woman is admitted to hospital, where the diagnosis is established by means of an ultrasound scan. A planned Caesarean section will then be performed about two weeks before the expected date of delivery of the baby. A good outcome can be anticipated for mother and baby, provided there has been prompt admission to hospital.

PLASMAPHERESIS

A technique in which the patient's plasma is removed (but not the blood cells) and replaced with plasma protein; also known as plasma exchange. During the process of plasmapheresis, blood is removed, red cells and white cells separated, plasma discarded, and then the red and white cells are suspended in fresh plasma and re-transfused. By removing the plasma (the fluid component of blood) many substances are eliminated from the body. Some of these substances have been implicated as the agents which cause damage in some diseases — for example, immune complexes in systemic lupus erythematosus (qv) and antibodies in myasthenia gravis (qv). Plasmapheresis is used in the management of such conditions. The technique can be very effective, if only temporarily.

PLASTER OF PARIS

Calcium sulphate hemihydrate; after soaking in water, it sets like concrete, giving out heat. Special bandages impregnated with it are used to make 'plaster casts'. Once fractured bone is 'set' to the bone's normal shape (a procedure called reducing or

P

manipulating the fracture, it needs to be held in the correct position to allow healing and prevent movement of the fracture, which is very painful. The cast is therefore closely moulded to the joints above and below the fracture; skill is involved in doing this without causing chafing and sores to form beneath it. Plaster of Paris is heavy and has the disadvantage of softening in water. New lightweight, waterproof casts can be made from epoxy resins, but these are difficult to use and expensive.

PLATELET

Platelets are components of blood, made in the bone marrow by breaking off from a large cell called a megakaryocyte. Their main function is to assist in clot formation when a blood vessel is injured. The platelet can stick to the damaged vessel wall, change its shape to stick to other platelets, and discharge its contents to make further platelets stick together. A useful indicator of how well the platelets are functioning is the bleeding time, the time taken for a small skin cut to stop bleeding.

The normal platelet count is 150,000–400,000 per cu mm of blood ($150-400 \times 10^9$ per litre). An insufficient number of platelets causes a tendency to bleed, or thrombocytopenia (qv). A high platelet count is frequently a feature of bone marrow disease such as myeloma (qv).

PLEURISY

Inflammation of the pleura or covering of the lungs; it is usually a sign of underlying lung disease, but is occasionally due to injury. Causes include pneumonia, pulmonary embolism, lung tumours and abscesses.

Pleurisy is signalled by a characteristic stabbing pain, often felt just below the nipple, which is provoked by deep breathing, coughing and movement of the chest. It is often so severe that breathing is quick and shallow. There may be a dry cough and fever. The doctor may hear a noise through the stethoscope caused by the inflamed coverings rubbing against each other with each breath.

An X-ray may reveal a collection of fluid in the space between the coverings; this is known as a pleural effusion. Sometimes a sample of this fluid is drawn off through a fine needle in order that it may be examined for bacteria or cancer cells.

Treatment depends on the underlying cause.

PMS/PMT

see *Premenstrual tension*

PNEUMOCONIOSIS

A lung condition caused by inorganic dusts. The term includes many occupationally related diseases. There are two main groups, defined according to the type of dust involved: first, the inactive dusts, which accumulate in the lung but are harmless and thus do not really cause disease; and, secondly, the active dusts which may cause fibrosis of the lung and emphysema.

Coal miner's pneumoconiosis (anthracosis) is the best known example of 'active-dust' pneumoconiosis. In some cases it co-exists with silicosis, which appears to increase the severity of the disease. As well as developing emphysema, a small proportion of miners go on to develop large patches of fibrous tissues (progressive massive fibrosis), which are clearly visible on chest X-rays. The symptoms are those of any chronic lung disease, principally cough and shortness of breath. Somewhat surprisingly, however, patients with the most striking X-ray abnormalities often have fewer symptoms and less impairment of lung function than do some with less marked X-ray abnormalities. Other 'active dust' pneumoconioses include those due to exposure to aluminium powder, hard metals (eg tungsten carbide), kaolin, beryllium and asbestos. There is no treatment.

PNEUMOCYSTIS CARINII PNEUMONIA

A form of pneumonia; pneumocystis is the most common opportunistic infection in patients with AIDS. It was formerly classified as a protozoan (a primitive unicellular organism), but has more recently been included in the fungi. It is present in most adults, but only multiplies and causes symptoms when immunity is depressed. Pneumocystis is signalled by a dry, persistent cough with breathlessness, often accompanied by fever. The diagnosis is made by bronchial lavage, and identifying the organism in the lung secretions. It can be readily treated by large doses of the antibiotic co-trimoxazole, or by inhalation of pentamidine. Preventative treatment is now given to patients at risk in the form of inhalations of pentamidine every 2 or 4 weeks.

PNEUMONECTOMY

Surgical removal of a lung. Today this is usually a part of the treatment of cancer of the bronchi or airways (bronchial carcinoma). The lung is removed by dividing the pulmonary artery and veins to the lung, together with the main bronchus. A chest drainage tube is placed into the cavity for a few days after the operation. Postoperative recovery is surprisingly rapid and patients are usually allowed home within 7 to 12 days of surgery.

Careful pre-operative assessment is necessary to ascertain that the remaining lung is sufficient to allow the patient to breathe adequately. This is particularly important, as most patients undergoing pneumonectomy have been smokers and are therefore likely to have other lung diseases.

PNEUMONIA

A respiratory infection involving lung tissue; it is distinct from the generally less serious bronchitis, in which disease is limited to the airways. A small number of bacterial species are responsible for most pneumonias (pneumococcus and haemophilus in particular) but 'atypical' pneumonias caused by relatively unusual organisms are becoming more common (see, for example, Legionnaires' disease, Psittacosis and Pneumocystis pneumonia). Tuberculosis may cause fatal bronchopneumonia if not treated early, and pneumonias caused by viruses, though relatively rare, may also have a poor outcome. Symptoms include a rise in temperature and pulse rate, shortness of breath and a cough which produces thick, discoloured phlegm (yellow or green). Pain in the chest on breathing in may occasionally be felt.

Bronchopneumonia, which results from infection of the bronchi (the major airways leading to the lungs), occurs most frequently in children, in whom it is often a complication of viral illness such as measles or whooping cough, and in the elderly. In adults it may occur 2–3 days after the onset of acute bronchitis; it is often a complication of chronic bronchitis or emphysema. Bronchopneumonia is associated with an increased death rate in the very young and old and remains a common and relatively gentle mode of death in those terminally ill from other causes.

Lobar pneumonia affects a specific segment (or lobe) of lung and is usually found in those without a pre-existing respiratory disease; it is therefore sometimes known as primary pneumonia. The bacterium-like mycoplasma is an important cause of this type of pneumonia.

Aspiration pneumonia results from the inhalation of vomited stomach contents and has serious consequences, both because of infection and from the presence of gastric acid which partially digests the inflamed tissue.

Most patients with pneumonia can be diagnosed from clinical examination and chest X-ray, with blood and sputum tests to confirm which organism is causing the infection. Treatment is with injected antibiotics, oxygen and physiotherapy to aid expectoration of phlegm. The outcome depends on the type of pneumonia and on the previous health of the patient. Most patients recover from the condition.

PNEUMOTHORAX

Partial or complete collapse of the lung due to air entering the space between the lung and the chest wall. The commonest form is spontaneous pneumothorax, which occurs in young, healthy adults, and usually results from rupture of an air-containing 'blob' on the surface of the lung. The condition can recur in 50 per cent of cases. Chest pain and breathlessness are the usual symptoms. Patients with asthma, emphysema and other chest diseases are predisposed to pneumothorax. Chest injury, such as stabbing, is frequently complicated by pneumothorax. If the leak from the lung is one-way (ball-valve effect), a build-up of air pressure may follow, giving rise to a tension pneumothorax. This can cause a severe reduction in output from the heart and is a medical emergency. It is treated in the same way as an uncomplicated pneumothorax, by releasing the air trapped in the cavity. This is achieved by inserting a needle through the chest wall and into the air-containing cavity; the needle is attached to a rubber tube which ends in a container of water so that air is slowly released to bubble out through the water but cannot be sucked back in again because of the water seal.

POLIOMYELITIS

An infectious viral disease which occurs in epidemics in some developing countries. In developed countries, the number of cases has dramatically decreased following the introduction of routine immunization. Transmission is via saliva and faeces. The incubation period is 1–3 weeks. Early symptoms are mild and non-specific, with fever, diarrhoea and a headache. These subside after a few days to be followed by the major illness with signs of viral meningitis, vomiting, stiff neck, headache and aversion to bright lights. This may progress to paralysis, but fewer than 10 per cent of those infected develop paralysis, the remainder recovering completely after the initial febrile or meningitic illness. If paralysis does progress, any muscle group may be involved. Bed rest is advisable in the early stages of poliomyelitis, followed by physiotherapy. Recovery may not be complete and some cases are fatal, despite intensive treatment.

P

POLYARTERITIS NODOSA

A rare inflammatory condition affecting particularly the medium and small arteries in which damage to the vessel wall may result in localized dilatation of the vessels. The cause of the condition is unknown, although abnormalities of the body's immune system which cause antibody-antigen complexes to be deposited in vessel walls may be involved. Most cases occur in those aged between 40 and 60 years, with men affected more frequently than women. The condition is usually signalled by fever, malaise (a general feeling of being unwell) and weight loss, together with symptoms relating to the particular organs involved, which may be the skin, kidneys, heart, joints, gastro-intestinal tract or nervous system.

The condition requires vigorous treatment with agents that suppress immune responses, such as steroids, and sometimes also with more toxic immunosuppresive drugs. The outlook depends on the extent and severity of organ damage.

POLYCYSTIC KIDNEY DISEASE

An inherited condition in which normal kidney tissue is replaced by innumerable cysts. There are two types of polycystic kidney disease: adult and infantile. The first type is inherited in an autosomal dominant manner, and the second in an autosomal recessive manner (see both *Dominant* and *Recessive patterns of inheritance*).

The adult form is the more common and usually becomes apparent between the ages of 30 and 50, although it can appear earlier or in the elderly. Symptoms include blood in the urine (haematuria), high blood pressure, bacterial infection of the kidney (pyelonephritis) or chronic kidney failure. The kidneys may become grossly enlarged and loin pain is frequent. An ultrasound scan will show up the renal cysts; liver cysts, which occur in about one-third of patients, will also be revealed in this way. Treatment aims at clearing up urinary infections, controlling blood pressure and dealing with the complications of chronic renal failure. Rarely, removal of the kidney (nephrectomy) may be required if the bleeding cannot be stopped. Kidney failure is progressive and many patients require dialysis or transplantation, although the age at which this occurs is very variable.

The infantile form of polycystic kidney disease is much rarer. In addition to renal cysts, liver fibrosis is found. Progression of the disease is very variable. Severe cases may die from renal failure in the first few months of life. The older the child when the disease becomes apparent, the less severe the renal disease but the more severe the damage to the liver. Symptoms and treatment are the same as for the adult form of the disease. Antenatal diagnosis may be available in the near future.

POLYCYTHAEMIA

An increase in red blood cells and haemoglobin (the red pigment in blood) above 175 grams per litre in men and 155 grams per litre in women. There are a variety of causes. Polycythaemia can occur in order to compensate for low oxygen in the body (for example, at high altitudes or in people who smoke); as a result of the over-production of a chemical called erythropoietin, which stimulates the red cell precursors to grow in the bone marrow (primary poly-cythaemia); or as a feature of chronic alcoholism (secondary polycythaemia).

In primary polycythaemia there is an underlying proliferative disorder in the bone marrow which can result in a high white cell and platelet count as well as an increase in red cells and haemoglobin. In secondary polycythaemia a reduction in the volume of plasma (the fluid component of blood) − in prolonged vomiting, for example − leads to an increase in haemoglobin. Both primary and secondary polycythaemia cause thickening of the blood with reduced blood flow, resulting in a tendency to clot. The condition may be signalled by venous thrombosis or a stroke. The simplest form of treatment of the primary form is removal of blood by venesection (qv). In other cases treatment is that of the underlying cause.

POLYMOSITIS

see *Myositis*

POLYMYALGIA RHEUMATICA

An autoimmune disease characterized by aching and stiffness in the shoulder and hip girdles, particularly in the morning. The condition is found predominantly in patients over 60 years of age, women being affected more often than men. Onset may be insidious over several weeks, or may be sudden; it is often associated with symptoms such as fatigue, loss of appetite, weight loss and depression. Blood tests may help in the diagnosis; in particular, the erythrocyte sedimentation rate (ESR), measuring the 'sinking rate' of red blood corpuscles, is invariably raised, indicating disease activity. The condition may be associated with giant cell arteritis (qv).

The symptoms of polymyalgia rheumatica usually respond dramatically to steroid therapy, which may have to be continued for several years. The condition may be debilitating, often with marked pain and stiffness in the limbs; difficulty in getting out of the bed or bath is common.

POLYNEUROPATHY

see *Neuropathy*

POLYP

A growth attached by a stalk to the surface from which it arises. The term refers only to the shape and not to the nature of the growth. Some polyps, such as those found in the bladder, are true tumours, while others (those arising inside the nose and ears, for example) are caused by inflammation. Some polyps found inside the womb may be due to a hormonal imbalance. Bowel polyps may be tumours or may arise as a consequence of inflammation. Polyps may be either single or multiple. Only a minority of tumour polyps are cancerous. Most polyps can be removed and cured by surgery.

POLYPOSIS

The presence of a very large number of polyps. Familial polyposis coli is the most important condition of this type. In this hereditary disease (1 in 8000 births) the large bowel is studded with numerous polypoid tumours. A child born to an affected parent has a 50 per cent chance of developing the disease. The condition is not apparent at birth and the polyps develop gradually during childhood. These invariably become cancerous with time. The treatment consists of surgically removing the affected part of the bowel around the age of 20 years, when growth is complete.

P

In another, rarer, form of familial polyposis (called Peutz-Jeghers syndrome), polyps are found throughout the gut together with brownish pigmentation around the mouth. These polyps do not become cancerous and are left untreated.

PORPHYRIA

A rare group of inherited and acquired disorders affecting the metabolism of haemoglobin (the red pigment in blood). These disorders can be due to a defect in metabolism of either the liver or the bone marrow. Acute intermittent porphyria is characterized by severe attacks of abdominal pain and neuropsychiatric symptoms (tingling in the limbs and acute psychosis); drugs such as barbiturates, and alcohol and the contraceptive pill can set off an attack. Variegate porphyria also involves neuropsychiatric symptoms, and a severe skin sensitivity to sunlight and injury; sufferers were thought to be the original werewolves, because the skin reaction caused severe disfigurement, they were more hairy than unaffected people and had psychiatric symptoms. Porphyria cutanea tarda also has a skin reaction associated with it; those affected also invariably have liver disease.

Diagnosis is by detecting the abnormal byproducts of blood metabolism (porphyrins) in either the urine or faeces; often the urine has a typical 'port-wine' colour. At present there is no cure.
SEE ALSO *Idiosyncrasy*

PORTAL HYPERTENSION

A sustained increase in the blood pressure in the veins running between the intestines and the liver (portal vein).

Food products which are absorbed by the intestines are transported to the liver via this system. Portal hypertension is due to disease which causes scarring to the liver (cirrhosis), a block in the main portal vein before it gets to the liver, or blockage of the veins leading from the liver.

The increased pressure in the portal vein leads to a swelling of veins in areas where the portal system joins the systemic system (that is, the oesophagus, rectum and umbilical regions). These swollen veins are similar to the varicose veins normally seen on the lower leg. The most serious problems arise in oesophageal varices, which are engorged abnormal veins at the lower end of the oesophagus.

Their tendency to bleed can often be life-threatening. Emergency treatment includes controlling the bleeding with drugs (such as vasopressin), or injecting the veins with an agent to block them. Also, a balloon swallowed by mouth (Sengstaken tube) can be blown up in the oesophagus to press on to the veins for a short period of time.

PORT-WINE STAIN

An uncommon form of birth mark or haemangioma composed of capillaries (the smallest blood vessels). It is present at birth and is often extensive. Common sites are the face and limbs. The mark is usually pink at birth and darkens with age (like port, hence the name). Unlike some other birth marks, it does not disappear. Occasionally a facial port-wine stain is accompanied by abnormal blood vessels in the brain, leading to epilepsy (Sturge-Weber syndrome, qv). Very rarely, an arm or leg may grow larger than normal because of abnormal blood supply associated with a mark on the limb.

The skin discoloration caused by a port-wine stain cannot be treated surgically, but skilful make-up is effective for disguising any unsightly facial blemishes.

POSTPARTUM HAEMORRHAGE

Vaginal blood loss as a consequence of childbirth. The haemorrhage may be primary or secondary. Primary postpartum haemorrhage is vaginal blood loss in excess of 500 ml (1 pint) occurring within 24 hours of child-birth. Excessive bleeding after this time is less common but similarly caused and is termed secondary post-partum haemorrhage.

Primary haemorrhage may be a result of injury (vaginal or cervical tears) or failure of the uterus (womb) to contract after delivery of the infant. The latter means that blood vessels fail to constrict in the area where the placenta (afterbirth) is/was embedded. This phenomenon may occur sponta-neously (uterine atony) or may be caused by failure to separate and expel the placenta.

Haemorrhage may be severe and lead to shock; in this situation the rapid correction of blood loss and treatment of the cause of bleeding are essential.

Several conditions may predispose to post-partum haemorrhage. These include uterine overdistension (caused by twins, or excessive amniotic fluid), uterine fibroids, failure of the bloodclotting mechanism, several previous pregnancies, and antepartum haemorrhage.

The drug ergometrine is used to induce uterine contraction in cases of atony and also to assist in expelling the retained placenta. Only very rarely nowadays is manual removal of the placenta required. The introduction

of this drug and the provision of properly equipped delivery facilities have contributed significantly to the prevention of maternal death due to postpartum haemorrhage.

POTT'S FRACTURE

A group of fractures of the ankle joint associated with a degree of dislocation of the joint surfaces; the ligaments around the ankle joint may also be ruptured. Pott's fractures are caused by injuries that turn the ankle in or out and leave the joint itself very unstable. They may be associated with a 'twisted' ankle, when the foot is fixed in one position and the leg is forcibly rotated at the ankle joint.

There are many types of Pott's fracture, so no single treatment is ap-propriate. All require immobilization, either in a plaster cast or else by internal fixation using plates, wires or screws (see *Fixation*). Pott's fractures take six weeks or longer to heal.

PRE-ECLAMPSIA

see *Eclampsia*

PREMATURE BABY

Premature or pre-term babies are born before the thirty-seventh week of pregnancy (term being from 37–42 weeks, with an average of 40). Some-times there is an obvious reason for pre-term birth, such as infection of the uterus (womb), bleeding from the placenta (afterbirth) or pre-eclampsia (qv) but it often remains unexplained. With rare exceptions, babies born before 24 weeks do not survive, because their lungs are too immature to inflate.

The extent of problems experienced by pre-term babies depends on the degree of prematurity. Generally,

P

those less than 30 weeks (usually weighing less than 1.5 kg (3 lb 5 oz) have major problems and require neonatal intensive care facilities. Problems include heat loss through thin, poorly insulated skin, and this requires nursing in an incubator; immature lungs (respiratory distress syndrome); feeding difficulties, which sometimes can only be overcome by the giving of nutrition intravenously; infection, which needs antibiotic treatment; and haemorrhage into the brain or its lining (detected by ultrasound).

Most pre-term babies remain on a neonatal unit until close to their expected date of delivery. Babies weighing more than 1kg (2 lb 3 oz) have about a 90 per cent chance of survival. Under 1 kg (2 lb 3 oz) the outlook is not so good.

PREMATURE BEAT

see *Ectopic beat*

PREMENSTRUAL TENSION (PMT)

Premenstrual tension or syndrome (PMT or PMS) may be defined as any combination of emotional or physical features which occur cyclically in a woman before menstruation (period) and which disappear during menstruation. Symptoms vary from culture to culture, but this represents different attitudes towards 'women's problems' and different ways of communicating both physical and emotional complaints.

Psychological symptoms include irritability, depression, anxiety, fatigue, headache, low sex drive, and reduced confidence and concentration. Physical symptoms include the swelling of fingers, legs, abdomen and breasts, breast tenderness, skin greasiness and acne, and a change in bowel and bladder function. Certain disease processes, including hay fever, asthma, migraine or epilepsy, may be activated by PMT.

Patients are often required to keep a chart of their symptoms over several months to provide conclusive evidence of premenstrual tension. Discussion of the symptoms is important in the treatment. It is also important for a woman's partner to realize that the symptoms are not imagined. Various drug treatments have been used with varying success. These include minor tranquillizers, progesterone, vitamin B6 (pyridoxine) and the oral contraceptive pill.

PRENATAL DIAGNOSIS

see *Antenatal diagnosis*

PRESBYOPIA

Natural changes in the eye which occur with age and as a result of which progressive hypermetropia (long-sightedness) develops. From the late teens onwards the lens of the eye gradually becomes less pliable and able to adapt itself to different focal lengths. This is not noticeable until the forties by which age the refractive power of the eye cannot be sufficiently increased to enable near objects to be seen clearly. Small print too appears blurred unless it is held at arm's length.

Presbyopia can be corrected with a convex lens. Distance vision, for which the higher refractive power of the lens is not required, remains unaffected. The lenses are placed in 'half-moon frames', as they are only required for close work.

PROCIDENTIA

Prolapse of the uterus (womb). There

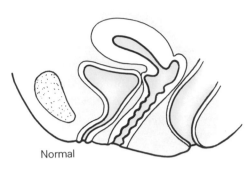

Normal

In the early stages of procidentia the uterus (**1**) may fall into the vagina (**2**) causing it to bulge. In a complete prolapse, the uterus protrudes through the vaginal opening (**3**).

are three types of uterine prolapse. The first is called a cystocoele, which occurs when the front wall of the vagina is weak, allowing the bladder to bulge into the vagina. The second is called a rectocoele, in which the back wall of the vagina is weak, allowing the rectum to bulge into the vagina. The third type is called an enterocoele, in which the top part of the vagina is weak, allowing the bowel to bulge into the top of the vagina. These abnormalities may be present singly or there may be a combination of two or more. All are associated with a sensation of 'something coming down'. Prolapse may also be associated with difficulty in emptying the bladder or bowel.

Prolapse is more common in elderly women, especially those who have had large families. The treatment is usually surgical and consists of vaginal hysterectomy (removal of the uterus through the vagina. The front and back walls of the vagina are usually repaired at the same time (colporrhaphy). If surgery is not recommended, because the patient's general health is poor, a ring pessary (qv) may be inserted into the vagina to support the womb and prevent it prolapsing.

PROCTITIS

Inflammation of the rectum (the last part of the large bowel). Proctitis has a number of causes, including diseases such as ulcerative colitis, Crohn's disease, venereal or sexually transmitted disease (particularly Herpes simplex infection) and infective diseases. Sufferers may get diarrhoea, often with blood, pus and mucus. They also sometimes experience pain on passing a motion and a feeling of incomplete emptying of the rectum (tenesmus). Sensation in the rectum may be impaired and sufferers may therefore experience what is called 'urgency', with little warning that they will pass a motion.

Diagnosis depends on the outcome of sigmoidoscopy (qv); in this a small rigid tube is introduced through the anus to look at the lower bowel and take samples for microscopic examination. Treatment may involve the use of prednisolone suppositories or creams, or the specific treatment of an infection.

PROGNOSIS

The estimation of the future course of a disease. It is often used to describe malignancy. Prognosis is considered poor in cases in which the growth of a tumour is rapid and response to treatment poor. The prediction of prognosis depends on the observation of a number of other individuals with a similar condition.

P

PROGRESSIVE BULBAR PALSY

Degeneration of the nerves that normally control the muscles of the lips, tongue, palate, larynx (voice-box) and pharynx. The condition usually occurs as part of motor neurone disease (qv). The onset is insidious but the condition invariably gets worse. The tongue becomes wasted and shrunken and shows obvious fasciculation (random contractions of groups of muscle fibre). Eventually it cannot be stuck out of the mouth. Speech becomes slurred because of paralysis of the lips, tongue and palate. At first the sufferer occasionally chokes on fluids but this progresses until he or she is unable to swallow; food is regurgitated through the nose or inhaled into the lungs, causing aspiration pneumonia.

PROLACTINOMA

A tumour of the cells in the pituitary gland at the base of the brain which produce a hormone called prolactin; this hormone initiates the production of milk for breast feeding. Raised levels of circulating prolactin are a symptom of prolactinoma, and as well as causing milk production can also interfere with the normal process of ovulation and menstruation, leading to infertility. The tumour itself can cause pressure on nearby structures such as the optic nerves and can thus lead to impairment of vision.

Treatment usually involves oral medication, although in some cases surgical removal of the tumour together with most or all of the pituitary gland may be necessary.

PROLAPSE

The slipping down of some organ or structure. The term is chiefly applied to downward displacements of the rectum and womb (uterus); for details of the latter, see *Procidentia*. It is also used to indicate protrusion of part of an intervertebral disc into the spinal canal (intervertebral space or foramen), see *Slipped disc*.

Prolapse of part of the rectum can occasionally occur in children as a result of a bowel movement. Treatment involves replacing the prolapsed part and, if necessary, retaining it in position by means of a soft pad. The condition tends to diminish as the child grows older. Prolapse of the bowel may also occur in elderly people with lax anal musculature, and is treated surgically.

PROPHYLAXIS

Any procedure which prevents disease. Examples include vaccination and the use of antimalarial drugs for travellers to countries where such disease is endemic. Prophylactic treatment with antibiotics carries a theoretical risk of allowing resistant bacteria to develop, but is of clear benefit in high-risk situations; for examples, when used in a patient with valvular heart disease who needs to undergo dental treatment or some surgical procedure.

PROSTATECTOMY

Surgical removal of the male prostate gland, which lies at the neck of the bladder; the urethra, which drains the bladder, passes through it. This used to be an 'open' operation involving an incision in the lower abdomen. With the advent of fibre-optic endoscopic equipment and the transurethral resectoscope, it is now routine to perform a transurethral resection (removal) of the prostate by passing the instrument along the urethra. This

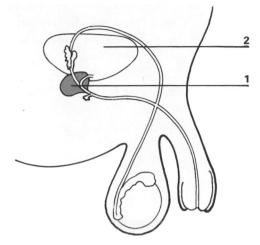

In later life the prostate gland **(1)** is apt to increase in size and change in shape. This can obstruct the flow of urine from the bladder **(2)** and cause great difficulty in urinating. Removal of the gland (prostatectomy) is the most effective treatment for the condition.

allows a more rapid recovery than the traditional operation.

Prostatectomy is most commonly performed for benign prostatic hypertrophy in elderly men, which causes difficulty in urination. It is also performed for prostatic cancer.

PROSTHESIS

An artificial spare part used to restore the function or appearance of a natural part. For example, the replacement of blood vessels and heart valves with functional plastic materials or total hip replacement using metal, with plastic or ceramic components. Cosmetic prostheses are used to disguise defects such as a lost ear or eye, or may be implanted (like a breast implant after mastectomy). Artificial limbs are specially tailored to each amputee and are highly sophisticated, particularly for the arm and hand, with functional joints and motors with variable power, which are modified according to requirements.

PROTEINURIA

An excessive amount of protein in the urine; a normal amount is defined as less than 0.15 g per day. Small amounts are common and do not necessarily indicate kidney disease; they can occur, for example, with febrile illnesses, urine infections or after heavy physical exertion. Proteinuria of between 1 and 2 g per day usually indicates kidney disease (most often glomerulonephritis, qv), but does not cause the complications of heavy proteinuria, exceeding 3 g per day, in which nephrotic syndrome (qv) may develop. Important systemic diseases that produce glomerulonephritis and proteinuria include diabetes mellitus, amyloidosis, systemic lupus erythematosus and arteritis. Proteinuria during pregnancy may indicate the development of pre-eclampsia (see *Eclampsia*).

The investigation of proteinuria requires assessment of renal function, imaging the kidneys for structural abnormality and searching for evidence of systemic disease. Screening tests for proteinuria with so-called reagent strips are very sensitive and a positive test should always be confirmed and quantified on a 24-hour urine collection. In many cases a renal biopsy is performed to establish the exact cause. Treatment depends on that underlying cause.

PSEUDOGOUT

A condition which derives its name from the fact of its clinical similarities to gout. Like gout, it is caused by deposition of crystals in the joints and the surrounding soft tissues, but whereas in gout the crystals are of uric acid, in pseudogout they are of calcium pyrophosphate. Pseudogout is usually signalled by acute arthritis, often

P

affecting only one joint. It commonly affects the elderly, particularly women. Often there is no obvious cause for an attack, but sometimes it follows a minor injury or another illness. Inflammation in the joint (most commonly the knee but also sometimes the ankle, shoulder, elbow or wrist) develops over a 24-hour period.

The natural course of the condition is to clear up over a few weeks but in the acute stages treatment with an anti-inflammatory drug (see *NSAID*) may be of benefit.

PSITTACOSIS

A chlamydial (see *Chlamydia*) infection of parrots and budgerigars which is occasionally transmitted to humans. Some infected birds may show no obvious illness but others have diarrhoea and a nasal discharge. Psittacosis causes pneumonia in humans, who become infected by inhaling contaminated dust or by direct contact. Symptoms include fever, aching, a headache and a cough. The diagnosis is confirmed by blood tests. The treatment consists of tetracycline antibiotics. Generally the patient improves after 1–2 weeks. Only in a few cases does psittacosis develop into a serious illness, when inflammation of the heart and death may follow.

PSORIASIS

A common skin condition the exact cause of which remains unknown. About 2 per cent of the population are affected; Those most likely to suffer have a family history of the disorder. The typical skin lesions are red, scaly plaques varying in size from 0.2 cm to many centimetres in diameter. The scalp is a common site. The nails may become deformed. The condition tends to wax and wane, sometimes going into spontaneous remission (perhaps for prolonged periods) and at other times being particularly resistant to treatment. Usually the patient remains in excellent general health and the disorder has no internal associations, although occasionally arthritis occurs. Sometimes the disease seems to be precipitated by infection or drugs, but in most cases there is no obvious cause.

Treatment usually consists of direct applications of substances such as tar or the drug dithranol, although occasionally systemic treatment is required for particularly severe cases. Both natural and artificial sunlight treatment may lead to considerable improvement. Most of these treatments work, at least in part, by slowing down the rate at which the skin proliferates, because in psoriasis this rate is substantially accelerated. There is no known cure for psoriasis and all treatments are effective only in the sense that they bring the patient some relief.

PSYCHOSIS

A term used to describe major mental illnesses and often contrasted with neurosis. In psychosis severe symptoms of psychiatric disorder, such as delusions and hallucinations, are likely to occur. Unlike the patient with neurosis, though, the psychotic patient retains little or no insight into the morbid nature of his experiences and he may act on them. A distinction is sometimes drawn between organic psychosis, in which delusions and hallucinations arise as a result of an identifiable cause of brain malfunction (such as delirium tremens or dementia), and functional psychosis in which no external cause is evident. In practice the term psychosis is often used as a synonym for the latter group, of which schizophrenia (qv), manic-depressive psychosis (qv) and severe depression (qv) are the commonest examples.

PSYCHOSOMATIC DISEASE

A physical disorder which is viewed as being caused by or associated with psychological factors. Diseases which have in the past been viewed as having a psychosomatic element include asthma, diabetes mellitus, ulcerative colitis, peptic ulcers and hypertension (high blood pressure). Because it has proved difficult to describe specific psychological or personality characteristics associated with particular illnesses, the term psychosomatic has become less popular in medical circles. It nevertheless remains plausible to suggest that the course of recurrent illnesses, such as diabetes mellitus and asthma, may in some sufferers be influenced by psychological and social circumstances.

PSYCHOTHERAPY

A form of psychological treatment generally used for milder forms of mental illness. The two best known types are psychodynamic (or psycho-analytic) psychotherapy and cognitive psychotherapy.

In psychodynamic psychotherapy a patient sees a therapist once or more each week for at least a year. As in psychoanalysis (from which this form of treatment derives) the goal is to help patients achieve an insight into the origins of their behaviour and feelings, and thereby help them to change. Psychodynamic psychotherapy is used mainly in mild cases of neurosis and depression.

Cognitive psychotherapy is less intensive than psychodynamic psy-chotherapy, with patients seeing a therapist once weekly over a period of several months. This type of therapy views psychiatric problems as arising from maladaptive attitudes and from the expectations patients have of themselves and others. It focuses on helping a patient develop new attitudes and new ways of dealing with problem situations. Cognitive psychotherapy is used as a treatment for less severe depression, neuroses, and bulimia nervosa.

PTOSIS

Drooping of the upper eyelid. This may occur as a congenital maldevel-opment of the muscle of the upper eyelid, or as an acquired lesion of either the nerves supplying the muscle or a muscle disease itself. In the congenital condition treatment is aimed at preventing defective vision (ambly-opia). Acquired nerve disorders affecting either the third cranial nerve or the cervical sympathetic nerves will cause ptosis, usually in one eye only; in this case the underlying cause is found and treated as appropriate. Muscle diseases such as myasthenia gravis also cause ptosis and need appropriate treatment.

PUBERTY

A phase in human development during which sexual maturity is reached; it is associated with a growth spurt. It usually occurs between 12 and 15 years of age. In boys puberty is ac-companied by a rise in the male hor-mone testosterone. The penis, prostate, seminal vesicles and epididymis mature, and the muscles grow. In girls, menstruation and ovulation begin, the breasts and vagina mature, and subcutaneous fat grows. Some-times puberty occurs either earlier or later than the norm. Rarely this is abnormal and due to a variety of diseases affecting the hypothalamus and pituitary gland of the brain, or the ovaries or testes.

PUERPERAL FEVER

A temperature of 38°C (100.4°F) occurring on any two days within fourteen days after abortion or delivery. The underlying cause is an infection. The principal sites which give rise to the fever are the chest, urinary tract, breasts, legs and any surgical wounds.

The genital tract is particularly vulnerable to infection after delivery as the normal protective barriers are temporarily weakened. Predisposing factors include blood loss and the presence of retained placental tissue or bruising of the tissues as a result of delivery. Before the introduction of antibiotics, postpartum (postnatal) or puerperal sepsis was a common cause of maternal death but now more frequently it occurs as a low-grade infection. Such pelvic infection needs to be diagnosed and treated quickly to prevent the risk of chronic pelvic inflammation and subsequent infertility. The treatment of puerperal fever essentially involves locating the source of infection and then treating it appropriately with antibiotics.

PULSE

The pulse wave from a heart beat, felt in the arteries of the body. It is felt wherever a medium or large artery lies near the surface of the skin. The radial pulse is felt in the wrist, carotid pulse in the neck, brachial pulse at the bend of the elbow, and femoral pulse in the groin. By 'taking the pulse' abnormalities in rate, strength, rhythm and character can be assessed. This gives important clues to diseases of the heart. The normal rate is between 65 and 80 beats per minute.

The main venous pulse is the jugular venous pulse in the neck, which is examined for its rise and fall (wave form) and the extent to which it can be seen above the level of the heart. It reflects function in the right atrium, one of the upper chambers of the heart. Abnormalities in venous pulse are caused by heart failure, disease of the tricuspid valve in the heart, and by electrical conduction defects in the heart.

PURPURA

Easy bruising and spontaneous bleeding from the small blood vessels of the skin. It can occur in infections, particularly if there is toxic damage of the cell walls of the small blood vessels. A particular type of purpura, called HenochSchönlein purpura, may occur in children following acute infection. In this type a rash is found on the limbs, knees and elbows, and there may also be lesions in the gut and kidneys, resulting in bleeding. Purpura can also occur in vitamin C deficiency (scurvy) when the capillaries become abnormally fragile, and in any condition in which the blood platelets are reduced in number (thrombocytopenic purpura and leukaemia, for example). Treatment with steroids may also result in purpura.

PUS

A complex mixture of proteins and cells suspended in fluid and the result of some form of infection. Usually the predominant cell type is the neutrophil, a white blood cell whose particular function is to eradicate bacterial infection. Pus which is yellow or greenish-yellow in colour, depending upon the nature of the infecting organism, is found in abscesses, on ulcers and any suppurating surfaces.

PUSTULE

A small (0.3–0.5 cm/$\frac{1}{10}$–$\frac{1}{5}$ in) skin lesion containing small amounts of pus. Pustules do not usually have any serious significance. They appear in greater numbers in people with acne vulgaris and may sometimes be associated with widespread folliculitis (infection of the hair follicles). If they are particularly numerous or unusually frequent, then bacterial culture of the pus they contain should lead to identification of the cause and the prescribing of appropriate antibiotics. Failure to improve may be associated with underlying diabetes mellitus.

PYELONEPHRITIS

Bacterial infection of the kidney(s). The condition may be acute or chronic. Acute pyelonephritis usually results from the spread of bacteria up the ureters (the tubes leading from the kidneys to the bladder) in cystitis, and is more common in pregnancy when the ureters are dilated. The symptoms are fever, shivering and pain over the affected kidney(s); the symptoms of cystitis, such as frequency of urination and burning sensation on passing water, may also be present. Prompt treatment with antibiotics is usually successful, and serious complications are therefore unusual. Pyelonephritis is more likely to occur in those who have a kidney abnormality, such as malformation, stones or hydronephrosis, and so an investigation of kidney structure and function is usually carried out.

Chronic pyelonephritis is characterized by small, scarred kidneys and is usually diagnosed in patients who are being given tests for high blood pressure or kidney failure. There are often no symptoms. Active kidney infection is rarely found, and the disease is most often the result of previous kidney damage (usually in childhood) from a combination of vesico-ureteric reflux (urine flowing back from the bladder into the pelvis of the kidney during urination) and urine infection. The treatment of chronic pyelonephritis consists of dealing with the complications, such as high blood pressure and kidney failure, and any urine infections; appropriate antibiotics are given for the latter.

PYLORIC STENOSIS

Narrowing of the outlet of the stomach, or pylorus. In adults it is a complication of diseases such as stomach ulceration or stomach cancer. In infants it is caused by enlargement of the ring-shaped pyloric muscle, which surrounds the junction between stomach and duodenum (the first part of the intestine).

The diagnosis is usually made by observing the baby during a feed, when excessive stomach activity can be seen as waves crossing the abdomen (visible peristalsis) and the thickened muscle mass can be felt. Treatment is

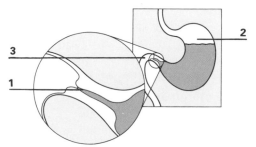

In pyloric stenosis there is narrowing of the pylorus **(1)** where the stomach **(2)** joins the duodenum **(3)** preventing it from emptying. In infants the condition causes vomiting by about three weeks of age; this becomes projectile and milk may be shot several feet.

initially by intravenous fluids to correct dehydration, and then by the surgical procedure of muscle-splitting (Ramstedt operation) to relieve the obstruction.

PYURIA

The presence of pus in the urine as a consequence of inflammation in the kidney, bladder or other part of the urinary tract (for example, pyelonephritis or cystitis). It is rare in men who do not have structural abnormality of these parts. Infection may be symptom-free and is confirmed by finding more than 100,000 organisms per ml of urine. The usual cause is *Escherichia coli*, a bowel organism. Other organisms may be associated with structural abnormality and re-infection, or previous catheterization.

Infections normally settle quickly after treatment with the appropriate antibiotics. Surgical correction of structural abnormalities may be necessray for recurrent and chronic infection.

Q FEVER

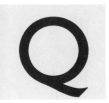

An illness caused by a rickettsia-like organism. 'Q' stands for Queensland, in Australia, where the disease was first described. The disease is spread among animals by ticks. Humans contract it after handling infected material from sheep and cattle, and infected placentas. Infection may also result from the ingestion of infected raw milk and the inhalation of contaminated dust.

The illness starts with a severe headache, high fever, chills and generalized aches. Pneumonia and enlargement of the liver and spleen are common symptoms. Q fever is occasionally complicated by infection of the heart.

The condition responds well to antibiotics and in most cases recovery is complete.

QUADRIPLEGIA

Paralysis of all four limbs. The most common cause is injury in the upper neck region of the spinal cord: this means that messages from the brain can travel no further. Similarly, sensation from the body to the brain is blocked. Paralysis can also be brought on by rough or unnecessary handling at the time of the accident, with damage to the spinal cord occurring subsequent to rather than as a result of the initial injury. Another cause of quadriplegia is disease involving the upper spinal cord; poliomyelitis and multiple sclerosis are examples.

Once paralysis is established it is permanent and treatment is directed at the prevention of complications. Bowel and bladder control is lost and a urinary catheter is usually necessary. Urinary tract infection is always a risk. Spasticity or stiffness of the muscles below the lesion develops slowly after the initial flaccid phase of spinal shock and can result in contracture of the limbs, making handling and positioning of the patient more difficult. The loss of skin sensation means that pressure sores can develop over poorly padded skin, such as that found over bony prominences, if the position of the patient is not altered regularly. Psychological support and rehabilitation have important roles to play in the management of these unfortunate patients. SEE ALSO *Hemiplegia, Paraplegia*

QUINSY

An old-fashioned term for peritonsillar abscess, which forms between the outer layer of the tonsil and the adjacent side wall of the pharynx as a result of an attack of tonsillitis that does not clear up.

The patient has severe pain in the throat, fever and difficulty in opening the mouth (trismus). This, coupled with pain on swallowing, leads to dribbling. There is swelling of the tonsils and palate with the uvula (the small flap of soft palate which protrudes) being pushed to the un-affected side. The tonsil itself may be almost completely obscured or covered with mucus.

In the early stages of inflammation prompt treatment with systemic antibiotics in large intravenous doses may cure the infection. Drainage is advisable when there is considerable swelling; for this the patient sits upright and the quinsy is lanced with a sharp blade under general anaesthetic. Tonsillectomy (removal of the tonsils) is advised six weeks after recovery in order to prevent further attacks.

RABIES

An acute virus disease of the nervous system which can affect all species of warm-blooded animals; also known as hydrophobia. It is transmitted by the bite of carnivorous animals, the dog being the commonest source of infection for man. The symptoms are those of a profound disturbance of the nervous system: excitement, fear of water and of swallowing, aggressive-ness and madness, followed by para-lysis and death. The incubation period varies from one week to several. During this time a specific vaccine can be given which may prevent the disease from developing. However, once the symptoms appear, treatment has relatively little influence on the outcome. Until recently the illness was almost universally fatal. The mortality rate remains very high, but some few patients treated in intensive care with curare-like drugs and assisted ventilation now recover.

RADICULOGRAPHY/ MYELOGRAPHY

An examination of the base of the spinal cord and the nerve roots in the spinal canal in the lower back by means of an injection of contrast medium, and X-rays. (Contrast medium is an organic, iodine con-taining liquid which is opaque to X-rays and will therefore highlight the internal structure of any cavity or tube into which it is placed.)

In this procedure, performed under local anaesthetic, a fine needle is in-troduced into the space between two vertebrae and the membrane sur-rounding the spinal cord and nerve roots is punctured. The correct position of the needle is verified by using X-ray screening and by observing that cerebrospinal fluid, which bathes the brain and spinal cord, flows freely from the needle. Contrast is then introduced and X-rays taken. The lower spinal cord and nerve roots are outlined by the con-trast and any compression — from a slipped disc, degenerative changes or, rarely, a tumour — highlighted.

By tilting the patient headdown, it is possible to run contrast into the chest and neck region and examine the spinal cord. Called myelography, this is usually performed if cord com-pression is suspected from a slipped disc in the neck region, or on the diagnosis of tumours or spondylosis (degenerative changes in the spine) in the neck.

RADIOTHERAPY

The use of ionizing radiation to treat

malignant tumours. Many, but not all, types of tumour are more sensitive than the surrounding normal tissue to radiation because of their fast rate of cell multiplication. This property is exploited by several techniques.

Traditional radiotherapy utilizes high-energy X-rays from an external source. The X-ray beam is carefully aimed so as to irradiate only a certain amount of tissue. X-rays generated at 50–150 kilovolts (kV) are used for superficial lesions. Higher-energy X-rays, generated at 200–500 kV, are required for deeper lesions; the body is irradiated from several different angles so that only the tumour receives the full radiation dose, where the X-ray beams overlap. The dose is often delivered in stages (fractionation).

Gamma rays generated by a Cobalt 60 source and high-energy electron beams produced by linear accelerators are useful alternatives to X-rays in the treatment of relatively superficial tumours. Electrons produce a very uniform distribution of the dose and so cause less radiation damage to bone than do conventional X-rays. Low-energy electrons can be used to treat certain types of skin cancer.

A relatively recent type of radiotherapy, called neutron therapy, is claimed to have an advantage over deep X-ray therapy (DXT) in that both poorly oxygenated and well oxygenated tumour cells are sensitive to it. Even partial damage by the neutrons will cause cells to die.

Internal radio therapy techniques involve the introduction of sealed radiation sources into the target organ (for example, radium pins inserted into the uterus) or intravenous injection of a radio isotope that will collect at the target organ (for example, iodine 131 concentrated in the thyroid gland).

RASH

Any skin eruption which is not confined to one location but is rather more widespread; a small cluster of warts, for example, is not a rash, but widespread psoriasis (qv) is. The form of dermatitis found in the nappy (diaper) area in infancy is a very common rash. In nappy rash the skin is irritated by the interaction of chemical breakdown products from urine with organisms contained in the faeces. Treatment is by increasing the frequency of nappy changes and physically protecting the skin by applying a barrier paste (such as zinc and castor oil) and perhaps a weak steroid ointment. Candida infection is common in nappy rash. If it is suspected, treatment with an anti-candidal cream may be necessary.

RAYNAUD'S PHENOMENON AND DISEASE

Raynaud's phenomenon is a condition in which intermittent constriction of blood vessels (particularly the small arteries) in the fingers and toes leads to a characteristic sequence of changes. The area affected (usually the hands) initially goes white and numb, then painful and blue, and finally red as the blood supply returns and the attack subsides. The precise mechanism which causes the vessels to constrict is not known, but the stimuli include cold, pressure and sometimes emotion. Women are more commonly affected than men. The condition is called Raynaud's phenomenon when there is an underlying cause and Raynaud's disease when there is not.

Underlying causes of Raynaud's phenomenon include several rheumatic conditions such as systemic sclerosis (thickening and hardening of tissues) and systemic lupus erythematosus. Rarely it may be associated with arterial disease such as atherosclerosis, pressure on the blood vessels supplying the ribs, perhaps caused by an extra cervical rib, the use of vibrating machinery, or smoking. Treatment of the phenomenon is that of the underlying disease; in severe cases of Raynaud's disease, sympathectomy (qv) may be helpful.

Gene carrier   Affected   Normal

RECESSIVE (PATTERN OF INHERITANCE)

Inherited characteristics are determined by information stored on genes, and may be passed from generation to generation in one of three manners: dominant, recessive or sex-linked. A recessive gene is only expressed (produces a clinical effect) if its counter-part, inherited from the other parent, also codes for the same characteristic. A couple are at risk of having children with an autosomal recessive inherited disease (for example, cystic fibrosis, sickle cell disease or thalassaemia major) if both parents are carriers for the abnormal gene. In such a case, on average 1 in 4 children will inherit an abnormal gene from each parent, 2 in 4 will be carriers (that is, inherit only one abnormal gene) and 1 in 4 will inherit the normal gene from each parent. Most recessive gene carriers are clinically normal, but may be identifiable if specialized investigations are carried out. The risk of two individuals both carrying an abnormal gene for the same recessive disease is increased if they are blood relatives or from an inbred population.

RECOVERY POSITION

The position in which people are placed when their level of consciousness is impaired. This is particularly important after a general anaesthetic, an epileptic fit, a head injury or after an excess of alcohol, when there is danger of the semi-conscious patient choking on his or her own secretions or vomit.

For the recovery position the patient is placed on his or her side **(1)**, usually the left, with the lower leg held straight and the upper leg flexed at the hip and knee **(2)**. The lower arm is raised and the upper arm is placed alongside the chest with the elbow bent **(3)**. The head is kept on its side so that secretions drain out of the mouth **(4)**; this position also keeps the tongue from falling to the back of the mouth and blocking the airway.

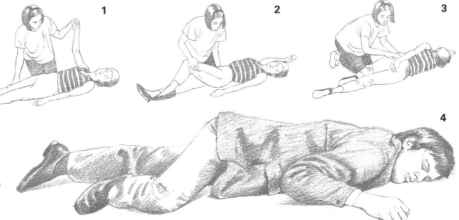

1

2

3

4

REFERRED PAIN

Pain felt in one part of the body but arising in another area where the cause of pain resides. Sensory or autonomic nerves leading from the part of the body where pain is being caused (for example, by ischaemia (bloodlessness), inflammation or cancer) transmit sensation to other sensory nerves at the point where they meet at the spinal cord and in this way refer pain to another area of the body. For example, pain in the chest and left arm may arise in the heart, that in the upper part of the abdomen may be due to diseases in the chest, shoulder-tip pain may signal a disease affecting the diaphragm (the sheet of muscle separating the abdomen from the chest or thorax) and abdominal pain may result from inflammation of the testicles.

REFLUX OESOPHAGITIS

A condition in which the oesophagus becomes inflamed as a result of acid from the stomach refluxing or regurgitating up it. The inflammation may be severe enough to cause a stricture, or narrowing, of the oesophagus. The condition is thought to be due to abnormal relaxation of the valve (sphincter) at the junction of the stomach and oesophagus, and is usually found in those suffering with hiatus hernia (qv), but can also occur in some patients without obvious evidence of such a hernia. The reflux of acid is intermittent, hence the symptoms are variable but include heartburn, pain and difficulty in swallowing (dysphagia). Coffee, alcohol, smoking and obesity aggravate the tendency to reflux. Treatment is to lower the acid secretion by the stomach using drugs such as ranitidine or cimetidine. An operation on the junction of the oesophagus and the stomach, to stop reflux, can be performed in troublesome cases.

REITER'S SYNDROME

A clinical syndrome comprising arthritis, conjunctivitis and urethritis (inflammation of the urethra, the tube that transports urine away from the bladder). There is a strong genetic predisposition to the condition, which is associated with the inheritance of a cell-surface antigen known as HLA B27. Men are affected more commonly than women. Development of the condition is usually triggered by an infection of the genital tract with chlamydial organisms or of the bowel with shigella, salmonella, yersinia or campylobacter bacteria. Symptoms usually develop within three weeks of infection. The arthritis found in Reiter's syndrome is termed 'reactive', meaning that it has been induced by infection at a site distant from the joint itself, and shows no evidence of live micro-organisms in the tissues of the joints. It is often asymmetrical in distribution, with the knees and ankles commonly affected; the sites at which tendons and ligaments join bones may also be inflamed. Conjunctivitis is only severe in about one-third of patients. Urethritis may cause a mild discharge of pus and in women patients may lead to cystitis. Skin and mouth lesions may also be present.

The syndrome is usually self-limiting, clearing up without treatment after several months, but in some people recurrent or chronic joint disease, particularly spondylitis (qv), may develop.

REJECTION

Rejection occurs when the recipient of

a transplanted organ becomes allergic (sensitized) to antigens from the donor of the organ; the transplanted organ (such as a kidney, liver or heart) is invaded by lymphocytes from the recipient. These cells are responsible for immunity and they begin to destroy the transplanted organ. The latter contains antigens not only on the cells of the organ itself but also on 'passenger' white cells within the organ. They are recognized as 'non-self' or foreign by the immune system of the recipient and a reaction ensues which damages and rejects the transplanted organ. Three types of rejection occur:

- Hyperacute, which is rare if donor and recipient antigens are accurately matched, occurs a few hours after transplantation
- Acute rejection may occur within a few weeks or months. It is relatively common and thought to be due to the action of the recipient's sensitized lymphocytes
- Chronic rejection occurs after months or years of normal functioning of the organ.

The cause is unknown, but is thought to be due to an accumulation of antibodies and antigens within the transplanted organ.

To prevent rejection, drugs which suppress the immune response — corticosteroids and cyclosporin A — are used. The chances of rejection are minimized by matching both the blood groups and the tissue antigens of donor and recipient. National and international registers of the blood groups and tissue antigens of people waiting for transplants are kept.
SEE ALSO *Transplantation*

RESISTANCE (ANTIBIOTIC)

Resistance to antibiotics is a constant problem in the treatment of infections and occurs in a number of ways. Some strains of bacteria have a natural resistance to antibiotics; others may acquire it either by producing drug-destroying enzymes or by developing alternative metabolic pathways which bypass the mechanism of bacterial growth and proliferation upon which an antibiotic acts. Bacteria can undergo mutation and the new strains that result may be unaffected by the antibiotic, emerging as one or more resistant strains. Antibiotic resistance is transmissible from strain to strain. This is achieved by plasmids (pieces of DNA outside the normal chromosomes) which possess the code for antibiotic resistance and can be transferred from an antibiotic-resistant strain of bacteria to a sensitive strain, conferring resistance on the latter.

Injudicious use of antibiotics promotes resistance. The use of a new broad-acting antibiotic instead of an appropriate specific one, or even the unnecessary use of antibiotics, encourages the emergence of multiple resistant strains that may render future treatment ineffective.

RESPIRATORY DISTRESS SYNDROME

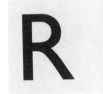

A disease of newborn premature babies with immature lungs; also known as hyaline membrane disease or surfactant deficiency. The normal lung consists of millions of interconnected air bubbles (alveoli) separated from the tiny blood vessels (capillaries) by lung tissue (alveolar wall). The tendency for alveoli to collapse because of surface tension is overcome by a detergent-like substance called surfactant, which is produced by the cells of the alveolar wall. Without this surfactant, the lungs cannot expand. It is produced by the fetus from 22 weeks of pregnancy, but only in small quantities until 32 weeks. Babies are thus more susceptible to respiratory problems the earlier in pregnancy they are born.

In respiratory distress syndrome breathing becomes progressively more difficult within a few hours of birth, and oxygen has to be given to prevent cyanosis (blueness). The illness worsens over the first 36 hours of life until enough surfactant is produced, and then gradually improves over the next five days. Severely affected babies need ventilation. Most recover and their lungs are normal, but some suffer damage to the lungs as a result of the ventilation (bronchopulmonary dysplasia), and need prolonged oxygen therapy. A few die of complications in the first few days.

RESPIRATORY FAILURE

The result of inadequate transfer of gases between the air and the bloodstream. As carbon dioxide is produced and oxygen consumed by the body the level of carbon dioxide in the blood rises and the oxygen level falls. Respiratory failure is virtually synonymous with 'ventilatory failure', which is defined as raised levels of carbon dioxide in the blood (hypercapnia), and the affected patient is usually, but not necessarily, breathless. It is commonly the result of chest diseases, but also occurs in patients with neurological disease, such as Guillain-Barré syndrome, motor neurone disease and poliomyelitis, and is a frequent result of poisoning by drugs such as opiates (see *Narcotics*), which inhibit the brain's control of respiration.

Where there is a treatable cause of respiratory failure — such as pneumonia — appropriate treatment of this cause is given. In some severe cases, artificial respiration using a ventilator is necessary, but this may be inappropriate in the elderly patient with chronic bronchitis, since it can prove impossible later to wean such patients from the ventilator; this subjects them to a protracted, undignified and uncomfortable death. Some patients with chronic respiratory failure are helped by continuous home oxygen therapy, and others by use of a ventilator while sleeping. Very rarely is lung transplantation an option.

RETINAL DETACHMENT

The retina is the light-sensitive layer of rods and cones that lies at the back of the eye. The retinal layer depends on blood vessels for its nutrition and function. These are found in the choroid layer which lies next to the retina. If a small hole develops in the retina, the fluid behind the lens (called the vitreous humour) escapes between the retina and the choroid. The retina rapidly dies without its nourishment and the sight is lost. This can occur after a severe blow to the head or in old age. It also occurs when the retina is stretched, as in very shortsighted people (whose eyeball is elongated), or may be due to a growth. The visual loss is usually described as a curtain falling across one edge of the visual field.

Retinal detachment is treated by laser or phototherapy. In both methods light rays cause a very small burn to coagulate the hole and seal the tear. This prevents any further escape of the vitreous humour, with its associated destruction of the retina.

RETINITIS PIGMENTOSA

An hereditary disease of the retina (the

light-sensitive lining of the back of the eye) due to a degeneration of the pigment. It usually begins in childhood and progresses slowly to result in serious visual impairment or blindness in middle age as the field of vision gradually narrows. Night blindness is often the first symptom.

Retinitis pigmentosa may occur as an isolated disease but is often part of some rare disease of the nervous system. Although methods now exist to identify carriers of the disease and to detect the disease in children before symptoms occur, there is no effective treatment for the disease itself.

RETINOPATHY

Any disease process involving the retina (the light-sensitive membrane at the back of the eye). The term may also be used more specifically to describe the retinal symptoms that may accompany high blood pressure and diabetes mellitus as a result of damage to the arterioles (small branches of the arteries), and hypoxia (lack of oxygen in the vessels leading to the retina). These symptoms involve degenerative changes to the small blood vessels, which may be directly observed in the retina and nowhere else in the body. Examination of the eye by means of an ophthalmoscope will reveal these changes. In hypertension these symptoms are narrowing and irregularity of the arterioles, exudates with a fluffy appearance like cotton wool, and flame-shaped or blot haemorrhages on the retina. Papilloedema (swelling of the optic disc as a result of a build-up of pressure within the skull) may be present in some cases of severe hypertension but without the other signs. In diabetes mellitus an early indication of hypoxia is the appearance of tiny, round red dots (microaneurysms) on the retina. Later,

blot haemorrhages and hard well-demarcated discharges may be found. The presence of cottonwool discharges is a sign of worsening retinal hypoxia. In this situation, the retina may form fragile new vessels in an attempt to supply the ischaemic, or bloodless, retina. If this occurs laser therapy is urgently needed to prevent sudden blindness due to haemorrhage from these vessels.

Exudates may also rarely be found in other diseases that cause either arteriolar damage or hypoxia (such as severe anaemia and kidney failure).

RETROLENTAL FIBROPLASIA

An abnormality of growth of the blood vessels in the immature retina (the light-sensitive inner lining of the back of the eye); also known as retinopathy of prematurity. The condition may progress to scarring and, if severe, to retinal detachment or distortion. The condition is virtually confined to premature babies who have been given excessive amounts of oxygen. It affects about 10 per cent of those weighing less than 1 kg (2 lb 3 oz) at birth (born before 30 weeks), but 50 per cent of those less than 1 kg (2 lb 3 oz) at birth (before 28 weeks). Fortunately, few have significant visual impairment.

RETROVERSION

A term applied to any structure that is turned 'backwards' but which usually refers to cases in which the womb (uterus) is tipped backwards instead of forwards. Retroversion occurs in 10–20 per cent of normal women in whom, nevertheless, the organ can change position; for example, in pregnancy. In some women no cause is found. In others retroversion may result from a prolapse (see *Procidentia*).

Endometriosis (qv), infection, or rarely, cancer, may cause the womb to become retroverted.

The two principal symptoms or complications that may arise from retroversion are painful intercourse (dyspareunia) and the womb very occasionally becoming stuck in the pelvis at around 12 weeks of pregnancy (incarceration). If symptoms are thought to be due to retroversion, a 'pessary test' is usually applied; in this a pessary is inserted to correct the position of the uterus and to see whether the symptoms are relieved. If the symptoms are relieved with the pessary and recur on its removal, then a pessary is inserted permanently. The retroversion may also be corrected by an operation to shorten the ligaments that support the womb.

RETROVIRUS

A virus which works backwards. It contains ribonucleic acid (RNA) and an enzyme reverse transcriptase (which can convert its own RNA into deoxyribonucleic acid or DNA). When the virus has entered a cell, the enzyme reverse transcriptase can copy the RNA into a segment of DNA, which can then be inserted into the nucleus of the cell. Copies of the virus can then be manufactured using the cell's own DNA. Thus, a retrovirus is capable of converting a cell into its own viral factory. The human immunodeficiency virus (HIV — see *AIDS*) is a retrovirus, and for this reason it is difficult to find an effective treatment.

RHESUS FACTOR

The rhesus factor refers to the rhesus blood group system and an antigen that was first detected, in rhesus monkeys, in 1937. Most people (85 per cent in the UK and USA) carry this rhesus D antigen on their red cells (rhesus positive) while the remainder do not (rhesus negative). The principal problem with the rhesus antigen occurs in rhesus negative pregnant women who are carrying a rhesus positive fetus. Antibodies against the antigen do not develop naturally in the rhesus negative mother but may be stimulated to do so if a few red blood cells from the rhesus positive fetus cross the placenta and enter her circulation. Any antibodies formed in the mother against the rhesus antigen can result in problems in subsequent pregnancies with rhesus positive babies, as the antibodies will then cross the placenta from the mother to the fetus and cause severe haemolytic anaemia (haemolytic disease of the newborn, qv). Rhesus negative mothers of rhesus positive babies are therefore routinely given anti-D vaccine, which destroys any rhesus positive cells before they have a chance to stimulate the maternal immune system.

RHEUMATIC FEVER

A very rare inflammatory disease which occurs most commonly in children aged between 3 and 15 years and affects predominantly the heart, joints, nervous system and skin. It results from a reaction to a type of streptococcus bacterium. Onset is usually about eighteen days after a sore throat caused by the bacterium. The main symptoms are fever, with joint pain and swelling migrating between different joints. The most serious complication is inflammation of the heart, which develops in about half of affected children in the first attack. This causes a raised pulse rate and, if severe, may lead to heart failure; the heart valves may also be damaged. Less commonly, involuntary movements (chorea) may be noted. A characteristic rash with red rings may develop and then disappear rapidly. An attack of rheumatic fever usually lasts about three months and may recur after further exposure to the streptococcus.

Treatment involves rest, penicillin to fight any residual infection and paracetamol to reduce fever. Penicillin therapy should be continued until adult life to prevent recurrence.

RHEUMATISM

see *Rheumatoid arthritis*

RHEUMATOID ARTHRITIS

The commonest form of chronic inflammatory joint disease; in the United Kingdom it affects up to 3 per cent of the population. It is clear that there is an inherited susceptibility to the disease, which affects women more than men. Environmental factors, such as certain bacteria or viruses, are thought to trigger the disease, though none has so far been definitely implicated. The inflammation is maintained by cells and antibodies of the immune system, one of the best documented antibodies being termed 'rheumatoid factor'.

Inflammation of the lining of the capsules (cavities) of joints (synovial membrane) is the main feature of the disease, which leads to painful swelling. This inflammation may damage the cartilage overlying the bones and eventually the bone itself may be eroded, resulting in considerable joint deformity and disability. The disease may also be associated with characteristic nodules or hard lumps around joints, tendons or at other sites in the skin and soft tissues.

Rheumatoid arthritis is classically signalled by symmetrical inflammation of the small joints of the hands in a young woman. Other joints subsequently affected may include those in the feet, ankles, knees, wrists, the elbows and shoulders. The disease may also affect the jaw and neck. Pain is associated particularly with early morning stiffness, which then improves during the course of the day.

Arthritis may be associated with inflammation in other organs and tissues, and with anaemia, lymph gland enlargement, thinning of bone and wasting of muscles.

The condition is characterized by periods of attack and remission. The course is unpredictable and newly diagnosed patients should not assume that they are going to develop a severe deforming and crippling disease. Indeed, most patients remain fit for normal activities or find that function is only moderately impaired.

Treatment depends on the severity and distribution of inflammation. It may involve rest in the acute stages, and painkillers, nonsteroidal anti-inflammatory drugs (see *NSAID*) and local steroid injections into joints may be required. In those more severely affected, more powerful but toxic 'second-line' drugs (with known side-effects) may be used and in some patients surgery may be necessary.

RHINITIS

Inflammation of the lining of the nose. Acute rhinitis is usually due to the common cold and is often followed by secondary bacterial infection. This may spread throughout the whole respiratory tract, including the middle ear. Acute rhinitis may also accompany illnesses such as chickenpox and scarlet fever.

Chronic rhinitis may result from a series of attacks of acute rhinitis in rapid succession. In most cases the inflammation is maintained by neighbouring infections (for example, sinusitis or chronic tonsillitis); sometimes disease of the adenoids is responsible. Persistent irritation from dust or tobacco can also lead to chronic rhinitis.

Treatment is directed at clearing up the cause. Topical steroids are often helpful; so too are mild vasoconstrictors (drugs that constrict the blood vessels), which may be used in conjunction with antibiotics. Prolonged use of vasoconstrictors can, however, lead to a rebound phenomenon of further swelling (rhinitis medicamentosa).

RHINOPHYMA

A cosmetically unsightly lesion of the nose caused by fibrosis and hyperplasia of the sebaceous tissue of the skin of the nose. This is usually a consequence of acne rosacea (qv), and the result is swelling of the tip of the nose and the nostrils, making them look not unlike a strawberry. Rhinophyma is treated by shaving off the excess tissue under anaesthetic.

RHYTHM METHOD

see *Safe period*

RICKETS

An abnormality of growing bones usually related to lack of vitamin D. It may be caused by a dietary deficiency of the vitamin (which is present in dairy products) or by a disease of the intestine which interferes with its absorption. Vitamin D is also manufactured by the skin under the influence of ultraviolet light, and lack of exposure to the sun may be a contributory factor. Other rarer causes of rickets include inherited abnormalities of bone metabolism, and chronic kidney failure. Rickets is now uncommon in

developed countries, and tends to occur only in high-risk groups such as premature babies and some immigrants from developing countries. Lack of vitamin D leads to reduced absorption of calcium from the intestine, adversely affecting growing bones and leading to characteristic structural and biochemical changes. Signs of softened bones include bowing of the legs in toddlers, and knock knees in older children. Ultimately growth is disturbed, and if the condition is untreated, short stature and bone deformity will result.

Prevention consists of giving vitamin D supplements to babies and children at high risk. In those already affected, treatment is by large doses of vitamin D, which must be given under medical supervision to avoid overdosage.

RICKETTSIA

Micro-organisms named after an American pathologist, Howard Ricketts. Although rickettsia multiply in the same way as ordinary bacteria, they are smaller in size and can only survive inside animal cells. In some ways they are intermediate between bacteria and viruses. Rickettsia is transmitted to humans by fleas, lice, ticks and mites, and causes diseases such as typhus fever, encephalitis, and Q fever. These infections normally respond well to tetracycline antibiotics.

RIGOR

A very high fever associated with shivering and shaking, and a feeling of cold. It commonly occurs with septicaemia (qv), or when a bacterial organism is circulating freely in the blood. Rigors can also occur after a mismatched blood transfusion, or during an allergic reaction to one.

RODENT ULCER

A term for basal cell carcinoma, a common skin tumour occurring in areas of the body exposed to the sun. The prime cause is long-term cumulative exposure to sunshine; the tumour is particularly common among elderly whites living in sunny climates. Rarely, multiple basal cell carcinomas may arise in an individual who received arsenic-containing medication many years earlier. The tumour is slow-growing and eventually ulcerates, although this may not occur for many months or years. Initially it is likely to have the appearance of a small pink nodule with a rolled edge which gradually grows outwards; pigmentation may vary between individuals and may be dark or light.

Treatment usually consists of surgical removal but radiotherapy is sometimes necessary. Occasionally the ulcers recur after treatment. Systemic spread is extremely unlikely, and there are no internal associations.

ROTAVIRUS

A virus identified in Australia in 1973 which is now known to be responsible for up to 50 per cent of cases of infantile gastro-enteritis. Most victims are under 1 year of age, and suffer vomiting, watery diarrhoea and fever. The virus is shed in the stools from the third to the tenth day of the illness, so scrupulous hand-washing is needed to prevent the infection from spreading. The virus can be identified in the stools by electron microscopy, a technique capable of magnifying objects thousands of times. Rotavirus diarrhoea is more common in winter, and may occur in outbreaks in nurseries. There is no specific treatment, and the illness responds to the general measures employed for gastroenteritis (qv).

ROUNDWORM

see *Worms*

RUBELLA

Also known as German measles, rubella is a mild viral illness with an incubation period of 14–21 days. Symptoms include a mild fever and a characteristic diffuse rash, which usually appears first on the face and then spreads to the body. Infection with rubella during the first three months of pregnancy may result in congenital malformation, blindness, mental retardation or deafness in the fetus. Vaccination is available, and is now recommended by many to all children around the age of 2 years, though others believe that only girls who have not had the illness by 12–14 years of age need to be vaccinated. There is no specific treatment.

RUPTURE

see *Hernia*

SAFE PERIOD

A natural method of family planning which aims to limit sexual intercourse to those times during the menstrual cycle when pregnancy is unlikely to result. This is achieved by identifying the time of ovulation, when intercourse should be avoided. There are three methods of identifying the safe period:

- Calendar (or rhythm) method. By keeping accurate records of the length of the cycle, the time of ovulation can be estimated (fourteen days before menstruation). The method is unreliable, especially if periods are irregular
- Temperature method. There is usually a slight rise in body tem-

S

perature at the time of ovulation (0.5°C) and this method depends upon taking the temperature daily to identify this time

- Mucus inspection method. At the time of ovulation the consistency of the mucus produced by the cervix (neck of the womb) changes from the thick and viscous to watery and profuse as a result of hormone changes. This method depends upon being able to recognize these changes.

Natural methods are not as effective as artificial methods of contraception but combining the temperature and mucus methods (symptothermal) can produce good results. Effective use of the safe period requires detailed knowledge of the method, accurate recordings, a period of abstinence and guidance from the doctor or family planning clinic.

SALMONELLA

The group name of a number of closely related bacteria that are responsible for several important human gastro-intestinal infections. The most sinister species is *Salmonella typhi*, which is responsible for typhoid. Other species cause many of the more serious forms of food poisoning. *Salmonella typhimurium* used to be the principal causative agent of all outbreaks of food poisoning due to salmonellae, but it has in recent years been eclipsed to some extent by *Salmonella enteritidis*, which has caused major contamination of the poultry industry, resulting in its presence in chicken flesh and eggs.

Salmonella gastro-enteritis (excluding typhoid) is very rarely a fatal condition in the previously healthy, although it can be most unpleasant; it may lead to rapid death in the sick, particularly the immunosuppressed. In general, infection follows some hours after the consumption of contaminated foods: insufficiently thawed frozen poultry which is then cooked is often to blame. Eggs may also be infected. The elderly and infirm should not consume eggs raw, but thorough cooking should kill bacteria.

Diagnosis is confirmed by finding salmonella in the stools. The treatment of salmonella gastro-enteritis is usually as for other forms of gastro-enteritis (qv). Antibiotic therapy is necessary in seriously ill patients although it involves the risks both of prolonging the infection and of the patient becoming a chronic carrier. Patients with any salmonella infection must avoid food preparation until clearance of the bacterium is confirmed.

SALPINGITIS

Infection of the Fallopian tube; also known as pelvic inflammatory disease. Salpingitis is commonly caused by bacteria and other harmful organisms gaining access to the Fallopian tube via the vagina. Usually both Fallopian tubes become infected. It is very uncommon for infection to occur prior to the onset of sexual activity and only in rare cases does the condition result from infection in another site (appendicitis or tuberculosis, for example).

Salpingitis usually causes lower abdominal pain, sometimes quite severe, with accompanying vaginal discharge and fever. The Fallopian tubes become swollen and filled with pus, chronic tubal abscesses may develop, and the tube can become permanently scarred, damaged or even blocked, to cause infertility. Not all infections cause pain or fever and a woman may not be aware that salpingitis has occurred until she discoves that she is infertile.

Treatment depends upon recognizing the infection and identifying the infecting agent; once this has been done the appropriate antibiotics can be prescribed. The accuracy with which the condition is diagnosed can be enhanced by performing laparoscopy (qv), a simple technique in which a special telescope is used to visualize the Fallopian tubes. If it is found that the infecting agent can be sexually transmitted, the woman's partner should also be examined and, if necessary, treated, in order to help prevent further infections.

SARCOIDOSIS

A disease of unknown cause that usually affects the chest but may be noticed at a variety of places in the body; also known simply as sarcoid. Typically it affects young adults. Acute sarcoidosis causes the lymph nodes to enlarge (lymphadenopathy) in the areas of the lungs near the heart and major blood vessels (hilar regions). The usual symptom is shortness of breath (dyspnoea); transient raised red blotches may be found on the legs (erythema nodosum) and there may be accompanying fever. Diagnosis is confirmed by chest X-ray, respiratory function tests, blood tests, bronchoscopy and the Kveim test (in which an injection of a specific sarcoid antigen is made into the skin and a skin biopsy taken from the same site six weeks later).

The outlook is generally good in mild cases and treatment may not be necessary. In more serious and in chronic cases, the disease has many possible manifestations, including hypercalcaemia (increased calcium in the blood), uveitis (inflammation of the middle coat of the eye), arthritis, meningitis, and tumerous lesions within the skull. Perhaps the most serious of all, however, is lung fibrosis, which may progress to cause chronic respiratory failure. Patients with any of these signs of severe sarcoidosis need treatment with steroids and regular hospital review to prevent progression of the disease.

SARCOMA

A malignant tumour arising from bone, muscle, fat or body sinews. It is much less common that carcinoma (see *Cancer*) in the proportion of 1 to 20. Sarcomas are named according to the tissue of origin – for example, osteosarcoma comes from bone, and liposarcoma from fatty tissue.

Sarcomas occur in all age groups and grow very rapidly to bulky size; early, blood-borne metastasis to the lungs is common. Sarcomas tend to occur in the limbs and abdomen.

Osteosarcoma is the commonest of all sarcomas and one of the most malignant bone tumours. It often affects children and young adults and usually occurs around the knee joint, causing pain and swelling. This tumour is resistant to radiotherapy and so treatment consists of surgery and chemotherapy.

Kaposi's sarcoma begins as purple nodules and occurs in East Europeans, and South and East Africans. It is now increasingly affecting patients with AIDS (qv).

SCABIES

An itchy, infectious condition affecting the skin. It is caused by the mite *Sarcoptes scabei*. Scabies commonly affects any age group. Transmission is by close bodily contact, such as sharing a bed. Sites frequently involved include the spaces between the fingers, the folds of the armpits, the nipples, penis and scrotum. Scratching rapidly leads to the skin becoming inflamed. The mite burrows through the outer layer of the skin (epidermis), causing an irritant reaction as it goes; characteristically, the track of the mite may be found at one of the usual sites. Frequently it is difficult to identify the mite and the diagnosis may be made presumptively in the presence of the other typical features. Often there will be a history of itching or rashes in close associates (such as brothers or sisters) of the affected individual.

Treatment is with one of a variety of lotions; these must be carefully and liberally applied to the whole of the skin from the neck down and not just to the areas apparently affected. The lotion should be applied at least twice, and all clothing and bed linen should be washed and tumble-dried on maximum heat. In addition it is important that other potentially affected individuals at home (although perhaps not showing any symptoms) should be treated at the same time, otherwise crossinfection and perpetuation of the problem may occur. Even after successful treatment the itch may persist for as long as 3—4 weeks, but will then gradually settle. A weak steroid cream may be used, if the itch is severe, as long as the initial treatment has been correctly applied.

SCARLET FEVER

Also called scarlatina, this is a highly infectious disease caused by a strain of streptococcus; these are airborne organisms but infection may also be acquired from contaminated milk or inanimate objects. It can be caught from contacts or from a healthy carrier. Children are mainly affected although adults may also suffer if they have not had scarlet fever in childhood. One attack usually confers immunity.

The symptoms are mild, beginning with fever, headache, then tonsillitis. By the second day there is a generalized redness, (erythema), this progresses to a scarlet rash, which peels. The tongue resembles a strawberry. The rash is at its height after two days, and then begins to fade; it is gone after a week. However, a close watch should be kept on the urine output in case of the complication of acute glomerulonephritis (inflammation of the kidneys), and on the pulse and temperature in case of rheumatic fever. There is no immunization programme.

Treatment is with penicillin.

SCHISTOSOMIASIS

A very common tropical infection affecting millions of people in Africa, the Middle East, Latin America and the Far East; it is caused by a special type of fluke known as schistosoma. Long tadpole-like worms, the fluke are found in freshwater snails contaminated by human urine and faeces. People are infected by bathing or wading in water containing the fluke, which then penetrate the skin. Once inside the body, they lie deep in the veins of the abdomen, grow larger and produce eggs. These eggs penetrate the walls of the bladder or rectum, depending on the type of schistosoma. Symptoms include cystitis, bloody urine (haematuria), diarrhoea and blood in the stools.

Several drugs are available for the successful treatment of this condition.

SCHIZOPHRENIA

A syndrome of major psychiatric disorders in which certain symptoms are likely to be present during acute episodes. Sufferers commonly describe delusions, which may concern interference with thought (for example, that thoughts have been taken away or implanted by another person), a feeling of being not in control of their bodies (that movements are being controlled by another, for instance), or that someone is trying to harm them. Hallucinations are common, particularly involving hearing, with a sufferer describing voices talking about him or her. A sufferer may behave in odd ways, laugh or cry at inappropriate times and speak in an unintelligible way. The disorder commonly begins in adolescence or young adulthood and pursues a variable course, some sufferers having one episode, others going on to develop a chronic disorder in which there is usually a deterioration of personality, with sufferers becoming withdrawn, less able to work and likely to neglect themselves.

The cause of schizophrenia is unknown, though genetic factors appear important. Emotional stress (such as within the family) is likely to have an adverse effect on a sufferer's state of mind. Tranquillizers are used to treat acute schizophrenia and to prevent further episodes.

SCIATICA

A term generally applied to pain radiating from the lower back to the buttock, thigh or leg, usually on one side but occasionally on both. Strictly the term should only be used for pain felt in the area served by the sciatic nerve along the back of the leg, but it may sometimes be loosely used for more diffuse pain originating from a disordered joint or ligament in the lower back. Although sciatica is usually associated with low back pain, in some individuals the most disabling symptoms may be felt in the leg.

Acute severe sciatic pain is usually due to a slipped disc (prolapsed intervertebral disc) in the lower back, rarely to other causes such as growths in the pelvis or on the sciatic nerve itself in the buttock. Discs are non-bony cush-

ions between the bones of the spine (vertebrae); disc material may press on the site where the nerve roots and spinal nerves that ultimately form the sciatic nerve leave the spinal cord, resulting in sciatica.

Treatment of acute sciatica usually involves a period of bed rest and pain-killing medication. After the acute stage, or in more chronic sciatica due to a chronic disc prolapse or spondylosis (degenerative changes in the spine), other forms of treatment such as physiotherapy may be beneficial. Rarely surgical treatment is necessary.

SCLERODERMA

An uncommon condition in which the small blood vessels are destroyed, resulting in the wasting of tissue and its replacement with fibrous or scar tissue. When this is localized, giving patches of white atrophic skin on the trunk or limbs and occasionally involving the underlying muscle, it is called morphea. The more severe generalized form of scleroderma is known as systemic sclerosis. Scleroderma chiefly affects middle aged women. Its cause is unknown. The skin is commonly affected; in the hands and feet and later the face, neck and trunk it becomes smooth, waxy, tight and thin. These changes produce a typical masklike appearance of the face, and inelasticity of the skin causes difficulty with movement, initially of the fingers but later of other joints. Skin ulcers and abnormal deposits of calcium just beneath the skin (subcutaneous calcinosis) may occur. In the gastro-intestinal tract fibrosis produces dysphagia (difficulty in swallowing), malabsorption and steatorrhoea (abnormal amounts of fat in the stools). Involvement of the renal blood vessels can lead to progressive kidney failure.

S

The CREST syndrome is closely related to systemic sclerosis and consists of calcinosis, Raynaud's phenomenon (numbness and pain in the hands or feet), oesophageal immobility, scleroderma of the fingers and telangiectasis (blood vessels appearing as red bumps on the skin). The outlook for this condition is generally better than for systemic sclerosis.

No treatment is available for the localized form of scleroderma which, in any event, is usually benign. Transient improvement can occur in systemic sclerosis as a result of treatment with steroids, and penicillamine (which inhibits fibroblastic proliferation) is sometimes helpful.

SCOLIOSIS

Lateral curvature or tilt of part of the spine. Scoliosis may be structural or non-structural. Structural scoliosis is due to spinal deformity, and may be congenital in origin (as in spina bifida or cerebral palsy). There are several forms. Infantile idiopathic scoliosis develops during the first three years of life; 90 per cent of children get better spontaneously as the spinal column straightens with growth, but in the remainder the condition get worse. In adolescent idiopathic scoliosis (the cause of which is unknown) the curve is first noticed around the age of 10 years. It usually affects the thoracic region and may cause serious deformity with compensatory curves lower in the spine and distortion of the ribcage; the latter is particularly prominent on bending. Scoliosis may also develop as a consequence of muscular weakness as, for example, in muscular dystrophy.

Treatment is difficult; it may not be possible to prevent progression completely, but several types of operation are now available either to correct scoliosis or to prevent early deformity from worsening. The basis of management is to hold the spine by an external splint at first and then to fuse it surgically when the child is older (8–12 years of age).

A short leg, hip deformity or spasm of the spinal muscles associated with a slipped disc can produce what is termed non-structural scoliosis, which is corrected once the person lies flat or the cause is removed.

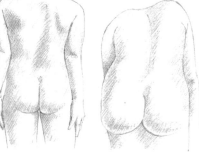

Adolescent idiopathic scoliosis usually affects the thoracic region of the spine. It is particularly noticeable when the child bends forwards.

SCOTOMA

Loss of part of the field of vision of one or both eyes. If the loss is at the edge of the visual field, it may not be apparent until formal testing is performed. If the loss is central, vision will be seriously affected. Scotomata may result from damage to the retina (the light-sensitive lining at the back of the eye), optic nerve or visual pathways within the brain. In the last type both eyes may share approximately matching visual field defects.

SCURVY

A disease resulting from a chronic dietary deficiency of vitamin C, leading

S

to reduced formation of collagen (an important structural protein in skin and connective tissues). Man, unlike most other mammals, is unable to synthesize this vitamin and is entirely dependent upon his diet or vitamin supplements for a satisfactory intake. The daily recommended requirement of vitamin C is 45 mg for adults; fresh fruit and vegetables are particularly rich sources, but care should be taken when preparing the latter as prolonged cooking will destroy the vitamin.

Typical signs of scurvy include spontaneous bruising of the skin and petechial haemorrhages (see *Petechia*) around hair follicles. Gingivitis is an accompanying symptom with hallitosis (bad breath) and loosening of the teeth, which may fall out. Haemorrhage around the long bones, usually in the legs, may cause pain and swelling. Wound healing is delayed. Symptoms regress rapidly after treatment with oral supplements of vitamin C.

Scurvy is now uncommon in the developed world. It is occasionally seen among the elderly, poor or demented who live on their own and subsist on wholly inadequate or bizarre diets.

SEBACEOUS CYST

A localized collection of sebum within the skin which forms a smooth, firm nodule, sometimes with a small hole at its centre through which the sebum may intermittently discharge. Sebum is an oily substance produced by the sebaceous glands in the skin and is important for maintaining the skin's texture. Small quantities of sebum are usually secreted onto the surface of the skin. A sebaceous cyst is caused by blockage of one of the sebaceous glands. The scalp is a common site. Treatment is by surgical removal. Antibiotic therapy may be required if the cyst becomes infected.

SEBORRHOEIC DERMATITIS

A skin condition of unknown cause which affects those areas presumed to produce the most sebum; the face, the area of the chest covering the breast-bone, the scalp and between the shoulder blades. The condition is characterized by scale and erythema (red eruptions). An alteration in the normal skin bacteria may be the cause in some cases, but the precise role of this change is not fully understood. Improvement usually initially follows treatment with locally applied corticosteroids (sulphur-containing ointments are often helpful as well), but the condition is difficult to eradicate completely and recurrence is common. A medicated shampoo containing a descaling agent may be required if the scalp is affected. A severe form of dermatitis resembling seborrhoeic dermatitis is found in some AIDS patients.

In infants a form of seborrhoeic dermatitis may occur which can be difficult to distinguish from atopic dermatitis (qv). In its mildest form this condition affects only the scalp (cradle cap). It usually clears up completely after treatment with a medicated shampoo and, perhaps, and oily descaling agent.

SEDATIVES

see *Tranquillizers*

SEIZURE

see *Convulsion*

SEMINOMA

The commonest tumour of the testis; it is cancerous. Seminoma occurs between the ages of 20 and 50 years. The testis becomes enlarged and hard;

S

it feels heavy but there is no pain. Seminoma spreads by metastasis to the lymph nodes in the abdomen and, in advanced cases, through the blood to the liver and lungs.

Treatment consists of removing the testis, followed by radiotherapy to the abdominal lymph nodes. Most cases of seminoma can be cured.

SEPSIS

An inflammatory reaction to bacterial infection. When micro-organisms such as bacteria invade and multiply in the body, the toxins they produce damage local tissues. The tissues respond to infection by means of the inflammatory response (or sepsis), which presents with redness, heat, localized swelling and pain. Pus may also form, and consists of cellular debris, fluid and inflammatory cells which are produced by the body to combat infection.

If the infecting organisms spread into the bloodstream, septicaemia may result. Treatment is with antibiotics and drainage of any abscess.

SEPTICAEMIA

A severe, life-threatening, generalized bacterial infection. Septicaemia can be caused by a large variety of organisms that penetrate the bloodstream, spreading infection throughout the body. It may also be caused by peritonitis or surgery, especially urinary tract operations, or a localized infection such as an abscess or boil. Antibiotics may be used during and after operations to try to prevent this complication, particularly if the operation has been for an infective process such as perforated appendix. The patient develops signs of shock and is pale, with a fast, weak pulse and low blood pressure. Often the skin is warm and dry and there is intermittent fever.

Clinical pointers may be found which help to determine the likely bacterium responsible; for example, a typical rash in acute septicaemia may suggest the cause is the meningococcus bacterium (see *Meningitis*).

Treatment of septicaemia involves large doses of intravenous antibiotics together with other supportive measures such as drugs to maintain blood pressure and kidney function.

SEX-LINKED (PATTERN OF INHERITANCE)

Inherited characteristics are determined by information stored on genes, and may be passed from generation to generation in one of three manners: dominant, recessive or sex-linked. Sex linkage is the mode of inheritance exhibited by genes located on the sex (X and Y) chromosomes. Diseases inherited in an X-linked recessive manner show up in males but not in females — for example, haemophilia and certain types of muscular dystrophy. An affected male cannot pass the disease on to his sons, but all his daughters will be carriers. For a female carrier, on average, half her sons will be affected and half her daughters will be carriers. Female carriers are usually clinically normal, but may be identified by special tests.

Diseases showing X-linked domi-

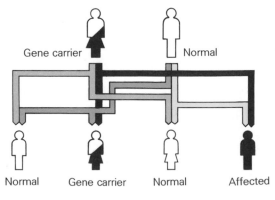

Gene carrier   Normal

Normal   Gene carrier   Normal   Affected

S

nant inheritance are rare — for instance, vitamin D-resistant rickets. In this pattern of inheritance, on average twice as many females as males are affected. An affected female transmits the disease to half her sons and half her daughters. An affected male transmits the disease to all his daughters but none of his sons.

SEXUALLY TRANSMITTED DISEASE (STD)

This term is now preferred to the older term 'venereal disease' (VD). STDs include gonorrhoea, syphilis, non-specific urethritis (NSU), genital herpes (simplex), genital warts and AIDS. (See individual entries for specific information.)

The symptoms may include discharge from the vagina or penis, burning when passing urine, ulcers of the penis or on the skin around the vaginal opening, abdominal pain and high temperature. However, in many cases some of these diseases do not cause any symptoms, particularly in women. It is important to have STDs treated in order to prevent them spreading to future sexual partners. Left untreated, some of these diseases cause damage to the Fallopian tubes, which can result in infertility or ectopic pregnancy. Some STDs are particularly serious during pregnancy and may infect the baby before or during childbirth.

SHIGELLA

The group of bacteria which causes bacillary dysentry. This is a highly contagious disease spread by food and water contaminated with faeces or by direct person-to-person transmission. Outbreaks of bacillary dysentry are more common in infant schools, geriatric wards and mental handicap units, where poor hygiene in the form of inadequate washing and drying of hands after opening the bowels may help to spread infection. The incubation period is about 2 days. In mild cases there is slight colicky pain and mild diarrhoea. In severe cases fever, chills, vomiting and profuse bloody diarrhoea occur. Treatment is with appropriate antibiotics.

SHINGLES

see *Herpes zoster*

SHOCK

General bodily disturbance as a result of severe injury. Shock is a clinical syndrome characterized by a lower than normal temperature, a fall of blood pressure (hypotension), a feeble rapid pulse (tachycardia), pallor and a cold moist skin, and often by vomiting, restlessness and anxiety. The causes are numerous: trauma, haemorrhage, severe burns, coronary thrombosis, perforation of an abdominal organ and profound dehydration. The end result of all of these is a lack of blood flow to the brain because of reduced blood volume, either due to massive blood loss (as occurs in haemorrhage), inability of the heart to pump adequately (coronary thrombosis) or loss of plasma volume in the blood (burns, perforated organ or dehydration).

Unless promptly treated, shock is fatal. It is the major cause of death in multiple injuries (road accidents and so on) and highlights the need for injured patients to be taken rapidly to hospital, or else to receive intravenous fluids at the scene of the accident.

SHORT SIGHT

see *Myopia*

S

SHUNT

An abnormal or surgically created passage between blood vessels which diverts blood. An abnormal shunt arises in some forms of heart disease, such as Fallot's tetralogy, in which a hole in the partition between the ventricles (lower chambers of the heart) allows blood to shunt from the higher pressured left side to the right. Sometimes the shunt is reversed (see *Eisenmenger's syndrome*) and venous blood travels from the right chamber to the left, without passing through the lungs. This unoxygenated blood produces a condition known as cyanosis, in which particularly the face and extremities are tinged blue. Shunts also occur between arteries and veins in arteriovenous angiomas (qv).

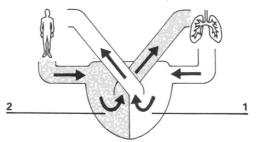

The left side **(1)** of the heart deals with fresh oxygenated blood and sends it to other organs. The right side **(2)** sends used deoxygenated blood to the lungs. A shunt disrupts the normal circulation of blood and allows the mixing of oxygen-rich blood with carbon dioxide-rich blood.

Surgically created shunts are used to make large veins for patients who need repeated haemodialysis (see *Dialysis*), by joining an artery to a vein. They are also employed in the treatment of liver disease, to reduce the blood pressure in the portal circulation (the veins leading from the gut to the liver) by means of a portocaval shunt. Temporary shunts are plastic tubes employed during open heart surgery.
SEE ALSO *Congenital heart disease*

SICKLE CELL DISEASE

An inherited form of haemolytic anaemia which occurs almost exclusively in people of African descent but is also found in people of Mediterranean origin. In sickle cell disease or anaemia, normal adult haemoglobin (the red pigment in blood) is replaced by sickle haemoglobin, an abnormal three-dimensional compound which results from a change in one of the amino acids making up the haemoglobin chain. Consequently, the red cell becomes sickle- or crescent-shaped. This can occur without cause but particularly when perfusion (blood supply through the small vessels) is poor — in infection, for example — or if oxygen is low in the blood and red cell production is therefore stimulated. The patient may then go into 'sickle crisis': further red cells become misshapen, the small blood vessels are blocked, and the oxygen supply is cut off. As a result, parts of the lung and bones may die.

The sickle cell trait is not a problem unless a person inherits the condition from both parents (the term for this is homozygous). People who have half sickle haemoglobin and half normal adult haemoglobin (heterozygotes) function normally.

'Sickle crisis' is managed with oxygen and painkillers (analgesics); often a blood transfusion is necessary.

SIDS

see *Sudden infant death syndrome*

SIGMOIDOSCOPE

An instrument used to examine the rectum and part of the sigmoid colon (the lower part of the large intestine). The sigmoidoscope is a hollow tube

S

20—30 cm (8—12 in) long and about 2—3 cm (about 1 in) wide, with a light to illuminate the bowel. The patient is placed on his or her left side and the instrument is passed through the anus to examine the lower bowel. Sigmoidoscopy is very useful for diagnosing the cause of the passage of blood and/or mucus in the stool and for biopsying polyps and tumours of the colon; sometimes these can be removed through the sigmoidoscope. It is also employed for diagnosing and monitoring the treatment of inflammatory bowel diseases, such as ulcerative colitis and Crohn's disease. SEE ALSO *Colonoscopy*

SILICOSIS

Fibrosis of the lungs caused by prolonged exposure to silica dust. Silica is present in many minerals, including sand, and individuals at risk are predominantly those whose work exposes them to stone dusts; the use of masks to prevent inhalation is strongly advised. Patients in the early stages of silicosis have no symptoms, but certain characteristic changes are present nonetheless which will be revealed by chest X-ray. In the later stages patients experience progressive difficulty in breathing (dyspnoea) and ultimately respiratory failure. Diagnosis is often made on the basis of the patient's occupational record and the result of the chest X-ray, but bronchoscopy and lung biopsy may be needed to confirm it.

The patient should avoid completely exposure to stone dusts in order to delay progression. There is no effective treatment; it is possible that lung transplantation will become an appropriate therapy in the future. As is the case with most other lung diseases, smoking makes the development of the condition more likely.

SINUS ARRHYTHMIA

An entirely harmless and indeed normal variation in the pulse rate encountered in most children and young adults. Sinus arrhythmia is caused by the heart's response to the normal respiratory cycle of inspiration and expiration (breathing in and out), which changes the pressure within the chest and thereby the ease with which blood returns through the veins in the chest to the heart. Thus in inspiration the heart rate slows, only to speed up again in expiration. The pulse therefore gets steadily slower, reaching its slowest rate at the end of a breath in and then steadily faster, reaching its fastest at the end of a breath out. The response of the heart is dulled with increasing age, and the pulse may then feel totally regular, but only in certain neuropathies is all sinus arrhythmia lost.

SINUSITIS

Inflammation of the membrane lining the paranasal sinuses. Small channels called ostia link this lining to that of the nose. Long and tortuous, these channels are not ideally sited for their principal functions of drainage and equalizing air pressure, because of man's upright posture, and do in fact help spread infection. Secretions from the sinuses are collected and wafted towards the nose by hair-like structures on the cell surfaces called cilia.

Acute sinusitis usually occurs as a result of infection from rhinitis (inflammation of the lining of the nose) which often spreads via an ostium after diving or swimming. Infection may also spread to the sinuses after a tooth has been extracted or after a nasal bone has been fractured. Pain is felt over the affected sinuses, usually the frontal sinuses over the eyes or the

S

maxillary sinuses in the cheekbones, due to a build-up of pressure as the ostium becomes blocked by swelling. The nose itself may also be blocked, or there may be nasal discharge or catarrh. Painkillers (analgesics) and antibiotics are the mainstays of treatment, coupled with measures to re-establish drainage. This is usually done by means of decongestants, which work by constricting the arteries and reducing the swelling. Irrigation (washing out with sprays) may also be necessary.

In chronic sinusitis the lining of the sinuses is irreversibly diseased. The condition requires an operation to strip the lining and enlarge the drainage channel.

SITUS INVERSUS

A condition in which all the organs within the abdomen and thorax (chest) are arranged in the reverse of normal, as a mirror image. Complete situs inversus is not usually associated with disease and tends to run in families. It is usually discovered either during a routine physical examination, when the apex beat (the contraction of the ventricles, or lower chambers) of the heart is felt on the right and the liver is found on the left, or on a routine chest X-ray when the heart shadow and gastric air bubble (an obvious bubble of air within the stomach) are seen on the right.

When the heart occupies its normal position but there is situs inversus of the abdominal organs, the heart is nearly always seriously malformed.

SJÖGREN'S SYNDROME

A chronic but generally benign inflammatory condition, occurring predominantly in women, which affects the salivary glands, tear glands and other tissues. The syndrome is associated with abnormalities of the immune system but its cause is unknown. The usual clinical sign is dry eyes and mouth (sicca syndrome); less commonly, the parotid glands behind the jaw may be enlarged, and there may be malaise (a general feeling of being unwell). The condition may damage the cornea (the transparent circular window at the front of the eye), and predisposes to recurrent infections. The syndrome may occur alone, but in half of cases is associated with other diseases, particularly rheumatoid arthritis.

Treatment may include the use of artificial tears in the form of eye drops; in more severe cases steroid or more powerful immuno-suppressive treatment may be necessary.

SKIN

The largest organ in the human body, forming not only an essential barrier between the body and the environment, but also containing cells which help to perform a host of complex functions such as regulating body temperature through sweating and interacting with the body's immune systems.

The skin is divided into an outer layer (epidermis) and an inner layer (dermis). The dermis contains blood vessels, nerve endings and cells; it produces connective tissue upon which the elastic characteristics of the skin are dependent. The epidermis contains none of these. Within the epidermis the vast majority of cells are keratinocytes, cells which produce a variety of important chemicals and which also form the closely adherent building blocks which provide the outer protective sheath of the human body. The keratinocytes multiply and grow

S

Structure of the skin: **1** epidermis; **2** dermis; **3** sebaceous gland; **4** hair follicle; **5** subcutaneous fat; **6** sweat gland.

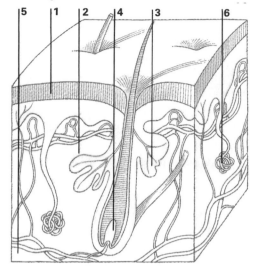

outwards towards the surface, where they die and form a protein coat (stratum corneum) which is slowly shed in an imperceptible fashion. Other cells contained within the epidermis are derived from the bone marrow and appear to function as an important peripheral component of the immune system. These Langerhans cells have a role in the recognition of foreign substances such as bacteria and viruses to which the skin is exposed.

SKIN GRAFTING

A form of plastic surgery, most commonly employed to treat patients with extensive burns. Usually, a partial-thickness graft is used. Skin from a donor site is carefully cut away and transferred to the burned area; for example, skin from the thigh may be transferred to cover a burned area over the chest. There is no problem with rejection because the skin is taken from the patient. Furthermore, since only the upper layers of skin are removed from the donor site, the skin at the donor site regenerates.

When extensive areas of burnt skin have to be grafted it can be very difficult to find large enough donor areas on the patient. So-called 'skin banks' have therefore been set up, although immune rejection may limit the use of these grafts.

Deep, full-thickness skin grafts are sometimes required for extensive burns, but have the disadvantage that the donor site may later need a partial-thickness graft. They take root much less readily than partial-thickness grafts.

SLEEPING SICKNESS

see *Trypanosomiasis*

SLIPPED DISC

The slipped disc, medically known as prolapsed intervertebral disc, is a common cause of temporary disability. Between each major bone (vertebra) in the spine there is a fibrous disc that helps to cushion the vertebrae from jarring during movement. If the disc (or its fibrous rim) degenerates, its softer core may protrude through the rim (prolapse) so that it presses on the nerves leaving the spinal cord at that level or less often, in the neck or upper back, upon the spinal cord itself. The exact symptoms depend on which disc has

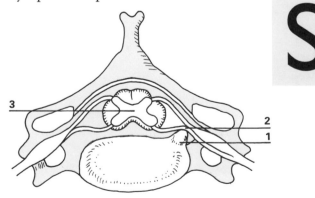

A slipped or eroded invertebral disc **(1)** may result in the soft core of the disc poking through the rim and pressing on the nerves **(2)** leaving the spinal cord **(3)**.

S

slipped, but there will always be problems involving one of the limbs on the affected side; for example, pain radiating down the arm when a disc in the neck is involved or in the leg when a disc 'slips' in the lower back. Lumbar prolapse is the commonest cause of sciatica (qv). Much less often a central disc prolapse in the neck causes spinal paralysis. Most low back pain is, however, unrelated to slipped discs, contrary to popular belief.

If the slipped disc continues to press on the nerves or spinal cord despite rest (and perhaps a collar or corset), surgical treatment will be required — traditionally by removing the troublesome disc or decompressing the spinal cord (laminectomy, qv) in extreme cases, but local treatments (injection under X-ray control) to destroy the part of the disc causing the trouble and/or osteopathic manipulation are possible in some.

SMALLPOX

A highly contagious and often fatal disease caused by the smallpox virus. The disease is now extinct as a result of an unprecedented international vaccination campaign begun in the 1960s. It was transmitted by the inhalation of infected particles, either directly from a patient or through contaminated articles. Symptoms started with a high fever, shivering and headache. A few days later eruptions appeared on the face and then spread to the trunk and limbs. The eruptions were filled with cloudy fluid and then yellowish material. About two days after the onset of illness these eruptions started to dry up. The scabs eventually fell off, leaving pitted scars on the skin. In severe cases death was usually caused by a combination of pneumonia and cardiac failure.

SMOKING

Cigarette smoking is one of the principal causes of preventable disease and premature death in the industrialized nations.

Data from large studies in several countries have shown that cigarette-smoking men have between 30 per cent and 80 per cent higher death rates than non-smokers, particularly in the age group 45–55. The principal cause is coronary heart disease; the risk of fatal or non-fatal coronary heart disease is 60–70 per cent greater in smokers than non-smokers. Women who smoke and use oral contraceptives increase their chances of suffering a heart attack by a factor of five. In both men and women a decrease in mortality from coronary heart disease begins within one year of giving up the habit, and within 5–10 years mortality is the same as in non-smokers.

Smoking also has an effect on other arteries, aggravating peripheral vascular disease (narrowing of the arteries due to atheroma, usually in the legs).

The cause-and-effect relationship between cigarette smoking and lung cancer is well known and the risk of cancer rises proportionately to the number of cigarettes smoked per day. Cancers of the mouth, larynx (voicebox), oesophagus and bladder are also more common in smokers. More recently, it has been demonstrated that the risk of cancer in non-smokers is increased by so-called passive smoking, in which cigarette smoke is inhaled from the atmosphere.

Smoking is the most important factor in the development of chronic bronchitis and emphysema and is associated with an increased incidence of chest infections and deaths from pneumonia and influenza.

Smoking in pregnancy may ad-

S

versely affect the fetus: there is an increased incidence of miscarriage, premature birth and death in the newborn period, and infants of smoking mothers weigh an average of 170 g (6 oz) less than those born to non-smoking mothers.

Gastric and duodenal ulcers are more common and cause more deaths in smokers than in non-smokers.

SOLVENT ABUSE

see *Glue sniffing*

SPASTICITY

Stiffness of the limbs due to an imbalance of the nervous stimuli acting on the motor nerve cells within the spinal cord. Spasticity results from disease of or injury to descending motor pathways from the brain. There are many causes, including damage to the fetus in the womb, injury at birth, and postnatal hypoxia (lack of oxygen in the blood), infection and metabolic disturbance. In the older child and adult, spasticity may result from damage to the central nervous system as a result of injury, such as to the spine, or stroke. Some cases result from diseases such as multiple sclerosis or primary degenerative disorders such as motor neuron disease which usually arise in middle life.

Generally this type of neurological damage tends to result in overactive muscles, causing the legs to extend and the arms to flex. Voluntary movement of the limbs is restricted to a varying degree. Depending on the underlying cause, spasticity is frequently associated with an inability fully to control the bladder and anal sphincter.

Treatment is based on intensive physiotherapy to prevent the permanent shortening of muscle or fibrous tissue (contracture) and to help the patient maximize any voluntary function that is retained.

SPECULUM

An instrument used to examine the parts of the body which are not accessible to visual examination without such an aid.

It is most commonly used to examine the inside of the nose, ears or vagina. The size and shape of the speculum varies according to which function it performs. A small electric lamp is required to light up the cavity and so aid inspection.

SPERMATOZOON (SPERM)

The fully matured male reproductive cell which fertilizes the female ovum to form the fetus. Spermatozoa are produced in the testicle by a specialized process that takes approximately 72 days; it is a continuous process, although the rate of production may be slowed down or halted by certain illnesses or drugs Many millions of sperm are released in each ejaculate. Only one sperm is necessary to achieve fertilization.

SEE ALSO *Contraception, Infertility, Ovulation, Sterilization*

SPHINCTER

A muscle which surrounds an opening or tube and serves to open and close it. There are several examples:

- The gastro-oesophageal sphincter, between the gullet and stomach. If this sphincter is not working well acid from the stomach will rise up into the gullet to cause heartburn or indigestion
- The anal sphincter, at the opening of the anus. This is composed of an

S

internal and an external sphincter. Only the external sphincter is under voluntary control and loss of control of this results in faecal incontinence

- The urethral or urinary sphincter. The emptying of the bladder is partly controlled by this sphincter. If the external sphincter fails, urinary incontinence will result.

SPHYGMOMAN-OMETER

Apparatus for measuring blood pressure, consisting of an inflatable cuff with a pump and pressure gauge. The cuff is placed around the upper arm (usually the right one) and then inflated so as to block the arterial pulse to the arm. Pressure is then gradually released so that the returning pulse can be heard through a stethoscope placed over the artery below the cuff. The pressure in the cuff is measured in millimetres of mercury by reference to a numbered scale. Two measurements are taken: the first and higher reading is the systolic blood pressure and reflects the maximum pressure in the arteries; the lower, diastolic, reading is the minimum arterial pressure. Normal values would be 120 and 80 mm of mercury (120/80 mmHg) respectively.

SPINA BIFIDA

Failure of the vertebral arches to close during fetal development so that the bones of the spine (vertebrae) remain incomplete towards the outside. The length of spine involved and the position of the abnormal segment vary, although spina bifida most commonly affects the lower back.

There are two types of spina bifida: occulta and cystica. Spina bifida occulta is the commoner of the two and consists of a small vertebral defect in the lower back, often with an overlying skin abnormality, such as a tuft of hair or a haemangioma (benign tumour composed of dilated blood vessels). The spinal cord and its coverings are usually normal and neurological abnormality is rare so that as a rule no treatment is needed.

Spina bifida cystica is much more serious that spina bifida occulta. It is found in two forms: meningocoele and myelomeningocoele. In meningocoele, which is relatively uncommon, the spinal cord is intact, and a sac consisting of meninges (the coverings of the spinal cord) containing cerebrospinal fluid projects through the bony defect and forms a soft lump under the skin. There is no neurological damage; the danger is that the sac will rupture, leading to infection. The defect is repaired during the first two weeks of life. Hydrocephalus (qv) is present to some degree in most cases and may require treatment with a shunt (qv) to direct cerebrospinal fluid from the cerebral ventricles to the peritoneal cavity. In myelomeningocoele the spinal cord has not formed properly but lies exposed together with nerves on the surface of the back. This leads to abnormal function of the body below the defect: the legs may be para-

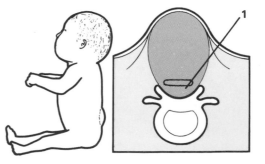

The usual site of spina bifida is low on the infant's back **(left)**.
In myelomeningocoele **(right)**, the malformed spinal cord **(1)** lies exposed together with nerves on the surface of the back.

lysed with loss of sensation; poor bladder function may lead to kidney damage; and abnormal bowel activity causes constipation. Hydrocephalus is present to some degree in most cases.

An operation to close the defect is possible, but the abnormal spinal cord does not recover. Antenatal diagnosis by ultrasound and alphafetoprotein screening is now practised. Therapeutic abortion has considerably reduced the number of newborn babies affected. It also seems likely that the incidence of these conditions is reduced by giving vitamin supplements during pregnancy.

SPINAL FUSION

A surgical technique to fix together the small bones of the spine (vertebrae). These bones are normally held in place by their interlocking joints, ligaments and muscles but they can shift out of alignment as a result of certain degenerative changes in the spine, such as spondylosis. In spondylolisthesis, for example, the spine in the lower back (the lumbar region) may shift forwards on the pelvis, causing pain in the back and the legs; and in adolescent scoliosis a curvature of the spine develops. In spondylosis and adolescent scoliosis the vertebrae involved can be fused together or in spondylolisthesis the lower lumbar vertebrae can be fused to the pelvis to prevent further movement. This is achieved by inserting bone chips (a bone graft) taken from the ilium (a pelvic bone) between the vertebrae to form new bone. Alternatively a metal rod may be used, particularly for scoliosis (see *Fixation*). Fusion is also used occasionally in the neck to treat cervical spondylosis, and to fix some types of unstable spinal fracture that may otherwise cause paralysis. SEE ALSO *Laminectomy*

SPIROCHAETE

see *Syphilis* and *Yaws*

SPLENECTOMY

Surgical removal of the spleen. (See next entry for details of site and function.) There are a number of reasons for performing a splenectomy: for example, to stop excessive bleeding as a result of injury to the spleen; to cure hypersplenism, in which an abnormally large spleen becomes over-active in removing red blood cells and platelets from the blood; or to remove a lymphoma, as in Hodgkin's disease.

The main long-term problem resulting from the operation is an increased risk of pneumococcal infection. This is more common in children, in whom it can cause a severe type of pneumonia. The risk of this type of infection is reduced by vaccination, and the use of long-term low-dose penicillin. Adults who have had their spleens removed should receive penicillin at the earliest sign of a common cold or influenza.

SPLENOMEGALY

Enlargement of the spleen, generally to an extent that is detectable by the doctor when he or she feels the patient's abdomen. The spleen is an organ situated in the upper part of the left side of the abdominal cavity, and it is normally covered by the ribs. In the fetus the spleen has a role in the production of blood cells. In children and adults it filters out old red and white blood cells from the circulation and destroys them. It also contains many cells of the immune system, and is important in defending the bloodstream against invading microorganisms, such as bacteria.

S

The spleen may become enlarged as a result of a number of disease processes: infections (for example, glandular fever, bacterial endocarditis (inflammation of the lining of the heart), tuberculosis, brucellosis, typhoid, and tropical infections such as malaria, trypanosomiasis and leishmaniasis); blood disorders (such as acute and chronic leukaemia, haemolytic anaemia and myelofibrosis); liver disease when there is portal hypertension; and other problems including lymphoma, storage diseases (in which, due to an inborn error of metabolism, abnormal fats or carbohydrates are stored in body cells) and autoimmune disorders.

Treatment depends on the underlying cause.

SPONDYLITIS

A characteristic inflammatory condition of the spine; its cause is unknown. The classic form is known as ankylosing spondylitis (qv). Another form of spondylitis, which is clinically very similar to ankylosing spondylitis in its effects, may also develop in a few individuals with psoriasis and inflammatory bowel disease (Crohn's disease and ulcerative colitis, for example), and in people with reactive arthritis or Reiter's syndrome.

SPONDYLOSIS

A term applied to degenerative changes in the spine which often occur with increasing age. These changes involve the bones of the spine (vertebrae), particularly in the neck and lower back (lumbar region), which develop osteoarthritis in the joints between them; and the soft tissue cushions (discs) between the vertebrae, which lose height and in some cases bulge into the spinal canal. Small bony out-growths from the top and bottom of the vertebrae may also develop. The changes characteristic of spondylosis are a very common X-ray finding and are present in many individuals without symptoms. The symptoms of spondylosis are limitations of movement, and pain in the neck, back or limbs, the latter as a result of pressure on the nerve roots and spinal nerves leading from the spinal cord. Sometimes there is pressure on the spinal cord itself in the neck giving slowly progressive spinal paralysis.

Treatment is with analgesics and supportive collars to relieve the pain. Surgery is performed only in severe cases of nerve root compression or in some cases of spinal cord compression in the neck.

SPRAIN/STRAIN

An incomplete rupture or tear of a ligament. Sprains are usually caused by injury which stretches the ligament involved; for example, twisting injuries involving the ankle joint may cause a sprain of one of the ligaments that connect the bones on either side of the joint. Local pain, swelling, tenderness and sometimes bruising may result from such strains. Pain is aggravated by movement, which tenses the affected ligament.

Treatment depends on the severity of the injury and which ligament is involved. A short period of immobilization may be necessary, but in general early activity is encouraged. Painkilling medication may be required. Sprays and creams containing local anaesthetics or anti-inflammatory agents may also relieve symptoms.

In some circumstances the term 'strain' may also be used to describe chronic stress on a ligament — for example, for strain induced by pro-

S

longed standing or walking or in a deformed limb in which a ligament is subjected to unusual stress. Physiotherapy, elastic supports or other appliances are sometimes helpful in these cases.

SPRUE

Chronic food malabsorption acquired in a tropical area (tropical sprue). (Non-tropical sprue is a collective term often used to identify other malabsorption syndromes, such as coeliac disease.) Tropical sprue is endemic in the Middle East, the Far East, India and the Caribbean, but is relatively uncommon in Africa. It may occur in the indigenous population of these areas or in travellers who have spent only a short time in the tropics. Symptoms include diarrhoea, anorexia and weight loss. In severe cases there may be vitamin and nutritional dificiencies. The lining of the small intestine becomes flattened (villous atrophy), thus reducing the area for the absorption of nutrients. The cause of tropical sprue is not known with certainty, but it probably results from an infection of the intestines. Folic acid deficiency, which results from chronic malabsorption, may in itself be responsible for some of the features.

Treatment is with antibiotics (for example, tetracycline) and folic acid for a period of at least six months. Relapses may occur.

SQUINT

Malalignment of the eyes, medically known as strabismus. Two types are recognized: concomitant and paralytic. Concomitant squints develop in childhood and are usually caused by muscle imbalance. The image from the squinting eye is suppressed by the young brain so that normal visual develop-

ment is prevented, resulting in a lazy eye with poor vision (amblyopia). In this type of squint the eyes move together and the degree of squint remains constant whatever the direction of gaze. The priority in the treatment of a concomitant squint is to allow normal visual development to take place in the squinting eye, by periodic patching (covering up) of the good eye. When the good vision of the squinting eye has been ensured, measures to correct the squint by orthoptic exercise or surgery can be considered. Early recognition and expert treatment of squints is very important.

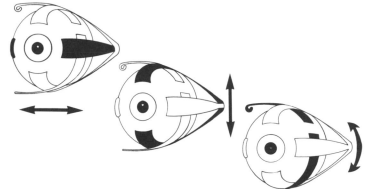

The six eye muscles are arranged in three pairs. Each pair moves the eye in different directions. Defects connected with the outer and inner recti, or straight muscles which turn the eye from side to side and enable coordinated movement produce inward or outward squints. Upward or downward squints are rare.

A paralytic squint is caused by damage to the nerves supplying the eye muscles, or to a disorder of the muscles themselves (for example, myasthenia gravis). In this type the degree of squint varies in different directions and is accompanied by double vision (diplopia). Treatment of a paralytic squint depends on the underlying disorder.

STAMMERING

A disorder of the rhythm of speech, probably due to a failure to syn-

S

chronize articulatory and respiratory movements during speaking; also called stuttering. Stammering may take a number of different forms: hesitation at the start of sentences, pauses in the flow of speech, or involuntary repetition of syllables or whole words. Some people have particular difficulty with certain syllables, and will often use long phrases and sentences to avoid attempting them. Stammers disappear when the person sings. The symptoms characteristically fluctuate with emotional stresses.

Stammering is a common disorder in children under 15 years, particularly boys. In a quarter of cases the problem will persist into adulthood.

Speech therapy in older, well-motivated children can be very effective.

STAPEDECTOMY

Surgical removal of the stapes (the small bone or ossicle in the middle ear which transmits sound from the eardrum to the cochlea), and its replacement by an artificial one.

The main reason for stapedectomy is otosclerosis (qv). The conductive deafness produced by this condition can be compensated with a hearing aid with good results but a successful operation means that this is unnecessary. However, stapedectomy is a difficult operation, and not without risk — there is estimated to be a 3 per cent chance of severe deafness due to damage to the cochlea during the operation and 3 per cent later (perhaps many years after the operation). For this reason European practice is not to operate on both ears, nor to operate on the ear which picks out speech sound more efficiently. The relative ability of the two ears is tested beforehand by audiometry.

STAPHYLOCOCCUS AUREUS

A small round bacterium which lives in grape-like clusters and can invade tissue to cause infection. It is golden in colour when cultured (hence its name 'aureus', Latin for gold); is carried in the nose of about half to three-quarters of the population; and is also usually present on the skin and sometimes in the throat.

Many species of staphylococcus are resistant to penicillin as the bacteria produce an enzyme called penicillinase which inactivates it. Staphylococcal infections can be cured by several different antibiotics.

STATUS ASTHMATICUS

An attack of asthma (qv) which has persisted for hours or days without remission, despite treatment.

Asthma attacks may occur minutes or hours after antigen exposure. They may be precipitated by exertion, inhaled irritants, emotional stress and chest infection. The person experiences tightness of the chest, with wheezing and breathlessness. The attack can usually be brought to an end by a bronchodilator drug, inhaled from an aerosol. If the attack progresses, breathlessness becomes worse, and the patient cannot lie down but feels more comfortable leaning forward with the arms supported. A bluish tinge to the complexion may be visible (cyanosis).

In status asthmaticus the patient is likely to be exhausted and dehydrated because of breathing through the mouth. The inflationary pressure developed by the labouring chest muscles is often sufficient to cause the lung wall to perforate, leaking air into the pleural cavity.

Treatment consists of the inhalation

of a bronchodilator drug through a nebulizer which humidifies the inspired, oxygen-enriched air. Intravenous corticosteroid therapy is given. It is usual for samples to be taken of the oxygen tension of blood in the arteries as an indication of progress. Assisted ventilation may be needed, especially if the patient is exhausted.

STATUS EPILEPTICUS

A series of epileptic seizures (see *Epilepsy*) without recovery of consciousness in between. Most seizures are usually followed by a gradual return to consciousness.

Status epilepticus is potentially life-threatening and requires urgent treatment. Benzodiazepines (such as diazepam) or barbiturates are commonly used. The drug is given intravenously for rapid effect, often in the form of an infusion over a short period of time so that the dose can be adjusted as necessary. As in the case of single seizure epilepsy, it is important to correct any underlying metabolic disturbance such as hypoglycaemia (deficiency of sugar in the blood). Anticonvulsant therapy will be considered in order to prevent further seizures.

STEATORRHOEA

The passage of greater than normal amounts of undigested fat in the stools. The condition results from the malabsorption of fat and is a feature of tropical and non-tropical sprue (qv). The stools are characteristically bulky, pale in colour, greasy, foul-smelling and difficult to flush down the lavatory. The normal absorption of dietary fat requires the presence in the intestine of bile salts made by the liver, fat-degrading enzymes made by the pan

creas, the maintenance of the absorptive function by the cells lining the intestine, and the presence of special channels (lymphatics) in the intestinal wall to carry fat away. Steatorrhoea may result from obstructive disease of the bile ducts (uncommon), chronic pancreatitis, intestinal infection, inflammation of the small intestinal lining and lymphatic channel blockage (rare).

Treatment depends on the underlying cause, but in all cases includes the restriction of dietary fat intake.

STERILIZATION

A means of rendering a person (male or female) infertile. In both sexes sterilization procedures impose a blockage so that sperm and eggs cannot come into contact, thus preventing fertilization.

In women the operation requires a general anaesthetic. Various methods are used to block the Fallopian tubes (the site where fertilization usually occurs): the tubes may be cut and tied, destroyed by heat, or blocked with bands or special clips. Such procedures ofter require an open abdominal

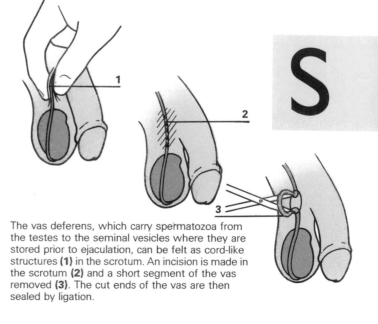

The vas deferens, which carry spermatozoa from the testes to the seminal vesicles where they are stored prior to ejaculation, can be felt as cord-like structures (1) in the scrotum. An incision is made in the scrotum (2) and a short segment of the vas removed (3). The cut ends of the vas are then sealed by ligation.

operation and a hospital stay of about 5–7 days. The operation can also be performed by means of an instrument called a laparoscope. This method has two advantages: only a short stay in hospital is required (1–2 days) and only very small scars are visible. The operation is effective immediately if it is performed before ovulation has occurred in that particular cycle.

Male sterilization involves cutting the vas deferens (vasectomy), the duct which carries sperm from the testis. The operation is performed through small incisions on each side of the scrotum. It is usually carried out under local anaesthetic. Male sterilization is not immediately effective because some sperm are stored beyond the site of the block. The patient should therefore have two negative sperm counts before he can assume that the operation has become fully effective.

Neither male nor female sterilization is 100 per cent effective, yet it remains the most efficient method of contraception with the lowest overall failure rate. Sterilization is a permanent method of family planning and is therefore only appropriate for couples who feel that their families are complete. In certain circumstances reversal of either operation is possible, although it is not always successful.

STEROID

One of a class of drugs closely resembling naturally occurring corticosteroid hormones in structure and function. Steroids are used for their anti-inflammatory and immunosuppressive properties in a wide range of medical conditions, including asthma, ulcerative colitis, eczema (see *Dermatitis*) and rheumatoid arthritis. They can be given intravenously, orally or rectally, inhaled, or applied locally as appropriate.

Short courses of oral steroids are usually without side-effects, but prolonged high doses may induce a condition resembling Cushing's syndrome (qv) and also suppress the individual's ability to produce corticosteroids naturally. Sometimes administration on alternate days is used in an attempt to reduce these problems, often after a period of daily therapy when the condition being treated has been brought under control. Once they have been given for a few days or weeks, steroids cannot be withdrawn suddenly or circulatory collapse can occur. The normal ability of the adrenal glands to increase output of corticosteroids at times of stress is lost in those receiving steroid medication. The dose is therefore temporarily increased for patients with serious illness or who require surgery. Giving the drugs by means other than the oral route in cases requiring long-term administration may minimize side-effects; smaller doses can be used if, for example, intravenous or intramuscular injection is used.

STILLBIRTH

A stillborn infant is defined as an infant born after the twenty-eighth completed week of gestation and who shows no sign of life. This definition can be vague, as in some cases the correct period of gestation is unknown. The stillbirth rate is calculated as the number of stillbirths per thousand births after 28 weeks. Usually the stillbirth rate is combined with the early neonatal death rate (deaths in the first week of life) to calculate the perinatal mortality rate.

The causes of stillbirth are varied but the principal factors can be categorized into three major groups:
- Congenital abnormality. About 20 per cent of all stillbirths have major

S

abnormality, those of the central nervous system (such as anencephaly and spina bifida) being the most common. Antenatal screening and appropriate termination can prevent stillbirths due to these causes

- Low birth weight. About 40 per cent of stillbirths are associated with low birth weight, which can be due to prematurity or growth retardation. These conditions can be precipitated by maternal diseases such as increased blood pressure (preeclampsia, by bleeding in pregnancy and by premature labour

- Hypoxia (lack of oxygen). Postmortem evidence of hypoxia is found in 50 per cent of stillbirths. This may happen suddenly or gradually and is usually the result of poor exchange of oxygen across the placenta (afterbirth).

Factors which may help decrease the stillbirth rate include higher living standards in all social groups, and prevention of maternal problems together with adequate antenatal supervision, guidance and education.

STILL'S DISEASE

A form of juvenile chronic arthritis (JCA) in which inflammation of joints is accompanied or preceded by a generalized illness; it is also known as systemic onset JCA. Most affected children are of pre-school age. The illness starts with fever, a pink rash, often most evident in the evening, enlarged lymph nodes and spleen and, in rare cases, pericarditis (inflammation of the smooth membrane surrounding the heart). The arthritis affects a number of joints, particularly fingers, wrists, knees and neck.

There are two other forms of JCA: the pauci-articular form (affecting few joints) which usually occurs in young children and involves up to four joints;

and the later-onset polyarticular form (affecting several joints) which occurs in older children and resembles rheumatoid arthritis in adults.

Diagnosis is confirmed by specialized blood tests and X-rays. Inflammation of the eye iritis is a possible complication, particularly of pauci-articular JCA.

Treatment involves the use of NSAIDs and sometimes steroids, in addition to rest in the acute phase, and physiotherapy, mobilization and exercise later on. Most children recover after several months or years, but in a few the condition develops into chronic debilitating arthritis.

STING, INSECT

see *Insect sting*

STITCH

see *Suture*

STOKES-ADAMS SYNDROME

A brief episode during which cardiac action stops as a result of an underlying disturbance in heart rhythm (arrythmia) such as asystole, ventricular fibrillation or, most commonly, heart block. During the attack the patient becomes pale and has no pulse, and unconsciousness and convulsions from cerebral hypoxia (lack of oxygen to the brain) may occur. Flushing of the face and skin elsewhere signals the return of cardiac output, as blood flows through the vessels dilated by hypoxia. Consciousness is usually restored rapidly, within 10–15 seconds. The attacks occur suddenly without warning, and can thus be distinguished from simple faints. They can be prevented by the provision of a pacemaker.

S

STOMATITIS

Inflammation of the mouth. There are a variety of causes of stomatitis. These include infections such as *Herpes simplex*, abscess of the gum and thrush (candida); diseases elsewhere in the body, including any chronic debilitating illness, leukaemia or vitamin deficiency; skin diseases such as pemphigus, pemphigoid and lichen planus; drugs such as antibiotics and cytotoxic medication; ulcers in the mouth (aphthous ulceration), cheek biting and ill-fitting dentures.

Treatment is of the underlying cause.

STONE

see *Calculus*

STORK MARKS

see *Birth mark*

STRANGURY

A condition in which urine comes out drop by drop and causes severe pain when it is passed. Strangury occurs when the urine is infected, especially during severe cystitis; occasionally it is due to the passage of blood or blood clots from the bladder. It causes spasm of the muscles in the urinary passage.

Treatment consists of antibiotics for the infection and increased fluid intake to dilute and 'flush out' the urine. SEE ALSO *Dysuria*

STRAWBERRY MARK

see *Angioma*

STREPTOCOCCUS

A group of bacteria which, when stained and viewed under the microscope, appear as chains of 'berry-like' organisms. Streptococci are responsible for a wide variety of infections involving many organs of the body. Common infections that may be caused by streptococci include sore throats/tonsilitis, pneumonia, cellulitis/erysipelas, impetigo, otitis media, sinusitis, meningitis, urinary tract infections and wound infections. If severe, any of these local infections can enter the blood-stream, leading to septicaemia. Glomerulonephritis (severe kidney disease) and rheumatic fever may occur following streptococcal infections. The incidence and severity of many of these infections have been reduced by the use of penicillin or related antibiotics; however, the increased use of these drugs has led to some strains of streptococci developing resistance to penicillin.

STRETCH MARKS

see *Striae*

STRIAE

White lines or streaks on the skin, sometimes resulting from skin disease, such as lichen planus (qv), but more often due to stretching of the skin such that the upper epidermis gives way. Striae are most often seen in pregnancy (striae gravidarum), when they appear over the abdomen and thighs. Increased steroid hormone levels in the bloodstream also contribute to the development of these stretch marks. When they first form they are usually pink or bright red. Gradually the colour fades until they become silvery white, but they never disappear completely. Striae also result from severe obesity.

STROKE

Bleeding from or blood clotting

S

(thrombosis) within a cerebral artery, leading to a disturbance of neurological function; known medically as cerebrovascular accident. Less common causes are haemorrhage into the brain due to rupture of an atheromatous artery in a person with high blood pressure or of an aneurysm lying close to the surface of the brain. The symptoms depend on the area of brain involved and the extent of damage caused by either tissue death or haemorrhage. The most familiar type of stroke causes paralysis of one side of the body (hemiplegia) together with hemianopia (loss of half the visual field). The onset is sudden, and weakness may increase over a period of several days. Provided this does not lead to severe cerebral oedema and mid-brain compression, some degree of recovery is common, and a complete return of function may occur, especially if tissue death has been limited. Recovery is usually less complete after a haemorrhage, which often produces substantial destruction of brain tissue and is much more often fatal than cerebral thrombosis. Strokes become more common with age.

Recovery mostly takes place within the first few weeks, but function may continue to improve with training. The diagnosis is not usually in doubt, and causes such as tumours and arteritis are rare. Tissue death and haemorrhage may be distinguished by a CT scan; this is important if anticoagulants (qv) are considered as treatment. Otherwise, treatment centres on providing support and help, involving physiotherapists, speech therapists, occupational therapists and home support workers. Early mobilization is encouraged.

STUPOR

A state in which a person is mute and unable to move yet maintains conscious awareness; the term 'akinetic mutism' is also sometimes used. For the most part sufferers are unresponsive to their surroundings though they may follow people in the vicinity with their eyes. The cause of stupor may be psychiatric or neurological in origin and distinguishing between them is sometimes difficult in the early stages. Psychiatric causes include catatonic schizophrenia, severe depression and hysteria. Neurological causes include brain tumours and, more often, cerebrovascular disease (disease of the brain or the blood vessels supplying it).

STURGE-WEBER SYNDROME

A developmental disorder of unknown origin in which there is an abnormality of capillaries over the surface of one of the cerebral hemispheres of the brain. The condition is often associated with calcification (deposits of calcium) which can be seen on X-rays, outlining the folds of the cerebral cortex. Almost invariably there is a port-wine birthmark or naevus on the same side of the patient's face, and the eye on that side may be enlarged (ox-eye). Most patients are paralyzed on one side of the body from birth and suffer recurrent convulsions, which require treatment with anticonvulsant drugs, and often have disturbed behaviour as well. Some with intractable attacks of epilepsy are helped by removal of part of the affected cerebral hemisphere (hemispherectomy). The operation may abolish the epileptic attacks and improve behaviour but its results are somewhat unpredictable.

STYE

Acute inflammation of the glands in the eyelid associated with the eyelashes.

S

It is caused by infection with the bacterium *Staphylococcus aureus*. Treatment is with antibiotic eye ointment, especially after the stye has burst, in order to prevent recurrence; sometimes if the ointment is applied when the stye is developing the formation of pus can be prevented. Surgical incision and drainage by means of a fine syringe needle may be required in occasional cases. If styes recur, then surgical removal of the skin containing the inflamed gland may be necessary.

SUBARACHNOID HAEMORRHAGE

Bleeding into the subarachnoid space that lies between the outer surface of the brain and the arachnoid component of the meninges (the series of membranes which covers the brain and lines the skull). In most cases the cause is rupture of a berry-shaped aneurysm (qv) within the arterial blood vessels at the base of the brain (the so-called Circle of Willis) but occasionally the bleeding comes from an arteriovenous angioma (qv). The risk of bleeding is increased with high blood pressure. The sudden onset of a severe headache is a typical symptom, often with loss of consciousness. The neck is very stiff and paralysis of one side of the body (hemiplegia) or other neurological signs, such as dysphasia, may be present. CT scan of the brain and lumbar puncture are the techniques used to confirm the diagnosis. An arteriogram (see *Arteriography*) is performed to identify and localize the causal lesion. If an aneurysm is discovered, surgery is required to prevent further bleeding; of the several techniques available, clipping the neck of the aneurysm is the best. The timing of surgery is variable, but is usually within two weeks, as the risk of re-bleeding from an untreated aneurysm is highest then; surgical treatment in the first week may carry an unacceptable complication rate due to vascular spasm. Subarachnoid haemorrhage is a serious disorder with a death rate of up to 50 per cent in the first three months after the episode.

SUBDURAL HAEMORRHAGE

Bleeding into the subdural space between the dura mater and arachnoid (two of the membranes covering the brain), usually as a result of a head injury tearing the veins in the subdural space. Subdural haemorrhage can occur at any age, but is more common in the elderly whose veins are fragile, alcoholics who commonly injure themselves and patients receiving anticoagulant drugs in whom bleeding can be a side-effect. The interval between head injury and symptoms is variable, but can be several months after a seemingly trivial injury. The symptoms are the gradual onset of headache, drowsiness and confusion. Subdural bleeding rarely occurs on both sides of the head. A CT scan of the brain usually highlights the collection of blood (haematoma), but sometimes other imaging techniques, such as a magnetic resonance scan (MRI), are required. The blood is evacuated through a hole drilled in the skull. If a subdural haemorrhage is treated early the outlook is good; left untreated the condition may be fatal.

SUDDEN INFANT DEATH SYNDROME (SIDS)

Sudden, unexpected death in infancy which cannot be explained by known disease. The diagnosis can only be made if the postmortem examination shows no evidence of relevant congenital abnormality involving the lungs, heart or nervous system, or serious infection (such as meningitis). Most cases occur between 2 and 6 months of age, 3 months being the most vulnerable age. SIDS is the commonest cause of death in infants between the ages of 1 month and 1 year in developed countries, and occurs in 2 or 3 babies per 1,000.

The cause of SIDS remains elusive, despite considerable research. Various theories have been put forward, including abnormal heart rhythm, decreased blood sugar, choking on regurgitated feed, over-heating and abnormal response to infection. Suffocation by bed-clothes or underneath a sleeping adult has long been disregarded as an explanation. The most promising area of research concerns the control of breathing. Babies who suffer SIDS appear to have recurring periods of irregular breathing with pauses (apnoea). SIDS occurs during sleep, often at night (hence its alternative name, 'cot death'). There is often a preceding mild illness such as snuffles. Distraught parents may attempt to revive the baby or rush him or her to hospital, but all efforts fail. The baby has often been dead for some time when discovered. As death is unexpected, the coroner is informed, and a postmortem is mandatory.

Since the cause is unknown, there can be no sure method of prevention. For babies at high risk (some premature babies, and brothers and sisters of SIDS victims) home apnoea monitoring (a device with some sort of alarm system) is used, but is not foolproof.

SUNBURN

Diffuse inflammation of the skin as a result of exposure to intense sunlight. Sunburn is caused by ultraviolet irradiation emitted by the sun. It can range from mild erythema (red eruptions) to severe blistering with systemic upset. In minor cases of sunburn the effects can be relieved by calamine lotion. Severe sunburn requires local treatment of the blisters with appropriate creams or lotions and dressings to prevent secondary infection, and adequate fluid intake.

If burns are to be avoided the skin's production of melanin (the substance responsible for skin pigmentation and for filtering sunlight of its harmful effects) needs to be stepped up; this can be achieved by gradually increasing exposure to natural or artificial ultraviolet light. Protection is also provided by suntan lotions, which prevent penetration of the skin by the ultraviolet rays which provoke sunburn.

Excessive exposure to sunlight predisposes to the development of certain skin cancers. In Australia, for example, early and prolonged exposure has been strongly linked to the development of malignant melanoma (qv). Protection of the skin against the sun through the use of sunscreen lotions and hats is particularly important in such an environment.

SEE ALSO *Photosensitivity*, *Heat stroke*

SUNSTROKE

see *Heat stroke*

SUPPOSITORY

A small, cone-shaped medicament which is inserted into the rectum. Thanks to its cocoa butter or gelatin base the suppository is solid and can be handled at room temperature but melts once it has entered the body, releasing its drug content. Suppositories were originally developed for the treatment of conditions of the rectum (typically haemorrhoids) and are still used for that purpose. As many drugs that can be absorbed when taken orally are also absorbed from the rectum, suppositories can also be used to administer medication where taking it by mouth is not appropriate (for example, pain-killers for people who are vomiting, or NSAIDs for those who develop indigestion when taking them orally).

SUTURE

This means to stitch, or a stitch. Suture is an important aspect of surgery of any type and is most commonly used to join cut edges of a wound together. There are two categories of material used:

- Absorbable, which includes catgut (made of the intestinal wall of sheep, not cats as the name implies) and synthetics, which were introduced more recently and have many advantages over catgut. These types of suture eventually dissolve and are generally used inside the body or in body cavities.
- Non-absorbic materials, such as linen and silk, which have been used since the beginning of surgery and are still in use; the synthetic material in this group is nylon. These types of suture do not dissolve and must be removed, usually 7−10 days after the operation. Traditionally they have been used on the surface of the body but are declining in use with the growth in development of absorbable sutures.

SWAB

There are two common meanings of this word in medicine. It can mean a mop used in a surgical operation to absorb body secretions, or a piece of cotton wool on the end of a stick used to sample various body sites for infection, such as the throat or vagina. In the second of these applications the swab is sent to a laboratory so that the germs or bacteria causing the infection can be identified and the correct antibiotic medication prescribed.

SYDENHAM'S CHOREA

see *Chorea*

SYMPATHECTOMY

An operation to divide the sympathetic nerves either in the neck or in the lumbar region. The sympathetic nerves control the size of the small blood vessels in the body and so regulate blood flow and the amount of sweat produced. Sympathectomy is performed when the nerves become over-active. The operation removes the control centre of the nerves (the ganglia), thus improving the circulation and reducing sweat production. A cervical sympathectomy involves dividing the nerves in the neck with the aim of improving circulation to the arms; it is used as treatment in Raynaud's disease (qv) when blood flow to the fingers is reduced. Lumbar sympathectomy (in the lower back) increases blood flow to the legs and is sometimes performed in cases of atheroma (qv) when poor circulation is causing pain at rest and there is a threat of gangrene. Sympathectomy can be carried out by injecting alcohol into the cervical or lumbar ganglia (chemical sympathectomy), or by surgery.

SYNCOPE

A brief loss of consciousness (blackout) resulting from lack of blood flow

S

to the brain. The two causes of syncope are a fall in blood pressure or an obstruction to blood flow in the large arteries in the head and neck.

The commonest form of syncope is fainting. This can occur as a result of standing for a prolonged period on a hot day. Gravity leads to a pooling of blood in the legs, and blood vessels in the skin dilate in an attempt to lose heat. Blood pressure then starts to fall, and fainting occurs when the vagus nerve causes a sudden slowing of the heart. Atherosclerosis (qv) predisposes to syncope by causing the arteries to narrow. Turning the head or straining to pass urine may then be enough to cause syncope by reducing the already precarious blood supply to the brain. A sudden abnormality of the rhythm of the heart leading to a drop in blood pressure is an uncommon cause of syncope. This form is diagnosed by ECG monitoring.

SYNDROME

A collection of symptoms and /or physical signs which occur together and form a characteristic pattern. Usually the nature of the problem or its cause is poorly understood, and often the syndrome is known by the name of the person who first described it; for example, Sjögren's syndrome.

Many syndromes refer to congenital deformities which have now been found to be due to specific enzyme defects. One well known example is mongolism, known as Down's syndrome, caused by the presence of an extra chromosome (number 21) in each cell. Often a syndrome is renamed as a disease once its specific cause has been identified; for example, McArdle's disease, once a syndrome of exercise-induced muscle pain, now known to be due to a deficiency of the enzyme phosphorylase in muscle.

SYPHILIS

A sexually transmitted disease caused by a spirochaete (a corkscrew-shaped bacterium) called *Treponema pallidum*. Man is the only natural host of this very strict parasite, which dies rapidly outside the human body. It can infect via the intact membranes of the body or a cut or graze. Primarily it is acquired by sexual intercourse but may be contracted through the handling of the lesions that accompany the disease. It is estimated that two-thirds of individuals exposed to syphilis will contract the disease.

There are four phases to this disease. Primary syphilis is characterized by solitary or multiple ulcers known as chancres (qv) which occur at the site where the disease entered the body. The incubation period averages 21 days. This phase of the disease may be painless and the chancre so small as to be invisible. Primary syphilis is curable and is best treated with penicillin. Without treatment the chancre will disappear spontaneously but progression to the secondary stage of syphilis will still occur.

Secondary syphilis appears 2–4 weeks after the primary chancre clears up; it is signalled by a generalized rash which may recur. This phase is systemic and may affect any organ in the body; like the primary phase of the disease it is infectious. Wart-like lesions may affect the genitalia and the glands in the neck may swell (lymphadenopathy). In the early stages of secondary syphilis (less than one year's duration) the disease is curable with penicillin.

Tertiary syphilis evolves from untreated secondary syphilis in approximately one-third of patients, between 3 and 20 years after the initial infection. This stage used to be characterized by the formation of 'gummas', inflam-

S

matory, slowly growing lesions that destroy natural tissues (particularly in the heart, brain and joints) and can lead to extensive heart disease and syphilitic madness. Gummas are now rare but tertiary syphilis may present with meningoencephalitis (inflammation of the brain and infection of the meninges – see *Encephalitis*). Once the effects of tertiary syphilis become apparent the disease cannot invariably be cured by treatment with penicillin; nevertheless this should again be given.

Quaternary syphilis, which may develop without an intervening tertiary phase (tertiary syphilis is now uncommon), affects the brain and spinal cord (neurosyphilis), producing psychiatric disturbances and dementia or locomotor ataxia (which leads to characteristic sensory disturbances).

Syphilis contracted in pregnancy can infect the fetus across the placenta (afterbirth), leading to a syndrome known as congenital syphilis, which can produce any of the above manifestations in children. Treatment is with penicillin.

The diagnosis of syphilis is based on the examination of tissue from the chancre under the microscope and on special tests of blood and cerebrospinal fluid (in neurosyphilis). Follow-up is long term and tracing the infected person's previous sexual contacts is important.

SYRINGOMYELIA

An uncommon neurological disease caused by a cavity (syrinx) within the spinal cord. It may be congenital due to a developmental defect at the base of the brain (usually a variant of the Arnold-Chiari malformation causing obstruction to cerebrospinal fluid flow so that the central canal of the spinal cord distends), or it can rarely occur as the result of a spinal cord tumour. The patient's perception of pain and temperature is impaired in the arms and neck, and scoliosis (curvature of the spine) is usually present, followed later by degeneration of the muscles in the legs which may be painful. Symptoms rarely occur before adolescence even in congenital forms of the disease. If the cavity extends upwards into the brain (syringobulbia), speech, eye and facial movements, and sensation in the face may be affected.

An operation to improve the flow of cerebrospinal fluid at the base of the brain may be beneficial if performed early in the course of the disease. Otherwise, treatment is often unsatisfactory.

SYSTEMIC LUPUS ERYTHEMATOSUS (SLE)

An uncommon inflammatory condition of unknown cause which particularly affects young women. A wide range of tissues and organs may be affected. The condition is associated with many abnormalities of the immune system, including antibodies that recognize parts of the body's own cells (autoantibodies) and attack them; classically present in SLE is the antinuclear antibody factor which binds to cell nuclei and attacks them.

The commonest signs are arthritis in the small joints in the hands, wrists and knees, and aching muscles (myalgia), often accompanied by mild fever, tiredness and weight loss. A characteristic butterfly rash may appear across the face, and loss of hair, mouth ulcers and Raynaud's disease (reduced circulation to the fingers) may also occur. Pleurisy, cough or breathlessness may denote lung involvement. Protein in the urine may indicate disease in the kidneys which, in a few patients, leads to progressive kidney damage. Headache and psychiatric disturbance are among the neurological problems that may be experienced by SLE patients. Other organs that may be affected include the heart (noninfective endocarditis) and eye (uveitis).

Originally SLE was considered a severe, progressive and often fatal disease. Recently, however, the evidence derived from sensitive blood tests designed to detect autoantibodies has revealed that the condition is much commoner than hitherto realized and that many patients (for example with mild arthritis) have a mild form of it. The course of the disease is often characterized by periods of disease activity and remission.

There is no cure for SLE. Treatment is aimed at improving symptoms and reducing inflammation in the affected tissues and organs and may involve rest and nonsteroidal anti-inflammatory drugs (NSAIDs). For suppression of symptoms and signs in severe disease, steroids or other powerful immunosuppressive drugs may be necessary.

SYSTEMIC ONSET JUVENILE CHRONIC ARTHRITIS (JCA)

see *Still's disease*

SYSTEMIC SCLEROSIS

see *Scleroderma*

SYSTOLE

Contraction of the heart muscle. The term usually refers to contraction of the muscles of the ventricles (the lower chambers of the heart) which produces the pulse wave in the arteries. Atrial systole occurs shortly before this (the atria are the upper chambers of the heart). The period between the end of ventricular systole and the beginning of atrial systole is known as diastole; this is when blood flows into the heart from the veins. Ventricular muscle contraction starts when the tricuspid (right atrioventricular) and mitral (left atrioventricular) valves are closed; only when the pressure created by the contraction is raised above that in the pulmonary arteries and the aorta beyond will the pulmonary and aortic valves open and the blood flow into the circulation. Similarly, during relaxation of the ventricular muscle, blood flow through the latter valves will stop when ventricular pressure drops below arterial. Ventricular systole therefore takes place in the period just before opening and just before closure of the valves.

TACHYCARDIA

A rapid heart rate, faster than 100 beats per minute. Tachycardia may have regular or irregular rhythm, and may be a normal phenomenon or may be a form of arrhythmia due to underlying heart disease. A regular (sinus) tachycardia occurs in normal individuals as a response to exercise, emotion or pregnancy, and may also be found in conditions that do not primarily affect the heart, such as anaemia, Paget's disease of bone, carbon dioxide retention, thyrotoxicosis (overactivity of the thyroid gland) and liver failure, when increased blood flow is required to abnormal organs. Heart failure, constrictive pericarditis and shock are other causes of a regular tachycardia, as are certain drugs.

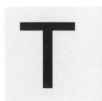

Cardiac arrhythmias that cause a regular tachycardia include atrial (supraventricular) tachycardia, ventricular tachycardia and atrial flutter (the atria are the upper chambers of the heart, the ventricles the lower). Atrial flutter is often regular, less often irregular, while atrial fibrillation is always irregular.

Treatment is directed at the underlying cause. In some cardiac arrhythmias drug treatment may slow the heart rate and improve cardiac function yet still leave the underlying irregular rhythm unaffected.

TACHYPHLAXIS

A tolerance or decreased effectiveness of a drug. Tachyphlaxis develops rapidly, sometimes within minutes of administration, and may follow previous exposure to only a few doses. It occurs not as a result of an immunological mechanism but because the body rapidly adjusts to and resists the effect of the drug; the reasons for this are unclear. Repeated administration of the drug produces a decreasing effect and alternative remedies may be needed.

TALIPES

see *Club foot*

TAMPONADE

A term most frequently used to describe an obstruction which prevents the ventricles (lower chambers of the heart) filling with blood due to an accumulation of pericardial fluid in the sac around the heart. This occurs most commonly as a result of cardiac surgery, injury and pericarditis (inflammation of the smooth membrane surrounding the heart). The amount of fluid required to cause cardiac tamponade is greater if the effusion accumulates slowly; this is because the body can absorb some of the fluid and because the heart is able to adjust to slow but not to rapid accumulation. Tamponade reduces the output of the heart and causes congestion of the systemic and pulmonary veins, giving the symptoms of heart failure. The accumulation of fluid may be detected clinically, by X-ray or, most easily, by echocardiography (ECG). Tamponade is a life-threatening disorder, especially if fluid accumulates rapidly. Treatment involves the pericardial fluid being drawn off by means of paracentesis (qv).

TB

see *Tuberculosis*

TEETH

see *Caries*, *Dentition*, *Wisdom teeth*

TELANGIECTASIA

Usually an inherited condition in which groups of blood vessels appear as red bumps on the skin and lips, and throughout the gut. Bleeding from the lesions causes iron deficiency anaemia. The condition may also occur in chronic liver disease, particularly cirrhosis of the liver. If the lesions are pressed the blood is pulsed out and they turn pale, but as soon as the pressure is removed the blood flows back and the colour returns.

The only available treatment is iron therapy and, if the anaemia is severe, blood transfusion.

TEMPERATURE

see *Fever*

TENOTOMY

The dividing or cutting of a tendon. The operation may be carried out 'closed' or 'blind', without exposing the tendon, or it may be an 'open' operation. In a 'closed' operation a fine knife is inserted through a small incision and passed under the tendon, which is then cut. In an 'open' operation the tendon is exposed and cut under direct vision. Which method is used is largely a matter of choice by the surgeon.

Tenotomy is usually performed to correct the shortening (contracture) which often results from neuromuscular disease. The calf muscles, for example, commonly shorten as a result of this type of disease and a tenotomy to lengthen the Achilles tendon behind the ankle is often performed to counter the effects of this. In sufferers from multiple sclerosis or muscular dystrophy deformity can be reduced by the release of soft tissue contractures through tenotomy. In ophthalmology the cutting of a tendon to one of the muscles that control eye movement is used in the treatment of some squints.

TERATOGENESIS

An abnormal development in the embryo and fetus as a result of environmental factors. These factors include ingested agents, usually drugs (for example, thalidomide), ionizing radiation (as in X-rays) and certain infections. Thalidomide caused abnormalities in limb development, resulting in a condition known as phocomelia (complete or partial absence of one or more limbs). Known teratogenic infections include rubella (German measles), cytomegalovirus, syphilis and toxoplasmosis. The range and severity of abnormalities caused by environmental factors is quite wide and cannot always be accurately predicted. For example, if rubella is acquired by the fetus in the womb, it can cause either mild or quite devastating abnormalities, the effect depending on the stage of development at which infection occurred. In general terms, the earlier in pregnancy that the infection occurs, the greater the degree of abnormality.

Despite the fact that many teratogens have been identified, no obvious predisposing teratogen can be detected in most infants born with abnormalities. In these cases the assumption is that abnormality occurred either as a spontaneous event or as a result of an as yet unidentified teratogen.

TERATOMA

A special type of tumour containing cells of a mixed variety (skin cells, muscle cells, thyroid cells, and so on). Traces of all the types of cell present in the body may be found in a teratoma. Teratomas can be malignant or benign and can occur in many areas of the body. The most common type is found in the ovary (dermoid cyst) and is nearly always benign. The cyst has the appearance of a soft waxy ball and contains thick sebaceous fluid together with other elements such as hair and teeth.

There is an equivalent teratoma in the male testis; this has a greater chance of being or becoming malignant.
SEE ALSO *Ovarian cyst*

TESTICULAR TORSION

Twisting of the spermatic cord and blood vessels leading to the testis. The normal testis is oval and lies in a sac in the scrotum with its poles

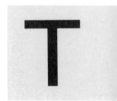

oriented 'up and down'. If the descent of the testis is abnormal (see *Undescended testis*), or the attachment of the blood supply and the tube that carries the sperm (the vas) is small, the testis may hang like a bell clapper (with the poles lying crossways). This narrow attachment permits the testis to swing around, and this puts a twist in the attachments. The twist cuts off the blood supply to the testicle. This is serious, since the testis becomes swollen and extremely painful, and begins to die. Within a few hours the testis is destroyed. Torsion can occur at any age, but is commoner during the teenage years, perhaps because the testis becomes less mobile with increasing age. The severe pain of torsion may be preceded by warning twinges, when incomplete twisting of the attachments occurs. Untreated, the testis becomes gangrenous, and so an urgent operation is needed to untwist the testis (orchidopexy). This is performed even when the diagnosis is in doubt, because of the consequences of missing a genuine torsion. The testicle on the opposite side is fixed down at the same operation, to prevent it from twisting. Occasionally the operation is too late to save the testis, and it is then necessary to remove it (orchidectomy).

TESTIS, UNDESCENDED

More properly known as testicular maldescent. During fetal life the normal testis develops by the kidney, just below the rib cage. It moves down the back of the abdominal cavity and passes through the abdominal wall in the groin. This tunnel is called the inguinal canal (it is here that inguinal hernias develop). The testis passes via the canal to the scrotum to reach its final position. If this journey is incomplete the testis can remain within the abdomen, or more usually it is held up at the inguinal canal. This is called maldescent of the testis.

Occasionally the testis ends up outside the normal pathway and can be found in the thigh or the perineum (between the legs), or at the base of the penis. This is an ectopic testis. A retractile testis is one which has safely made the journey to the scrotum, but can temporarily retreat to the inguinal canal.

The maldescended testis usually becomes infertile, and carries a risk of developing cancer (1 in 10 testicular cancers is associated with maldescent). It is also more likely to undergo torsion. The treatment is surgery to free the testis and its blood supply and deliver it to the scrotum (the operation is called orchidopexy). This is best done before 3 years of age, or as soon as the condition is diagnosed after that age. Occasionally it is better to remove the testis if it is in any way abnormal.

TEST TUBE BABY

The popular term used to describe in-vitro fertilization or fertilization of the female egg by the male sperm outside the body of the female partner.

The technique is used when natural fertilization is impossible; because of blocked Fallopian tubes, for example. The procedure entails collecting a mature female egg, either by laparoscopy (qv) or by sucking it out with a fine needle under ultrasound guidance, and mixing it with specially prepared male sperm. Under the correct conditions the two will fuse and begin to develop into an embryo by cellular division. After the fertilized egg has undergone several divisions so that a ball of cells is present (the very early embryo) it is replaced in the mother's uterus (womb) to allow further development to take place in the correct environment.

Successful pregnancies occur on 20–30 per cent of occasions. It is usual practice to fertilize more than one egg at a time and to implant up to three or four; this is felt to improve the chances of a viable pregnancy developing, as only a few of the embryo inserted into the womb will implant in its wall.

Eggs, sperms and embryos can be frozen and stored, although this practice is still relatively uncommon with human beings; veterinary medicine uses these techniques more often.
SEE ALSO *Infertility*

TETANUS

An infection caused by the toxin of the *Clostridium tetani* bacterium, which is widely present in soil and dust. The bacterium gains access to the body via an injury that has resulted in penetration of the skin; this may be as minor as a scratch from a thorn. Tetanus follows 2–14 days after the injury. Initially it causes stiffness and pain in the jaw and spine, and difficulty in swallowing. Later, 'lockjaw' develops and painful muscular spasms affect the entire body; the latter may be powerful enough to fracture vertebrae.

Without hospital treatment tetanus is usually fatal. Intensive care therapy comprising controlled paralysis using anaesthetic drugs, artificial respiration on a ventilator, penicillin and, most importantly, tetanus antitoxin, is now successful in most patients under the age of 50, and in about 50 per cent of older patients. Tetanus can be prevented by vaccination, which consists of a course of tetanus toxoid (an inactivated form of tetanus toxin) in childhood, with booster injections every ten years thereafter, or at the time of injury if the last booster was more than five years previously.

TETANY

Increased excitability of the nerves, leading to involuntary spasm of the muscles, characteristically of the hands, feet and larynx (voice-box). Tetany is brought on by insufficient calcium in the blood as a result of one of the following underlying causes: inadequate intake (malnutrition) or defective absorption of calcium, impaired function of the parathyroid glands which secrete calcium, chronic kidney failure causing calcium to be lost through the kidneys, or increased alkalinity of the blood as a result of overbreathing (with loss of carbon dioxide from the breath) or persistent vomiting.

Immediate treatment includes the administration of intravenous calcium; in the case of overbreathing, sedation may be required, and the patient is encouraged to 'rebreathe' his or her own expired air by slow breathing into and out of a paper bag clasped over the mouth as this restores the carbon dioxide level in the lungs and the bicarbonate in the blood. Longer-term treatment is directed at the underlying cause.

THALASSAEMIA

An inherited condition involving an abnormality of haemoglobin (the red pigment in blood). There are two forms of thalassaemia: alpha and beta (the more serious of the two), named after the protein chains that make up the globin part of the haemoglobin molecule. In alpha thalassaemia there is a reduced amount of the two alpha chains and in beta thalassaemia a reduced amount of beta chains. This results in chronic haemolytic anaemia which increases synthesis of red cells (erythrocytes) in the bone marrow, leading to deformity of the bones as the bone marrow cavities expand to accommodate this activity; the cheekbones, for example, are commonly affected and as a result are particularly prominent.

Treatment involves regular blood transfusions, although these produce the side-effect of iron overload which causes damage to some organs, particularly the heart and liver. Drugs to remove the iron are given intravenously. Thalassaemia may be diagnosed before birth, either by sampling fetal blood from the umbilical blood vessels or by sampling the chorionic villus (part of the placenta). The latter technique is difficult but has the advantage of making diagnosis possible earlier, at around 12 weeks of gestation, whereas the sampling of fetal blood vessels cannot be performed before 15 weeks of gestation and in centres with limited expertise it is not possible before 19−20 weeks. Abortion is offered only in cases of full-blown (homozygous) thalassaemia. Carriers of the disease may be mildly anaemic but lead perfectly normal lives. Indeed, such carriers are frequently encountered in Mediterranean countries such as Cyprus and Greece where thalassaemia is a major health problem.

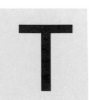

THIAMINE

Thiamine is vitamin B$_1$, deficiency of which is responsible for beriberi (qv) and diseases of the nerves (see *Neuropathy*). On a normal Western diet thiamine deficiency is most unusual, but unsupplemented ricebased diets are often deficient. The amount of thiamine needed is, however, increased in those on a predominantly carbohydrate diet and also in alcoholics, in whom thiamine is required for alcohol metabolism. Alcoholics are doubly prone to thiamine deficiency

because many of them also have a poor diet. Wernicke's encephalopathy (qv), the related 'Korsakoff's psychosis', and exacerbation of heart disease are the direct consequences of thiamine deficiency. The effects of this deficiency are curable only if it is recognized and treated early with high doses of vitamin B$_1$.

THROMBO-CYTOPENIA

A deficiency of platelets in the blood which may result in a bleeding tendency. Platelets are tiny cells without nuclei which are produced in the bone marrow and are essential for the clotting of blood. The normal platelet count is between 150,000 and 400,000 per cu mm of blood ($150-400 \times 10^9$ per litre). There is an increasing risk of bleeding if the platelet count falls below 20,000 platelets per cu mm of blood (20×10^9 per litre). Thrombocytopenia may occur as a result of impaired production of normal cells in the bone marrow, causing a fall in the number of platelets in the blood; for example, by anti-cancer cytotoxic chemotherapy, or by infiltration of the bone marrow with cancer cells from another site in the body. However, most cases arise as a consequence of platelet destruction (principally in the spleen) by the patient's own antibodies. Autoimmune thrombocytopenia, as this occurence is termed, is not uncommon in children, in whom it may occur after a viral infection. In adults, autoimmune thrombocytopenia may be picked up in an asymptomatic individual as a result of a routine full blood count. The main symptoms are spontaneous bruising, nosebleeds and, in the case of women, heavy menstrual blood loss. Numerous pinhead haemorrhages (petechiae) on the skin may accompany the bruises. In children, autoimmune thrombocytopenia is usually self-limiting and often clears up without specific treatment. If haemorrhagic problems are severe, a course of steroids is usually administered. In adults, the condition runs a more chronic course and the spleen may have to be removed to raise the platelet count.

THROMBO-EMBOLISM

The breaking off of a blood clot from its site of formation and its spread to block a blood vessel in a distant part of the body. Most commonly, the clot forms within the deep veins of the calf (a deep vein thrombosis) and spreads to the lungs (pulmonary embolus — see *Embolism*). Thrombi or blood clots can also form on the wall of the heart; when the heart beat is irregular (as in fibrillation, for example) the clot may pass to blood vessels further away. There is a high risk of thrombo-embolism after a heart attack and after heart valve and coronary artery bypass surgery. The anticoagulant drugs, (qv) which form the basis of treatment for thrombo-embolism can also be given as a preventative measure in the two at-risk situations just mentioned. The anticoagulants most commonly used are heparin, which must be given intravenously or subcutaneously (just beneath the skin), and warfarin. These drugs require regular monitoring with blood tests to ensure that enough is being given to prevent thrombosis, but that over-dosage does not occur to produce bleeding.

THROMBOLYTIC THERAPY

Treatment to dissolve blood clots.

The enzymes streptokinase or urokinase may be used for this purpose. Streptokinase is obtained from bacteria called haemolytic streptococci. It works by activating plasminogen, a protein in blood which dissolves fibrin (the main component of clots). However, it may cause unwanted severe bleeding. Furthermore, it produces allergic reactions in individuals who have antibodies as a result of previous streptococcal infections.

Urokinase used to be obtained from human urine but is now made from the growth of fetal kidney cells. It too activates plasminogen. It has an advantage over streptokinase in that it does not produce allergic reactions, but it too can cause bleeding.

Tissue plasminogen activator is a new synthesized form of thrombolytic therapy which is used to dissolve the clots after a heart attack. Its use is still largely experimental, but it may in time supplant the other agents.

THROMBOPHLEBITIS

Inflammation in and around the veins close to the skin (superficial veins) The condition is often seen in patients with deep vein thrombosis (clotting in the deep veins). The cause of thrombophlebitis is obscure but the clinical signs are dramatic. The vein involved is extremely tender, red, hot and swollen. A generalized fever is sometimes present. Thrombophlebitis is often provoked by the insertion of intravenous drips and the injections given through them, and it is almost universal among intravenous drug abusers. In these cases, removal of the cause and simple painkillers are usually adequate treatment. Thrombophlebitis is also associated with varicose veins. Unlike deep vein thrombosis, thrombophlebitis is superficial and is not likely to lead to serious complications such as pulmonary embolism.

Treatment is directed at measures to reduce the inflammation; these include the application of heat, elevation of the legs and the prescribing of anti-inflammatory drugs.

THROMBOSIS

Abnormal blood clotting in the veins (venous thrombosis) and arteries (arterial thrombosis). Venous thrombosis occurs particularly in the deep veins of the leg. These clots usually only present problems if they spread to the main veins and cause a blockage, which may cause the leg to swell. However, there is also a danger of fragments of the clot breaking off and spreading to the lungs (pulmonary embolism).

Arterial thrombosis results in the blood supply being cut off. Thrombosis of a brain artery is a common cause of stroke. A clot in one of the coronary arteries that supply the heart muscle produces a heart attack in the individual and death of the muscle tissue (myocardial infarction). This is always a potentially serious condition and may be fatal through ventricular fibrillation (qv) and cardiac arrest. However, many small and even some large infarcts may heal, leaving a scar on the heart muscle, and the patient can survive and live normally for many years; there is always, however, a risk of recurrence.

There are a number of risk factors which predispose to thrombosis: increasing age, obesity, immobility, varicose veins, cancer, major abdominal operations and pregnancy. Occasionally, there may be an inherited predisposition to thrombosis because of a lack of certain proteins that control clotting.

Treatment depends on the diagnosis.

THRUSH

see *Candida*

THYMUS

A gland in the chest which is large in children and becomes smaller in adults. It is a place where certain types of white blood cell or lymphocytes (T cells) mature and become able to recognize substances foreign to the body, such as viruses and bacteria. The thymus also produces hormones that regulate the development of peripheral lymphoid tissue. The auto-immune disease myasthenia gravis (qv) is the disorder most commonly associated with abnormality of the thymus. In severe cases the gland is removed bringing improvement by halting the manufacture of antibodies against the acetycholine receptor, a chemical neurotransmitter which passes impulses between the ends of nerve cells (neurones). Tumours of the thymus (thymomas) are present in some patients with myasthenia gravis.

THYROID

A gland consisting of two lobes connected to each other across the front of the windpipe (trachea) in the neck, just below the larynx. The thyroid is one of the endocrine or hormone-producing glands, and is under the control of the brain and pituitary gland via thyroid-stimulating hormone (TSH). TSH acts on the thyroid to promote the release of the iodine-containing hormones thyroxine (T4) and the more active T3 which have important roles in the control of metabolism and growth.

Disease of the thyroid may be signified by enlargement of the gland (goitre, which appears as a swelling in the front of the neck), and by signs of overactivity (sweating, tremor and weight loss). The many causes of thyroid disease include the very rare condition of congenital absence of the gland, over-stimulation by abnormal antibodies (Graves' disease — see *Thyrotoxicosis*), and various types of malignancy. Underactivity (hypothyroidism) is treated by oral replacement of T4, and overactivity (hyperthyroidism) by drugs, radioactive iodine or surgery.

SEE ALSO *illustration on page 144*

THYROIDECTOMY

Surgical removal of all (total) or part (subtotal) of the thyroid gland. Thyroidectomy is required in certain cases of benign and malignant swelling of the thyroid gland (such as thyroid cysts, certain types of goitre, thyrotoxicosis and various malignant conditions of the gland). It is performed under general anaesthesia through an incision in the neck. The patient who is undergoing thyroidectomy as treatment for thyrotoxicosis (a condition in which the thyroid is supplying an excess amount of hormone to the tissues) requires special preparation to return his or her thyroid to its normal state before the operation. This is done by giving the patient the antithyroid drugs iodine or propranolol. As the recurrent laryngeal nerve (to the vocal cords) runs behind the thyroid gland it is possible that it may be in advertently damaged during the operation and temporarily or permanently paralyzed leading to hoarseness of the voice but this complication, like injury to the panthyroid glands, is uncommon in skilled hands. After the removal of part of the thyroid gland the patient may suffer from underactivity of the gland (hypothyroidism). This is easily treated by one or two tablets a day of the hormone thyroxine.

THYROIDITIS

A generic term covering four inflammatory conditions of the thyroid gland. Pyogenic thyroiditis, giving pain, swelling and fever, is an extremely rare condition and is caused by infection from bacteria which, in many cases, are borne in the blood from another site. Reidel's thyroiditis is a rare disorder in which the thyroid gland and surrounding tissues become very firm and hardened. De Quervain's or granulomatous thyroiditis is probably viral in origin. The illness, which usually comprises pain over the thyroid and malaise (a general feeling of being unwell), frequently continues for several weeks or months if left untreated. In the early stages the patient may become thyrotoxic (see *Thyrotoxicosis*) due to leakage of thyroid hormone from the gland. Hashimoto's thyroiditis is an autoimmune disorder in which antibodies against thyroid tissue are produced. A chronic condition which may co-exist with other autoimmune disorders (such as pernicious anaemia), it is characterized by visible thyroid enlargement (goitre) and the gradual onset of hypothyroidism (underactivity of the thyroid). Pyogenic thyroiditis is treated with antibiotics. There is no treatment available for Reidel's thyroiditis. In the other two types, treating the associated hyper- or hypothyroidism (qv) appropriately is the priority. Steroids may also be helpful.

THYROTOXICOSIS

An excess supply of thyroid hormone to the tissues. The cause is Graves' disease (autoimmune inflammation of the thyroid gland). The clinical signs are varied and include a diffuse enlarged thyroid gland, fine tremor of the hands, excessive irritability,

T

anxiety, heat intolerance and weight loss (despite increased appetite). The condition can also lead to protrusion of one or both eyes (exophthalmos) and to paralysis of the muscles controlling the eye (exophthalmic ophthalmoplegia or ophthalmic Graves' disease), and ulceration of the cornea because the eyelids will not cover the eye. There may be skin changes, with raised thickened skin over the legs and feet, muscle weakness and irregularities in heart rhythm (particularly atrial fibrillation) and heart failure.

Treatment consists of blocking the release of thyroid hormone with drugs, or surgical removal of the thyroid gland (thyroidectomy, qv), or the use of radio-active iodine to suppress the activity of thyroxine-producing cells. The use of each is dictated by the patient's age and other factors such as his or her suitability for surgery and the severity of the condition. Usually the eye symptoms regress with treatment, but complicated eye disease is difficult to treat. In some cases treatment with high-dose steroids and irradiation may be required to relieve severe ophthalmoplegia.

TIC

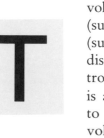

Irregular repetitive movements involving either a small group of muscles (such as in an eyelid) or a large group (such as in a shoulder). Tics usually disappear during sleep and can be controlled by the sufferer when he or she is awake, though the effort required to do so may have the effect of provoking anxiety in the affected individual. They usually begin during childhood, are particularly common in boys, and are for the most part transient although in some cases they persist throughout the sufferer's life.

Multiple tics occur in a comparatively rare condition called Gilles de la Tourette syndrome, the cause of which is unknown. In this, tics are accompanied by grunts or involuntary speech that may take the form of obscene expressions. Recovery is very rare, but some powerful neuroleptic drugs such as the phenothiazines may improve the condition.

TIC DOULOUREUX

see *Trigeminal neuralgia*

TINNITUS

The sensation of a sound in the ears. Many people have an experience of tinnitus, at least intermittently, which they find troublesome, and a significant number (about 200,000 people in the United Kingdom, for example) have such severe tinnitus that they are unable to work or function socially.

Like pain, it is a symptom, not a disease, and there are many causes. Some are simple, such as wax or fluid in the middle ear. In most cases, however, tinnitus is a reflection of damage to the cochlear nerve cells, and is usually but not invariably associated with deafness (qv); this may be the result of ageing or damage through noise exposure.

The use of a hearing aid which amplifies everyday background noise often suppresses tinnitus. Tinnitus maskers, which provide constant 'white noise' (similar to the noise you hear when a radio is not tuned in properly) are often of benefit too. Psychological techniques can also help in some cases where the origin seems to be emotional, especially in patients with depression who may be helped by anti-depressant agents. Overall, however, the benefit from drug treatment is still limited. Surgical treatment for tinnitus is now very rarely used as the success rate is so low.

TOLERANCE

A state of unresponsiveness. This state can occur naturally or it can be artificially induced. It can also be desirable or not, depending on the circumstances. Immune tolerance, for example, is an essential and naturally occurring phenomenon which safeguards the components of the body against attack by the immune system. Absence of this tolerance may result in autoimmune disease. In contrast, in transplantation operations the individual's immune response has to be suppressed in order to prevent rejection of the donor organ, and drugs are used to induce tolerance to antigent that would normally be recognized as 'non-self'.

Drug tolerance is used to describe the reduction in the efficacy of a drug which may occur with prolonged use. This leads to a need for an increased dose. An example of this is the ever-greater quantities of drugs of abuse, such as heroin, which are required to produce a constant effect. This form of tolerance may be due to increased metabolism or elimination of the drug, or to a process, poorly understood, through which the body becomes increasingly resistant to the effects of the drug. Blocking antibodies may occasionally develop in which case the resistance is autoimmune, but this is uncommon. The onset may be gradual, occurring only after many doses over a long period (compare *Desensitization*), or rapid, occurring after only a few doses in a short time (tachyphlaxis).

TOMOGRAPHY

A mechanical radiological technique designed to reveal more information about structures deep within the body than is possible using ordinary X-ray techniques; it should not be confused with computed tomography (CT scan, qv). In tomography the plane of interest remains sharply in focus while structures superficial and deep to this plane become blurred and indistinct as the X-ray tube and film are moved in an arc around the patient during exposure.

Many of the applications of tomography have now been superseded by computed tomography at centres where this expensive equipment is available. However, tomography is still useful in the investigation of lung abnormalities, and is still frequently used during urography to show detail of the kidneys, and in the assessment of bone problems.

TONOMETRY

The measurement of intra-ocular pressure — that is, the pressure of the fluid inside the eyeball. High pressure may indicate glaucoma. Low pressure is usually the result of injury to the eye.

A variety of different instruments is used, the most common being an applanation tonometer which takes only a few seconds to measure the pressure. Local anaesthetic eye drops are placed into the eye and the tonometer is placed on to the cornea (the transparent layer of tissue at the front of the eye), rather like a contact lens. The amount of pressure required to indent a small area is taken as the measurement of intra-ocular pressure.

TONSILLECTOMY

Surgical removal of the tonsils. There are still considerable differences of opinion as to the benefits of this operation, but in the past decade a more conservative attitude has prevailed. Repeated attacks of acute tonsillitis is

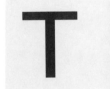

the usual reason for tonsillectomy, although ideally each case should be considered on an individual basis — severity and frequency of attacks, and how much schooling or work time is being lost are the main factors for consideration. Major obstruction to breathing and swallowing is recognized as a problem which tonsillectomy can benefit.

Tonsillectomy is almost invariably performed under general anaesthesia and the patient is usually allowed home within about two days. It is now thought best to encourage eating hard food to exercise the jaw muscles and prevent a build-up of residue of blood clot and granulation tissue in the tonsillar bed. Should this occur, there is a danger of secondary haemorrhage. Post-operative referred pain can often be felt in the ear, which shares a common nerve supply.

It is advisable not to have the operation just after an attack of tonsillitis or a cold as there is then an increased risk of post-operative bleeding.

TONSILLITIS

Inflammation of the tonsils. Tonsillitis may be a primary infection, usually caused by a strain of streptococci, or secondary to a generalized infection of the upper respiratory tract, in which case a virus is the most likely cause. The typical throat symptoms result from secondary bacterial infection. Streptococcal tonsillitis can occur in epidemic form in closed communities; if the infecting organism is a haemolytic streptococcus it may also produce the typical features of scarlet fever (scarlatina) and carriers may initiate infection in others while remaining symptom-free.

The features are sore throat, pain on swallowing, fever and earache from referred pain. The glands in the neck are swollen (lymphadenopathy), as are the tonsils, which are also reddened and covered with pus. The illness lasts about a week.

Complications are uncommon since the introduction of antibiotics. The most frequent complications are quinsy and chronic tonsillitis. Glomerulonephritis and rheumatic fever are very rare complications of streptococcal tonsillitis.

Treatment is with bed rest, ample fluids and antibiotics. Soluble aspirin (paracetamol for children) is usually effective. If patients have been subject to a number of severe attacks necessitating time off school or work, most otorhinolaryngologists (ear, nose and throat specialists) would consider tonsillectomy (qv).

TOPHUS

The formation of urate (uric acid crystals) in the joints and surrounding soft tissues as a result of gout. Deposits (tophi) may also develop over the elbow, ear and Achilles' tendon. Tophi can grow to several centimetres in diameter and are often surrounded by mild inflammation. Patients with newly diagnosed gout may have a few small tophi. In chronic tophaceous gout, however, tophi may be widespread; they may restrict movement, ulcerate through the skin (releasing the chalky urate), or may become secondarily infected. Fortunately, effective treatment is now available with the drug allopurinol, which reduces circulating uric acid concentrations. As a result, severe tophaceous gout is becoming rare.

TOPICAL

Treatment that is applied to the skin and takes effect once it has been absorbed by it. For example, a topical anaesthetic is applied to an area in order to numb it, and a topical steroid cream reduces allergic reaction by releasing its steroid compound through the skin.

TORTICOLLIS

An abnormal persistent contraction of the neck muscles, causing the head to be held in an unnatural position; it is also known as wry neck.

The commonest form of wry neck is called spasmodic torticollis. The pathological changes that produce this disorder are as yet not clearly understood but involve the basal nuclei or ganglia (nerve centres) of the brain; the condition causes repeated spasm of the sternomastoid muscle in the neck, resulting in a characteristic recurrent tilting of the head to one side.

Treatment is unsatisfactory: drugs may bring short-term benefit; and surgical treatment through division of various nerves and nerve roots produces very variable results.

TOTAL PARENTERAL NUTRITION

Intravenous feeding of a patient when enteral (gastro-intestinal tract) feeding is not possible. This is necessary when the gut cannot be used because of an inflammatory disease, such as Crohn's disease or pancreatitis. Parenteral nutrition is also required when oral and/or gastric tube feeding is not sufficient to prevent the marked muscle wasting that follows extensive burns, massive injury or major surgery.

Parenteral feeding replaces fluid and salts lost through perspiration and breathing, as well as providing an energy source and amino acids. Amino acids are the building blocks of proteins; enough are given to counteract the protein breakdown that inevitably occurs in any starved patient, especially after major trauma. Energy is provided by intravenous infusion of glucose, which is an immediately available energy source, and fats, which can be stored by the body for use when required. The intravenous diet also includes vitamins as well as trace elements such as zinc and copper which are essential for wound healing and normal blood cell production by the bone marrow.

TOXOCARA CANIS

A common, parasitic worm infecting the intestines of dogs and cats. Eggs of the worm are passed in the stool and incubate in soil for 2—3 weeks before they become infective. If they are then ingested by a human being they develop into larvae which penetrate the intestinal wall and are carried in the blood to the liver and lungs. Infection may not cause any symptoms, or the person affected may have a fever, skin rash and wheezy cough. Very rarely the infection causes blindness due to bleeding of the retinal arteries.

Most patients recover without any specific treatment and there is no proven effective therapy. However, anti-helminthic (helminths means worm) treatment with thiabendazole, mebendazole and diethylcarbamazine have all been used with some success.

Viable eggs have been found in 25 per cent of soil samples taken from British public parks; and 4 per cent of children who play in public parks have a positive reaction to toxocara antigens, indicating past infection.

TOXOPLASMOSIS

A disease caused by *Toxoplasma gondii*, a protozoan (primitive single-cell organism) which infects birds and

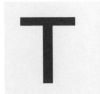

mammals. It proliferates within the cells of the host after ingestion, and its sexual cycle takes place within members of the cat family. Transmission to humans is through eating uncooked infected meat or brain, and through contamination with cat faeces.

Toxoplasmosis may be acquired or congenital. In most adults and in children (who acquire the infection after birth) it often produces no symptoms or causes only a mild transient illness. The exceptions are immuno-compromised patients in whom the immune system is deficient. In these individuals the symptoms that may occur are fever and inflammation of skeletal and heart muscle, and the brain may also be affected, causing toxo-plasmic encephalitis (qv), especially in AIDS sufferers. In congenital toxo-plasmosis the infection is acquired by a pregnant woman and then trans-mitted across the placenta to the fetus. The presence of specific antibodies in the blood may alert the doctor to this possibility and sometimes prophylactic abortion is advised. Affected infants who survive are often poorly devel-oped, with small eyes and brain, epileptic seizures and mental retar-dation. Effective antibiotic treatment for all but congenital toxoplasmosis is available.

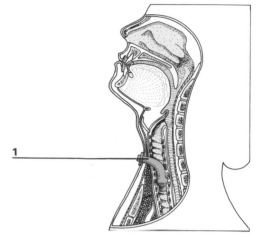

Tracheostomy involves making a temporary artificial hole in the windpipe (1) so that air passes directly down to the lungs, bypassing the normal route of mouth, pharynx and larynx.

hindrance to respiration (as in malig-nancy or serious injury, for example), laryngectomy (removal of the larynx) may also be required; the cut end of the trachea is brought to the surface of the skin.

Tracheostomy secures an airway at the price of temporary loss of speech. If the larynx is retained, closing the hole off with a finger or valved tube (tracheostome) allows air to be expelled via the normal route and speech to be produced. A bib which retains mois-ture is placed over the tracheostome to substitute for the humidifying effect of the nose, which would otherwise be lost.

TRACHEOSTOMY

A temporary artificial opening made into the trachea (windpipe). Tracheo-stomy is performed for a number of reasons: in cases of obstruction at this level caused by disease or a foreign body; to allow secretions retained in the lungs, for example in paralyzed patients, to be more easily cleared by means of suction; and in patients who are unconscious for a prolonged period and require artificial aids for breathing. If the larynx is non-functioning or is a

TRACHOMA

A viral infection of the conjunctiva (the front of the eye) and eyelids. It is contagious and spreads easily by direct contact, or indirectly on towels and handkerchiefs. An extremely common infection in Africa and Asia, it is re-sponsible for an estimated 400 million cases world-wide. The infection results in thickening and scarring of the con-junctiva, and eventually in blindness. It responds to treatment with the anti-biotic tetracycline or sulphonamides.

TRACTION

A method used either to hold the position of a fracture or to 'reduce' it (re-align the elements). Traction may be fixed, in which case it is applied against a counterforce applied to the patient's body; a Thomas splint is the best example of fixed traction used for fractures of the femoral shaft (thigh-bone). In sliding or balanced traction the patient's weight is balanced against an applied load. There are many ways in which this form of traction can be applied but essentially it allows the patient some movement in the bed while treatment continues.

Traction may be applied using adhesive strapping to the skin (skin traction); or, if traction is to be applied to the lower spine, through a firm belt or corset surrounding the lower trunk, attached to weights over a pulley at the foot of the bed which is tilted so that the trunk is higher than the head; or by a steel pin placed through a bone (skeletal traction). Skull traction can be applied to stretch the cervical spine through metal callipers fixed to both temples. Skin traction applied to the lower trunk or skull is used to treat slipped discs. Skeletal traction is used to treat fractures of the femur (a pin is placed through the upper tibia or shin-bone), and fractures of the tibia (a pin is placed through the calcaneum or heel-bone).

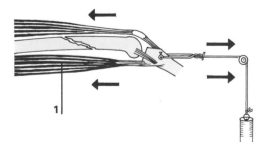

In fracture the elastic pull of the muscles **(1)** tends to cause the bone fragments to override. Continuous weight traction corrects this problem and maintains correct alignment.

TRANQUILLIZER

Tranquillizers are drugs which relieve anxiety and agitation. They are commonly divided into major and minor types; major tranquillizers may also be called neuroleptics, and minor tranquillizers anxiolytics, sedatives or narcotics.

Major tranquillizers are generally used in the treatment of psychoses such as schizophrenia and mania. Commonly used neuroleptics are chlorpromazine, trifluoperazine, thioridazine and haloperidol. In the treatment of schizophrenic patients, neuroleptics such as flupenthixol and fluphenazine may be given by a so-called depot injection which lasts 2—3 weeks.

Common side-effects of the major tranquillizers include sleepiness, weight gain, sensitivity to the sun and disorders of movement. Parkinsonism with slowed movement and limited facial expression, a common side-effect, can be treated with appropriate drugs. Akithisia (a state of extreme restlessness of the legs) and acute dystonia (in which a patient may have difficulty with neck, tongue and eye movements) may occur early in treatment. In the longer term, tardive dyskinesia (in which a patient develops involuntary movements of the tongue and lips) may result from continuous treatment with the major tranquillizers.

The minor tranquillizers most commonly prescribed are the benzodiazepines (such as diazepam and temazepam). These may be prescribed for the treatment of anxiety, insomnia and withdrawal from states of drug dependency. Generally they are prescribed with caution and for periods of not longer than a fortnight, as they are likely to cause considerable problems with sedation, tolerance, dependence and withdrawal symptoms.

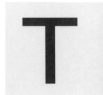

TRANSFUSION

The giving of blood into a vein, usually into the arm. Before blood can be given it must be cross-matched against the blood of the recipient. The blood to be transfused must be of the same A, B, O and rhesus blood group as the individual receiving it. Blood for transfusion is tested for the presence of the viruses hepatitis B and HIV (see *AIDS*); it is also tested for syphilis. At present, there is no readily available test for the virus or viruses which cause non-A, non-B hepatitis following blood transfusion; this is present in about 1 in 300 blood donors in the United Kingdom.

Autologous transfusion is sometimes used to avoid the risks of viral infection after transfusion: a person's blood can be taken and stored before an operation to be transfused back immediately afterwards.

TRANSPLANTATION

Surgical replacement of a diseased or failing organ with a healthy organ taken from a donor. Transplantation of the following organs/tissues is frequently performed in current clinical practice: kidney, heart, heart and lung, liver, pancreas, bone marrow, and cornea. Although the surgical procedures differ for each organ, all transplant operations require a donor and, except for the cornea, immunosuppression to prevent rejection of the foreign organ by the recipient's immune defences. Bone marrow transplants utilize living donors, as do some kidney transplants, but other organ transplants are performed from donors certified as brain dead (see *Brain death*).

The immune defences (antibodies and lymphocytes — a type of white blood cell) that protect against infections also recognize and attack foreign tissue and cause a transplanted organ to be rejected. The risk of rejection can be lessened by matching the tissue type of the organ donor as closely as possible to that of the recipient. For bone marrow and kidney transplants the best results are obtained when the donor is a close relative with similar tissue typing. Immunosuppression (with corticosteroids for example), is necessary to prevent rejection but increases the patient's susceptibility to infections (the leading cause of death in the early post-transplant period).

Transplantation is of proven benefit in prolonging and improving the quality of life in suitable patients with severe heart, lung and liver failure. Renal transplantation is superior to dialysis for patients with chronic kidney failure. Pancreatic transplantation is usually combined with renal transplant in diabetics with renal failure. Current success rates at one year for renal transplants are about 90 per cent for live related donors and over 80 per cent for unrelated donors who had just died before the organ was removed in order to be transplanted. Success rates for heart, heart-lung and liver transplantation are lower, but all offer a prospect of long-term survival. The indications for, and success rates of, bone marrow transplantation are both increasing. Future developments in producing more specific immunosuppression should further improve success rates, but the shortage of donor organs is likely to continue to be a problem.

TRAUMA

Trauma literally means a wound or bodily injury due to external violence, but the term has also come to embrace the physiological and psychological effects of such violence on the person involved. Shock (qv), for example, is a form of trauma. Trauma as a mental or emotional wound is recognized in psychiatry, where the term is used to describe any disturbing experience affecting the mind or nerves so as to induce hysteria (qv).

TRAVEL SICKNESS

A general term covering a group of syndromes such as seasickness, car sickness, train sickness, and so on; it is also called motion sickness. The disorder is caused by stimulation of the vestibular system (part of the inner ear apparatus concerned with balance) as a result of unusual motion, especially when this is relatively rhythmical as in the pitch or roll of a ship. People vary markedly in their susceptibility to travel sickness. The incidence of it decreases with age which suggests that the vestibular system adapts over time. Typical symptoms include nausea, vomiting, drowsiness, sweating and pallor. In severe cases the person may be forced to lie down.

The key to the treatment of travel sickness is prevention. Drugs, such as hyoscine, promethazine and cyclizine, which damp down the sensitivity of the labyrinth, are useful as preventatives and should be taken at least one hour before travelling. Dosages are usually reduced for children.

TREMOR

A regular, rhythmical, oscillating, involuntary movement usually described as 'shaking'. A small degree of tremor is normal (physiological tremor) and is usually imperceptible, but may be exaggerated and become noticeable with anxiety, in thyrotoxicosis (excess supply of thyroid hormone), and on taking drugs with adrenaline-like actions. Abnormal tremors may also be seen in alcoholism, Parkinsonism and in tumours or disease involving the brain. A tremor at rest which can be partially or completely suppressed by willed movements is characteristically seen in Parkinson's disease. Parkinsonian tremor most commonly affects the hands ('pill-rolling tremor') and less often the legs; like other abnormal tremors it disappears during sleep. Familial (autosomal dominant inheritance) tremor occurs in adult life, and is most apparent when the affected parts are held in certain positions (hands outstretched, for example) and throughout movement, but disappears at rest. Initially it affects the hands and head, but can progress to involve the jaw, lips and tongue. Characteristically it can be suppressed by alcohol or by drugs such as propranolol. Patients with tumours or diseases involving the cerebellum or its connections to the rest of the brain (multiple sclerosis, for example), may develop an intention tremor. This is absent at rest and in the initial stages of movement, but is particularly disabling because it worsens as fine adjustments necessary to complete a movement are demanded (for instance, touching an object).
SEE ALSO *Delirium tremens*

TREPHINE

This term can be used in two ways. First, to refer to the hole made in the skull by a neurosurgeon in cases of brain tumour. A trephine hole is larger than the usual small burrhole used, for example, to drain a subdural haematoma; a disc of the skull bone is removed in order to inspect the underlying brain and usually to take a biopsy. Second, it refers to a trephine biopsy in which a core of bone is taken in order to examine the bone marrow. This may be essential in establishing a diag-

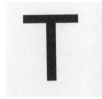

nosis of cancer involving the bone marrow or lymphoma. The biopsy is usually taken from the hip bone using a special needle. In most cases the procedure is performed under local anaesthetic. When the specimen has been obtained, the calcium has to be removed before the bone marrow can be examined. The advantage of a trephine biopsy of bone marrow over a bone marrow aspiration (qv) is that the 'architecture' of the bone marrow is preserved.

TRICHINIASIS

Infestation by the worm *Trichinella spiralis*. People are infected by eating raw or undercooked meat containing these parasites. Rats and pigs are the usual sources of infestation. The majority of cases are mild and unrecognized, but severe infection may cause serious illness or even death. Once swallowed, the larvae of the worm emerge and invade the bowel wall. The adult worm develops within 2−3 days. After mating, female worms discharge larvae over the next 4−16 weeks. Larvae penetrate the bowel wall and some are passed in the faeces. Others are carried within the bloodstream to the muscles, where they form cysts. In the early stages vomiting and diarrhoea may be symptoms, and sweating may be profuse. Later fever, rapid heart rate (tachycardia) and muscular pains begin. Rashes and facial swellings may be prominent.

Treatment is to expel larvae cysts in the early stages, or to destroy the adult female worms and larvae later using thiobendazole.

TRICHOMONIASIS

A sexually transmitted disease involving the lower genital tract. It is caused by an organism called *Trichomonas vag-*

inalis. The organism predominantly infects the vagina, urethra (the tube which drains the bladder), cervical canal, and glands around the opening of the urethra (for example, the Bartholins glands) and may be associated with other sexually transmitted diseases such as gonorrhoea.

Women patients usually complain of a green malodorous discharge and sometimes also of pain during sexual intercourse or urination. The external genitalia may become inflamed. The diagnosis is made by examining vaginal fluid under a microscope and identifying the organisms. In men, symptoms arc often few; however there may be evidence of inflammation beneath the foreskin and/or discharge from the urethra.

Treatment involves antibiotics (metronidazole), which should be given to both partners. Intercourse should be avoided until treatment is complete, as should alcohol, which in combination with this antibiotic may cause side-effects. A follow-up examination is important.

TRIGEMINAL NEURALGIA

A condition of unknown cause in which pain is felt in the face along the distribution of the trigeminal or fifth cranial nerve; also known as 'tic douloureux'. The pain is sharp, stabbing and of short duration, and is often precipitated by touching the face, cleaning the teeth, chewing or cold winds. It is usually felt in the area of the cheekbone, but can also occur in the jaw or forehead. Spasms may vary in frequency and may be felt over a period of several months, often with periods of remission. In most cases no abnormality of the nerve can be detected. The condition is rare under the age of 40 years.

Drug treatment with carbamazepine or phenytoin is often effective. In resistant cases, injection of the nerve with phenol or alcohol may be necessary, as may transection or cutting of the nerve. Permanent loss of sensation in part of the face will follow these procedures. In some cases of neuralgia the trigeminal nerve may be compressed within the skull by an artery lying in an unusual position. Surgical decompression of the nerve may then cure the condition.

TRUSS

An external appliance designed to control a hernia (qv). It consists of a padded steel disc held in place by a belt. The hernia, usually inguinal (of the groin), is firstly reduced (by lying flat) and then the plate of the truss is applied over the hernia and the belt tightened. The truss should then hold the hernia reduced on standing, walking, coughing and so on. Other types of hernia (umbilical, femoral, for instance) may also be controlled by a truss, but often less satisfactorily.

A truss is largely a short-term measure and its long-term use in the treatment of hernia is reserved for patients who are unfit for surgery.

TRYPANOSOMIASIS

An infection caused by organisms called trypanosomes, which are small, single-cell and transmitted by insects. There are two types of trypanosomiasis: African, also known as sleeping sickness; and American, also called Chagas' disease.

The African variety is transmitted by the tsetse fly. The person infected develops a high fever, with severe headache, insomnia and an inability to concentrate. If untreated the infection will progress to affect the central nervous system, resulting in the classic picture: a vacant expression, drooping eyelids and the patient gradually becoming comatose.

Chagas' disease is common in South America and is transmitted by a biting winged insect that lives in the cracks and thatches of poorly constructed dwellings. The infection may produce an acute, feverish illness initially. Later developments include signs of heart and gastrointestinal disease, such as cardiomyopathy (affecting the heart muscle), heart failure and chronic diarrhoea.

In its early stages African trypanosomiasis is treated with suramin or pentamidine isethionate. Once symptoms of central nervous system involvement develop, melarsoprol B (a highly toxic arsenical compound) is used, with variable effect. Eflornithine, an inhibitor of ornithine decarboxylese, has been shown to be more effective than melarsoprol B.

Chagas' disease is extremely difficult to treat. The drug nifurtimox is variably effective and highly toxic. The alternative, benznidazole, offers no advantages.

TUBERCULIN TEST

A skin test to detect previous exposure to tuberculosis. Tuberculin (a protein derived from tubercle bacilli) is injected into the skin and the degree of inflammation is then assessed. In subjects with a previous or current infection with tuberculosis, an immune response against the tuberculin produces inflammation at the injection site and a positive test. In the most widely used form, the Mantoux test, the result is positive if the area of hard swelling around the injection site after 48 hours is wider than 10 mm ($\frac{3}{8}$ inch). People with no history of tuberculosis or

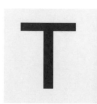

BCG vaccination produce no reaction to tuberculin and a negative result. False negative results can be produced in patients with tuberculosis who have a suppressed immune response.

TUBERCULOSIS

A chronic infectious condition (caused by the bacterium *Mycobacterium tuberculosis*) which usually affects the lungs but may also affect the skin, kidney, bowel, brain and lymph glands. The symptoms usually include a chronically persistent cough, perhaps with some coughed up blood (haemoptysis), fever, malaise (a general feeling of being unwell) and weight loss.

Once a very common disorder, it is now seen much less often in developed countries but is still very widespread in the developing nations. Under-nourishment and poor housing and sanitation are environmental factors important in causation and spread. Vaccination with BCG (qv) at an early age confers substantial immunity. Immunosuppressed individuals are at increased risk.

Diagnosis is ultimately dependent upon detection of the organism in the affected tissues, either in sputum or in a lymph node biopsy, for example; a useful screening procedure is the Mantoux skin test (see *Tuberculin test*) in which injection into the skin of protein derived from the bacterium responsible for TB may induce a reaction which indicates prior infection.

Treatment requires prolonged administration of antituberculous therapy, usually with several different drugs given simultaneously to minimize the risk of resistance. Residual scarring and damage of the affected bodily organ, usually the lungs but sometimes the kidney, frequently remains.

TUBEROUS SCLEROSIS

A dominantly inherited condition comprising epilepsy, eye abnormalities (white plaques in the retina), mental retardation and distinctive skin features. The condition may first be noticed as infantile epilepsy, and the presence of paler areas of otherwise relatively normal-looking skin ('ash leaf' spots) may be the only clue to the fact that the epilepsy is a result of tuberous sclerosis. Another symptom of the condition is adenoma sebaceum, a facial eruption superficially resembling acne vulgaris and consisting of erythematous nodules and papules scattered over the centre of the face; it does not occur until adolescence or adult life but is again typical. A further characteristic skin sign is the presence of small fibrous tags around the nails, called peri-ungual fibromas. Not all the various signs need be found in a single individual.

There is no treatment except anti-convulsant drugs for the epilepsy.

TUMOUR

From the Latin 'tumor', which means a swelling; the word is now generally used to denote an abnormal growth of cells and excludes swelling caused by inflammation.

A tumour is an abnormal lump of tissue, the growth of which exceeds and is uncoordinated with that of normal tissue. It serves no useful purpose, is unrelated to the needs of the body and may even be harmful. A tumour is dependent on the body for its blood supply and nourishment. Its growth may be enhanced or retarded by hormones, and drugs, as well as by the general condition of the patient. Tumours are named according to their tissue of origin and are subdivided

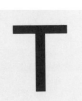

into benign and malignant. The suffix-oma is used to denote a tumour — for example, a neuroma is a tumour arising from nerve tissue.

Benign tumours very closely resemble their tissue of origin, grow slowly by expansion, remain localized and affect the patient primarily because of their size and location (perhaps by pressing on a vital organ, for example). Malignant tumours show a varying degree of cell abnormalities, grow rapidly and spread through the body so relentlessly that, unless treated, they eventually cause death. In most cases it is easy to decide whether a tumour is benign or malignant, because of factors such as its behaviour and appearance under the microscope. Sometimes, though, the dividing line between the two extremes is not clear and even an expert pathologist may experience difficulty in reaching a decision.
SEE ALSO *Adenoma, Cancer, Melanoma, Sarcoma, Seminoma*

TURNER'S SYNDROME

A sex chromosome disorder affecting 1 in 5,000 females. Affected individuals have only one sex (X) chromosome instead of the normal two. The main features of the condition are short stature, complete infertility and failure to develop secondary sexual characteristics, such as breasts, or to menstruate. A number of congenital abnormalities may be found, such as webbing of the neck and congenital heart disease (narrowing or coarctation of the aorta, for example). Intelligence and life span are normal. Sex hormone replacement therapy improves the development of secondary sexual characteristics, but the infertility is not remedied.

TWINS

There are two ways in which a twin pregnancy can occur. Two eggs (ova) may be released from the ovary at ovulation and each is fertilized by a different sperm. Alternatively, the single fertilized egg may divide completely at a very early stage and then two babies develop. The first kind of twins are fraternal twins, who may be of the same or different sex, and are no more alike than brothers and sisters. The second kind are identical twins who are always of the same sex, and are very similar in many ways. Fraternal twins occur more frequently in families with a history of twins, in older women, in women who have had several children previously, and after injections of fertility drugs.

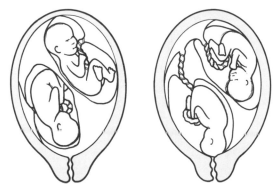

Fraternal or non-identical twins with separate placentas (**left**) make up 75 per cent of all twin pregnancies. Identical twins with shared placenta (**right**) make up the remaining 25 per cent. One pregnancy in 80 is a twin pregnancy.

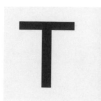

A twin pregnancy carries a slightly higher risk than a singleton pregnancy, but with regular antenatal care the outcome is usually good. Labour in twin pregnancy is no longer than in singleton pregnancy but an obstetrician usually assists the midwife with the delivery of the second baby. Twins often deliver prematurely, about a month earlier than expected. Each twin is usually lighter than a singleton baby at the same stage of pregnancy.

TYPHOID FEVER

The fever caused by the organism *Salmonella typhi*. Infection leads to symptoms after about 14 days. Headache, fever, malaise (a general feeling of being unwell) and constipation are common symptoms, and the spleen is enlarged and can be felt in half of the patients. During the second week of the illness the person has diarrhoea and abdominal tenderness. If untreated, the patient will become confused and dehydrated, and intestinal perforation or haemorrhage may occur. Blood and stool cultures will aid diagnosis, as will immunological blood tests to identify typhoid antibodies (the Widal reaction). Prompt antibiotic therapy with chloramphenicol in an isolation unit is the best treatment.

After treatment 5 per cent of patients may continue to carry the organism, and are potential sources of infection to others. Their faeces remain contaminated, although they themselves have no further symptoms. Public health measures are important to prevent the disease, and vaccination for travellers to endemic countries may offer a degree of protection.

TYPHUS

A disease caused by certain species of *Rickettsia*, not to be confused with typhoid. The typhus-causing *Rickettsia* are transmitted to man via arthropods (ticks), mainly from rodents. Typhus-like diseases occur world-wide. The organisms gain access via the skin, mucous membranes or respiratory tract. Incubation periods range from 3–20 days. Features include fever, rash, occasionally shock, liver and kidney disorders and sometimes involvement of the brain. Treatment is with antibiotics — chloramphenicol or tetracycline.

ULCER

Any break in a lining surface of the body; for example, the skin or the mucous membranes of the intestine. Ulcers may result from a number of disease processes: injury, infection, prolonged pressure, irritation by chemicals or malignant disease. Common examples of ulceration include duodenal ulcer, aphthous ulcer in the mouth, and varicose ulcer on the lower leg.

ULTRASOUND

The imaging of soft tissues using high-frequency sound waves. The sound waves are generated and received by a transducer, or scanner, in the probe. Ultrasound waves are reflected by soft tissues, especially where different soft tissues meet. Boundaries between bone and soft tissue and gas and soft tissue generate very strong echoes, preventing the transmission of sound to deeper tissues. The echoes received are computer-manipulated to produce an image of the plane scanned.

Medically the applications of ultrasound include imaging of the heart, abdominal organs, (liver, gall-bladder, pancreas, kidneys, spleen, uterus and ovaries), eye, thyroid, testes, breast and blood vessels in order to identify abnormalities of structure, including tumours. An unborn child may be screened for a number of congenital structural abnormalities; this is usually done at about 4–5 months of pregnancy. Imaging of the blood vessels can be combined with measurement of the rate at which the blood is travelling, and disturbances in flow can

T

be detected by the so-called doppler technique; this has proved useful in assessing the severity of arterial stenoses (narrowings).

Imaging of the brain is generally poor, as the skull gets in the way, except in infants less than 1 year old; in them the anterior fontanelle or soft spot (the depression on the top of the head where the three bones of the skull meet) provides an acoustic window; nevertheless CT scanning is more reliable. Ultrasound is being used in a few centres during brain surgery in adults when a flap of bone has been removed, allowing the probe to be placed directly on to the surface of the brain. However, this method is as yet still experimental and not widely-available.

There is no known hazard from ultrasound.
SEE ALSO *Brain scan*

URETHRITIS

see *Non-specific urethritis*

URINE RETENTION

An abnormal accumulation of urine in the bladder caused by an inability to pass water. It may be provoked by an obstruction to the bladder outflow tract, or a neuromuscular disorder affecting the bladder muscles or nerve supply. The commonest cause of obstruction is enlargement of the prostate in elderly men. This may produce acute retention of urine and require a temporary urethral catheter to relieve pain and discomfort. Ultimately the treatment will be to remove the obstruction — for example, by prostatectomy (qv). In cases of chronic retention the inability to empty the bladder completely may lend to over-distension and overflow incontinence.

Treatment is by removing the cause

of obstruction if one is present, or by manoeuvres to improve the emptying of the bladder in cases of neuromuscular disorder. Longterm urethral catheterization carries a risk of urine infection, but may be unavoidable in some patients.

UROGRAPHY

Radiological examination of the kidneys, ureters (tubes leading from the kidneys to the bladder) and bladder. The urinary tract cannot be seen on ordinary X-rays because its density is not appreciably different from that of surrounding soft tissue, hence the need for an intravenous urogram, or pyelogram.

In urography the kidneys are made opaque by intravenous injection of an iodine-containing organic chemical dye (contrast agent) that is taken up by the kidneys and excreted in the urine, thus making the ureters and bladder opaque too. X-ray films are taken before the contrast is given (control film) and at intervals after injection as the kidneys, ureters and bladder become dyed in their turn. Information is gained about the size and shape of the kidneys and the presence of any abnormalities, such as a tumour. The dye excreted highlights the urine-collecting system within the kidney and the ureters. Bright patches in the opacified urine may be due to non- or poorly- calcified stones, a tumour or a blood clot. If there is an obstruction to the urine flow, such as a stone in the ureter, then excretion is delayed and the renal collecting system and ureter nearest to the obstruction become distended.

UROLITHIASIS

The presence of stones (calculi) in the urinary tract. Up to 2 per cent of people may be affected at some time by urolithiasis; in half of these cases stones are recurrent. Most stones consist of calcium salts (oxalate and phosphate) and their formation is due to either high calcium levels in the blood (hypercalcaemia) or to high calcium levels in the urine without hypercalcaemia. Dehydration and infection increase the likelihood of stones forming. Many stones in the urinary tract are passed spontaneously and cause no problem. The complications that can occur include attacks of severe pain (ureteric colic), haematuria (blood in the urine), repeated urine infections, and hydronephrosis (dilatation of the pelvis of the kidney) due to obstruction of the ureter (the tube leading from the kidney to the bladder). Most stones are visible on plain X-ray because of the presence of calcium, but further investigations are needed to determine whether the underlying abnormality is metabolic or the ureter is obstructed. A diagnosis of urolithiasis therefore involves additional biochemical tests (to detect, for example, hypercalcaemia or hyperparathyroidism — overactivity of the parathyroid glands) as well as an intravenous urogram or ultrasound scan.

In recent years there have been major advances in the treatment of stones, particularly for those in the upper urinary tract (see *Nephrolithiasis* for further information). Stones in the bladder and lower ureters can be approached through a cystoscope and then either crushed or extracted surgically. If an underlying metabolic disorder is found, this is treated to prevent further stones being formed.

URTICARIA

A very common skin condition (also known as hives) consisting of raised, scattered patches of erythematous inflammation which are often extremely itchy and characteristically migrate from site to site over a period of hours. Individual lesions resemble nettle rash. Sometimes there is an easily recognized precipitating cause, such as a drug or unusual foodstuff, but usually there is none.

The vast majority of cases clear up spontaneously over a period of days or weeks. The only treatment required is with antihistamine, to control the itch. Very rarely, urticarial swelling may interfere with swallowing or breathing if the throat is affected (so-called angioneurotic oedema); in this instance the patient should be immediately taken to hospital for emergency treatment.

UVEITIS

Inflammation of one or more of the vascular structures in the eye. This can occur as a result of injury or surgery or be associated with a more widespread disease, such as sarcoidosis (qv), affecting other parts of the body. Often no specific cause can be found. Uveitis is characterized by blurring of vision, redness of the eye and pain which has been likened to toothache.

Treatment is by anti-inflammatory drugs, either as tablets, eye drops or a combination of both, and is usually successful with no residual loss of vision. Uveitis does, however, have a tendency to recur.

VACCINATION

A procedure to protect against specific infections by producing antibodies (or an immune response of the cells) against the causative virus or bacteria. It is also known as immunization. The vaccine is usually given by injection but oral vaccination, for example with the Sabin attenuated polio virus, may also be given. For viral diseases such as poliomyelitis, measles, mumps and influenza the vaccine consists of an inactivated virus or a live non-pathogenic virus (does not cause disease). Other viral diseases for which vaccines are available include hepatitis B, yellow fever and rabies, but, as yet, not human immunodeficiency virus (HIV, the cause of AIDS). Vaccines for bacterial infections such as whooping cough (pertussis), diphtheria, tetanus and pneumococcus consist of inactivated toxin (killed bacteria) or, for tuberculosis, a non-pathogenic strain of tubercle bacilli (BCG vaccine).

The side-effects of most vaccines are trivial, except for whooping cough vaccine which has on rare occassions been associated with brain damage. However, it is generally thought that the slight risks of this vaccine are outweighed by the benefits in preventing death and long-term complications from whooping cough. In the United Kingdom vaccination against diphtheria, polio, whooping cough, mumps, rubella (German measles), measles and tetanus are routinely performed during childhood and BCG vaccination during adolescence. Hepatitis B, influenza and pneumococcal vaccines are reserved for high-risk groups such as doctors and nurses working in dialysis units (hepatitis B), the elderly (influenza) and children (pneumococcus).

Second or subsequent doses (boosters) may be required several years after the first dose in order to ensure immunity, since the initial antibody level induced by the original vaccination may fall.

Travellers who are visiting foreign countries, especially under-developed ones, should check with their doctor or travel agent to establish whether vaccinations for diseases such as yellow fever, malaria, cholera, and typhoid are necessary or recommended.

VAGOTOMY

Cutting the vagus nerve or its branches; this is the nerve which controls the amount of acid that the stomach produces. Vagotomy is now rarely performed and is reserved for cases of duodenal ulcer that do not respond to treatment with powerful antacids or so-called H_2 receptor antagonist drugs such as cimetidine or ranitidine. If these fail to control the ulcer, a vagotomy is performed to reduce acid production by dividing the vagus nerve in the abdomen.

VALVULAR DISEASE

The common term used to describe diseases of the valves of the heart: the valves on the left side are called mitral and aortic, and those on the right tricuspid and pulmonary. The abnormalities that result from these diseases may be congenital or acquired. The commonest causes of valvular disease are rheumatic fever, endocarditis (inflammation of the lining of the heart) or a complication of a heart attack. Diagnosis involves physical examination, echocardiography (ECG), cardiac catheterization and angiography. Combined valve lesions are not uncommon.

Previous rheumatic fever is the commonest cause of narrowing of the mitral valve (mitral stenosis, qv), which develops gradually and often first becomes apparent months or years after the acute illness. Eventually, when the valve becomes very tight, the condition gives rise to increased pressure in the pulmonary circulation, decreased cardiac output and eventually to right-sided heart failure. A leaky mitral valve (mitral incompetence, qv)

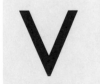

gives rise to left-sided heart failure. A tight aortic valve (aortic stenosis, qv) gives rise to an increase in the muscle bulk of the left ventricle and eventually to left-sided failure. Aortic incompetence also leads to failure of the left ventricle. Stenosis of the tricuspid valve is rare, whereas incompetence is frequently seen and is due to endocarditis in intravenous drug abusers. Pulmonary incompetence is usually due to raised pressure in the blood vessels of the lung. Pulmonary stenosis is rare.

VARICOCOELE

A collection of dilated (or varicosed) veins around the testis; it is commoner on the left side. The causes of varicocoele are similar to those responsible for variscose veins (qv) elsewhere in the body. In very rare cases a varicocoele may develop when drainage from the testicular veins into the renal veins is blocked by a growth in the kidney.

Varicocoele may cause a sensation of heaviness, and is said to be associated with lowered fertility; there is no evidence that treatment improves fertility. The scrotum is described as feeling like a 'bag of worms' when the patient stands, but on lying down the feeling disappears.

A varicocoele does not usually require treatment unless it becomes large and uncomfortable; surgical removal may then be considered.

VARICOSE VEIN

A dilated, tortuous vein, usually in the leg. Varicose veins are part of the price paid by humans for their erect posture; animals do not suffer from them.

In humans blood is pumped from the leg to the heart by the muscles of the calf. A series of valves prevents the blood, under the influence of gravity, from flowing in the opposite direction. Any weakness of these valves (which is usually congenital) gives rise to back pressure within the veins of the leg which eventually become varicose. The main veins affected are those of the calf, back of the knee and thigh.

Aching in the leg and bleeding from prominent varicose veins may occur. Treatment, in mild cases, is by injection sclerotherapy (injecting a substance to block the vein). In more severe cases ligation of the upper end of the long saphenous vein (Trendelenberg's operation), together with 'stripping', is necessary.

VASCULITIS

Inflammation of blood vessels. There are many causes of vasculitis, including bacterial and viral infection, drugs, autoimmune disease and connective tissue disorders (such as systemic lupus erythematosus). The actual mechanism by which vasculitis occurs is unknown, but it is thought that antigens and antibodies deposited in the blood vessel wall induce an inflammatory reaction. The symptoms of vasculitis depend on the severity of damage to the vessel wall and on the size of the blood vessels affected and the organ supplied. When those in the skin are affected a haemorrhagic rash (with bleeding into skin nodules), or purpura is seen. Other organs commonly affected are the kidneys, lungs, heart, and brain.

Treatment depends upon the underlying cause.

VASECTOMY

see *Sterilization*

VD

see *Sexually transmitted disease*

VENEPUNCTURE

The puncture of a vein. This is most commonly undertaken to withdraw small amounts of blood for laboratory analysis, but is also necessary for the withdrawal of larger amounts in blood donation, or rarely as a treatment for certain conditions (such as polycythaemia). Intravenous therapy with drugs and fluids requires venepuncture, as do several procedures used in investigation (pulmonary artery pressure monitoring, for example) or treatment (temporary cardiac pacemaker insertion). It is common practice for sampling and intravenous therapy to take place in the lower arm, although any site where veins are readily accessible may be used in venepuncture.

VENEREAL DISEASE

see *Sexually transmitted disease*

VENESECTION

The removal of at least $\frac{1}{2}$ litre (1 pint) of blood to reduce the blood volume. It is commonly used as a treatment for polycythaemia (qv). Venesection is also used as a treatment in iron overload and haemochromatosis (qv). It is performed with the patient lying flat on a couch; this is to avoid fainting due to low blood pressure. The skin of the elbow is anaesthetized and a large needle is inserted to draw out the blood, which drains into a plastic bag via a tube attached to the needle. It is usual for the patient to take a drink at the end of the procedure, and to remain lying down for at least fifteen minutes in order to allow the volume of blood to readjust.

VENOGRAPHY

see *Phlebography*

VENO-OCCLUSIVE LIVER DISEASE

Obliteration of the small veins that drain the liver as a result of the formation of scar tissue around their walls. The condition was originally found in children from the Caribbean, Israel and India who had ingested plant alkaloids used in the preparation of traditional herbal treatments (bush teas). It may also occur after bone marrow transplantation; the cause is uncertain in these cases. Features include enlargement of the liver; ascites (fluid in the abdominal cavity) and cirrhosis may also develop. There is no specific treatment.

VENTILATOR

A mechanical device for artificial respiration, or ventilation, used when a patient cannot breathe effectively on his or her own. In positive pressure ventilation, an endotracheal tube is placed in the windpipe and is connected to the ventilator by more tubing which delivers oxygen and removes expired gas. A bellows provides pressure to inflate the lungs. If ventilation is to be continued for more than 48 hours, a tracheostomy (qv) is usually necessary. A different form of mechanical artificial respiration is used if swallowing is unimpaired.

VENTOUSE

A piece of obstetric equipment used as an alternative to forceps to deliver the baby's head in cases of spontaneous delivery failing to occur. It consists of a metal cup attached by tubing to a vacuum pump. The cup is applied to the baby's scalp, and the pump is then used to create a carefully controlled vacuum, which sucks in the scalp. The cup is then pulled to ease the baby's head through the birth canal. The procedure may be less traumatic than forceps. The suction produces a lump on the baby's scalp, but this subsides after a few days.

VENTRICULAR FIBRILLATION

Chaotic twitching of the heart muscle of the ventricular wall. This phenomenon renders contraction of the ventricles (the lower chambers of the heart) impossible and causes the circulation to cease. The affected individual immediately loses consciousness and will die unless resuscitated.

The two major causes of ventricular fibrillation are ischaemia and heart block. Ischaemia means a lack of oxygenated blood; in the heart this implies coronary artery disease. When someone suffers a coronary blockage or thrombosis, then ventricular fibrillation is the usual mechanism of death. Heart block is when the electrical impulse which initiates ventricular contraction fails to pass from the atria (upper chambers) to the ventricles. Ventricular contraction then slows and this greatly increases the risk of ventricular fibrillation.

Ventricular fibrillation may also occur in hypothermia, prolapse of the mitral valve in the heart, and as a result of an overdose with one of the pherothiazine tranquillizers.

The treatment consists of cardiopulmonary resuscitation and restoring normal cardiac contraction by an externally applied electric shock.

VENTRICULAR SEPTAL DEFECT (VSD)

A congenital hole in the muscular wall or septum that divides the two lower chambers of the heart (the right and left ventricles) from each other. VSDs account for about 8 per cent of congenital heart disease. Small defects (maladie de Roger) do not usually produce symptoms, but a typical murmur may be heard. The hole often closes spontaneously in childhood.

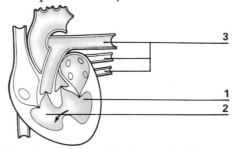

With each contraction of the heart, blood flows through the ventricular septal defect from the high-pressure left ventricle (**1**). This increases the pressure in the right ventricle (**2**) and in the pulmonary vessels (**3**), which take the blood to the lungs.

Large defects may cause problems as a result of the increased flow to the lungs, via the right ventricle, producing structural changes in the pulmonary vessels. This in turn produces an increase in pulmonary resistance, pulmonary venous pressure and right ventricular pressure. Eventually the back pressure may rise to a level above that of the left ventricle, causing a reversal of the flow: unoxygenated blood flows into the left side of the heart from the right, producing cyanosis. Surgery is, therefore, necessary to prevent this complication. Success rates are high.

VERRUCA

A viral infection of the sole of the foot which, unlike the common type of wart affecting the fingers, is forced into the skin due to the effects of constant pressure. Sometimes the lesions are single or alternatively there may be many which coalesce. The treatment is with keratolytic agents, which destroy the dead outer layer of skin where the virus resides. These agents may be applied in the form of a cream under an adhesive dressing or by soaking the affected area in the liquid; the resulting dead skin should be removed by abrasion before re-application of the keratolytic agent. Alternatively, if the lesions are few, surgical removal or destruction by freezing with liquid nitrogen may be successful.

VERSION

Obstetric term to describe the manual manipulation of a fetus to change the way it lies within the uterus (womb) of the mother. In late pregnancy the head of the fetus normally comes to lie within the mother's pelvis. Occasionally, though, the buttocks (breech presentation) or other parts of the fetal body engage in the pelvis, which can make subsequent labour difficult. Breech presentation is common in early pregnancy, but most babies turn spontaneously well before delivery. If the baby is still in breech presentation in late pregnancy, it may be deemed necessary to perform version to make labour easier and safer. External version is performed by manual manipulation of the fetus through the mother's abdominal wall. In effect, the baby is turned head over heels. No anaesthesia is required. Version is successful in at least 80 per cent of cases. Complications are rare, but include induction of premature labour, placental haemorrhage and twisting of the cord around one of the fetal limbs. As a precaution therefore, the fetal heart rate and rhythm are checked during and after version.

VERTIGO

see *Ménière's disease*

VESICLE

A small (less than 0.5 cm/$\frac{1}{5}$ in) blister. Certain skin disorders are characterized by the appearance of vesicles and include herpes simplex (qv), dermatitis herpetiformis and certain forms of hand eczema (see *Dermatitis*).

VIRILISM

Masculinization of women due to the overproduction of androgens (male sex hormones) from either the ovary or adrenal gland, or as a complication of drug administration. The main features are the development of hair in the male pattern of distribution, enlargement of the clitoris and loss of the normal female menstrual cycle, as well as frontal balding and deepening of the voice.

Ovarian causes include the polycystic ovary syndrome, in which too many weakly androgenic steroids are produced instead of the normal female hormone oestrogen; these become converted to the powerful androgen testosterone in the skin, lung and liver. Masculinizing tumours of the ovary also occur; these are usually benign.

Tumours of the adrenal glands may also cause the overproduction of androgens or androgen precursors. There are several congenital disorders of adrenal metabolism which result in increased androgen production; these conditions usually become apparent early in life. Treatment involves the giving of female sex hormones.

Some drugs can cause virilism. Phenytoin, used in the treatment of epilepsy, is one such; progestins, androgens and vitamin-hormonal compounds (anabolic steroids) are others.

VIRUS

Viruses are microscopic life forms responsible for a wide range of infections, ranging from ones without symptoms to the fatal. They contain molecular cores of either RNA (ribonucleic acid) or DNA (deoxyribose nucleic acid) but not both, unlike bacteria. The core is enclosed within a shell (capsid) and in some cases an outer membrane (envelope). Viruses can only grow and multiply within the cells of a host organism. The capsid and envelope allow the virus to attach to and then penetrate the host cell. Therein the RNA or DNA, the genetic blueprints for all life forms, causes the host cell to manufacture the proteins and nucleic acids necessary for the multiplication of the virus.

This may lead to the death of the infected cell and release of the virus, as in influenza, for example. In other infections the virus lies dormant in the cell and may re-activate on later occasions, as with herpes zoster, which causes shingles, or herpes simplex which causes facial cold sores. If the genetic material of the virus is incorporated into the DNA of the host cell, then malignant transformation may take place: for example, the Epstein Barr virus is implicated in the development of Burkitt's lymphoma.

VITAMIN B₁

see *Thiamine*

VITAMINS

A group of unrelated organic compounds essential for normal health. A minimum quantity is required in a diet to prevent deficiency disorders, but when taken in excess some vitamins (such as A and D) are harmful. Vitamins A, D, E, and K are all fat-soluble and may not be absorbed in patients with malabsorption syndromes.

Vitamin A (retinol) deficiency produces night blindness and dryness of the conjunctiva (the membrane covering the front of the eye).

Vitamin B complex is a mixture of essential substances, many of which are found in cereals. Thiamine (vitamin B₁) deficiency is seen mainly in alcoholics and produces beriberi (qv) and Wernicke's encephalopathy (qv). Rivoflavin (vitamin B₂) deficiency is usually mild and produces fissuring at the corners of the mouth (angular stomatitis). Niacin (vitamin B₃ — see *Nicotinic acid*) deficiency is uncommon but produces the skin disease pellagra. Pyridoxine (vitamin B₆) deficiency causes anaemia (qv) and neuropathy (qv). Vitamin B₁₂ (cyanocobalamin) deficiency can cause pernicious anaemia, a form of sensory neuropathy, and damage to the spinal cord. Deficiency as distinct from pernicious anaemia is usually due to gastro-intestinal disease. Other components in the vitamin B complex are biotin and pantothenic acid.

Vitamin C (ascorbic acid) is found in fresh fruit and vegetables. Deficiency produces scurvy. Claims that large doses of vitamin C protect against viral infections are unproven.

Vitamin D (cholecalciferol) is important in the normal growth and maintenance of bone. Deficiency produces rickets (qv) in children, and osteomalacia (qv) in adults. Some Vitamin D is manufactured in skin exposed to sunlight.

Vitamin E (tocopherol) deficiency is typically seen in low birth weight babies and adults with malabsorption syndromes who can develop a haemolytic anaemia.

Vitamin K is required for the manufacture of several blood clotting pro-

VITAMINS AND THEIR FUNCTIONS

Vitamin	Good sources	Needed for	Deficiency	Recommended daily intake Adults	Children (0–4 year)
A (retinol)	Carrots, tomatoes, spinach, apricots, liver, kidneys, oily fish, egg yolks, cheese, butter, milk	Healthy skin, bones, teeth and mucous membranes; night vision	Night blindness, conjunctival dryness, poor growth	1000 micrograms. Pregnant and breast-feeding women: 1200	500 micrograms
B_1 (thiamine)			Beriberi, Wernicke's encephalopathy	1.4 milligrams Pregnant and breast-feeding women: 2	0.7 milligrams
B_2 (riboflavin)		Carbohydrate metabolism	Cracked lips, fissures at corners of mouth	1.6 milligrams. Pregnant and breast-feeding women: 2	0.8 milligrams
B_3 (niacin)	Wholemeal bread and flour, yeast extract, cereals, milk, eggs, meat, vegetables, fresh liver		Pellagra, irritability, depression	18 milligrams. Pregnant and breast-feeding women: 21	9 milligrams
B_6 (pyridoxine)		Protein Metabolism	Anaemia; Neuropathy, insomnia	2.2 milligrams. Pregnant and breast-feeding women: 3	1 milligram
B_{12} (cyanocobal amin)		Red blood cell formation	Pernicious anaemia, neuropathy, spinal cord damage	3 micrograms. Pregnant and breast-feeding women: 3–5	3 micrograms
C (ascorbic acid)	Fresh fruit and vegetables	Healthy bones, teeth, connective tissue and red blood cell formation	Scurvy	30 milligrams. Pregnant and breast-feeding women: 50	20 milligrams
D (cholecalciferol)	Margarine, milk, butter, egg yolks, oily fish, sunlight	Absorption of calcium and phosphorous	Rickets, osteomalacia	2.5 micrograms. Pregnant and breast-feeding women: 10	10 micrograms
E (tocopherol)	Milk, egg yolk, cereals, green vegetables, nuts, liver	Wound healing	No clearly defined deficiency state	15 milligrams	5 milligrams
K	Green vegetables, nuts. Also synthesized by bacteria in the human gut	Blood clotting	Bleeding tendency	Deficiency unlikely	—

teins. Deficiency produces a bleeding tendency (see *Anticoagulants*).

A diet containing milk, eggs, butter, cheese, fat, fish, wholemeal bread, and fresh vegetables and fruit should provide vitamins in sufficient quantities for the average person. Meat and fish are not vital to a vitamin-adequate diet. However, vegans should be aware that B_{12} is found in very few vegetable sources; seaweed and some yeasts only. Elderly people do not absorb either minerals or vitamins as efficiently as younger people and so need to ensure that they have a good, nourishing diet and that they eat enough. Pregnant women and young children have special vitamin requirements.

VITILIGO

A skin condition characterized by white patches on the skin which are completely devoid of pigment. It is due to a total absence of cells called melanocytes in the affected areas. Melanocytes are the cells responsible for producing melanin, the skin pigment which gives a tan.

Other members of a family may be affected in about 30 per cent of cases. The depigmented patches often enlarge slowly during life so that in time nearly all the skin becomes white.

Most people with vitiligo are healthy but sometimes the condition is seen in patients with thyroid disease, diabetes (mellitus), Addison's disease and pernicious anaemia.

VOLVULUS

A twist in the bowel which results in obstruction at the base of the twist and dilatation of the trapped loop.

Occasionally a volvulus affects the ileocaecal region (the lower part of the small intestine, or the first part of the

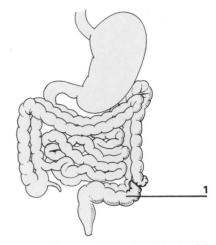

Volvulus commonly occurs in the sigmoid colon **(1)** at the lower end of the large intestine when the bowel is large, has a narrow base and is overloaded with faeces as a result of constipation.

large), and rarely the stomach. It can occasionally be deflated and untwisted by passing a rubber tube into the trapped loop, using a sigmoidoscope. If this fails, an urgent operation is needed to untwist the bowel and prevent gangrene and perforation (see *Peritonitis*). It is usual to anchor the bowel or remove the redundant loop to prevent a recurrence.

VOMITING

The forceful ejection of gastric contents, usually preceded or accompanied by nausea. It is a common symptom and occurs in many gastro-intestinal disorders. It may also be a symptom of non-gastro-intestinal conditions including infections, metabolic disturbances, migraine, travel sickness, pregnancy, heart attack, drug toxicity, an increase in pressure within the skull (intracranial pressure) and certain psychological disorders. Early morning vomiting is characteristic of pregnancy, alcoholism, and metabolic disorders such as those seen in kidney failure.

Peptic ulcers can induce vomiting soon after eating but sometimes this is delayed for an hour or more. Vomiting associated with psychological problems (for example, bulimia nervosa) usually occurs during or soon after a meal. Vomiting which is delayed after eating commonly accompanies gallbladder disease and intestinal obstruction or ileus. Projectile vomiting, the forceful ejection of vomit, is often seen in pyloric stenosis and in patients with raised intracranial pressure (as a result of intracranial haemorrhage or brain tumour, for example).

The cause of the vomiting can sometimes be deduced on inspection of the vomit. Undigested food suggests that there may be something preventing food from leaving the stomach. If intestinal obstruction or ileus is the cause the vomit may smell very offensive. If blood is present (haematemesis) medical attention should be urgently sought as life-threatening blood loss can follow.

WART

An extremely common form of viral skin infection usually affecting the fingers, although any body site may be involved. Warts are a common infection in children but, because the body frequently develops immunity to the virus, they usually clear up spontaneously. Certain individuals seem to have more difficulty than others in resisting wart-virus infection (for example, immunosuppressed patients and those with atopic dermatitis) and may require active treatment.

Treatment in mild cases may consist of a locally applied chemical which is capable of digesting the outer skin layer (the stratum corneum) in which the virus resides; the agent is usually applied daily, and the dead tissue is carefully abraded between applications. Alternatively the affected skin may be destroyed either by surgery or by the application of extreme cold in

the form of liquid nitrogen, which leads to tissue death and replacement by normal skin; these types of destructive therapy may sometimes leave scars.

Genital warts are sexually transmissible and are treated with an anti-viral compound under the direction of a specialist physician. There appears to be some statistical association between the presence of cervical warts (in the neck of the womb), which follow sexual intercourse with a man with penile warts, and the development of cervical cancer.

WERNICKE'S ENCEPHALOPATHY

A form of brain damage associated with alcoholism and caused by vitamin B₁ deficiency. The sufferer has difficulty in concentrating and responds to questions slowly. Symptoms include paralysis of the muscles controlling the movements of the eye, double vision and rapid movements of the eye from side to side (nystagmus). Movement and balance may be abnormal. Usually the condition is associated with the Korsakoff syndrome (a severe defect of recent memory in which the sufferer is unable to record and recall new information) and often with polyneuropathy (weakness and sensory loss in the extremities). There is usually a marked improvement after treatment with the vitamin thiamine.

WHITLOW

Acute inflammation of the nail fold due to infection with the herpes simplex virus. The inflammation and intact blisters characteristic of the condition are very painful.

Treatment is with acyclovir, an antiviral agent, but in many cases a

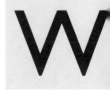

whitlow will clear up spontaneously.

The term is also sometimes used as an alternative to paronychia, indicating a small staphylococcal abscess at the edge of a nail.

WHOOPING COUGH

A highly infectious disease caused by the airborne bacterium *Bordetella pertussis*; known medically as pertussis. It especially affects the upper respiratory tract in infants under the age of 1 year. A child has no immunity as this is not conferred via the mother's antibodies, hence early vaccination is required.

There are three distinct stages to whooping cough:

- Catarrhal, when there is congestion of the nose and eyes, with a fever and dry persistent cough; ulcers may develop on the floor of the mouth
- Paroxysmal, when a whooplike cough is produced as the respiratory tract goes into spasm
- Recovery stage

The incubation period is 8–18 days. The child should be segregated for six weeks. Initial treatment is with antibiotics, primarily to cut down infectivity. The best treatment is prevention, by appropriate vaccination. Whooping cough vaccination received a set-back a few years ago when it was suspected that it might be associated with brain damage in a very small percentage of children who developed an encephalopathy (qv) or epilepsy. However, the danger is much less than the risk of getting whooping cough, which can be fatal, and vaccination is recommended for all healthy children.

WILM'S TUMOUR

The commonest kidney malignancy in childhood; also known as nephroblastoma. The tumour may be present at birth, and is usually recognized before the age of 5 years. The principal symptoms are fever, abdominal pain and swelling, and sometimes blood in the urine (haematuria). The tumour may be felt as a lump on one side of the abdomen. Diagnosis is by ultrasound and various X-ray procedures, which are also used to assess how far the malignancy has spread. Tumour deposits may occur in the lung, liver and bones. In rare cases both kidneys are involved.

Treatment depends on the degree of spread, and may include surgical removal of the tumour and kidney, chemotherapy and radiotherapy. The cure rate is over 90 per cent if the tumour is caught in the early stages.

WILSON'S DISEASE

An inherited (autosomal recessive) abnormality of copper metabolism, resulting from a deficiency in the blood of the protein which transports copper, called caeruloplasmin. In Wilson's disease, copper is deposited abnormally in the body tissues and causes damage to the brain, liver and kidney. The condition may become apparent in infancy when liver problems such as jaundice and cirrhosis are prominent, but may not be noticed until late childhood or adult life when neurological symptoms somewhat similar to those of Parkinson's disease become apparent. Severe dysarthria (slurred speech) is common. A characeristic finding and indication of Wilson's disease is a brown ring of copper laid down around the cornea of the eye (a Kayser-Fleischer ring).

Treatment with penicillamine is usually effective if given early enough, but if liver damage is severe the condition is potentially fatal and liver transplantation may be the only hope for the patient.

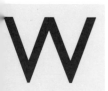

WISDOM TEETH

Wisdom teeth, or the third molars, are the last teeth of the permanent dentition to erupt into the dental arch. They usually appear after the age of 18 years. Depending on their position and size relative to the dental arch, they may cause problems during their eruption. If there is not enough room, pain is caused by the wisdom tooth pressing on the tooth in front. Sometimes there is space for the wisdom tooth to erupt only partially, causing a small flap of the overlying gum to be raised. This can be caught and rubbed against by the teeth, causing pain; this condition is known as pericoronitis. Both problems can be solved by removing the wisdom teeth, which can be performed either under local or general anaesthetic.

Very occasionally (in about 2 per cent of the population) the wisdom teeth may be absent from birth.

WOOLF-PARKINSON-WHITE SYNDROME

A congenital disorder in which an additional, and shorter, conducting pathway conducts the beat of the heart from atrium (upper chamber) to ventricle (lower chamber) faster than by the normal atriaventricular route (the so-called conducting bundle of His). The ventricle is therefore excited slightly before the normal impulse arrives, and the ventricular beat is thus a combination produced by the two impulses at slightly differing times. Diagnosis is by means of an electrocardiogram (ECG), which can detect the pattern of the two impulses.

It is also possible for impulses sometimes to travel backwards up the abnormal pathway to the atrium, creating a 'short circuit'. This may lead to arrhythmias, particularly paroxysmal tachycardia, atrial flutter and atrial fibrillation.

Treatment is mainly with drugs (such as amiodarone) or, rarely, surgery to divide the abnormal pathway.

WORMS

Worm infections are common worldwide, especially in tropical countries where there is poor hygiene. Children are particularly at risk. The severity of symptoms is related to the number of worms carried and a large proportion of infections pass unrecognized.

The two main types of parasitic worm infecting humans are roundworms and flatworms. Common roundworm infections in temperate climates, such as Britain's, are threadworms and toxocara (qv). Threadworms are white, about 1cm ($\frac{1}{2}$ in) long, and inhabit the large intestine. They emerge at night to lay eggs at the edge of the anus. The main symptom is itching (pruritus). Scratching leads to the transmission of eggs on contaminated fingers. Infection is harmless. Toxocara is a parasite of dogs which is transmitted by contact with urine or faeces, or contaminated soil. An infected child may suffer damage to the eyes, brain and lungs. Tropical roundworms include hookworms (which penetrate the skin and eventually settle in the intestine, where they suck blood and may produce anaemia and ascaris.

Flatworms include tapeworms (acquired from infected meat) and various types of fluke. The tropical blood fluke (bilharzia) is commonest, and is acquired by bathing in water contaminated by parasite-containing snails.

Drug treatment is available for most infections, but prevention is more important. Hygiene and control of animal hosts and vectors (animal or

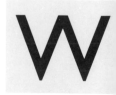

insect carriers such as mosquitoes) are useful measures.

XANTHOMA

A localized collection of fatty tissue. Xanthomas may occur almost anywhere in the body but are found most frequently in or just beneath the skin and around the tendons. They are usually signalled by yellow streaks round the eyelids (xanthelasmas — deposition of fatty tissue). As an isolated phenomenon, xanthoma (lipoma, as it is called in these circumstances) is entirely innocent and is usually left alone unless surgical removal is necessary because of its size. However, when xanthomas are multiple or they appear rapidly, then they require further investigation to measure the levels of cholesterol and lipoproteins in the blood. Certain types of elevation in the circulating fats, and especially high blood cholesterol, are associated with certain xanthomas (for example, those that appear in the creases of the palm of the hand). They are also associated with an increased risk of heart attack or pancreatitis. Treatment of these xanthomas involves drugs to lower the level of cholesterol in the blood.

XENOGRAFT

The transplantation of a tissue graft between animals of different species. Transplantations of whole organs (kidneys, for example) from animals to man have not been successful because of the strong immune response elicited and the inability to prevent rejection of the transplanted organ. Nevertheless, animal tissues (such as pig pericardium, the fibrous membrane which surrounds the heart) have been widely used to produce artificial heart valves with less risk of thrombo-

embolism than is produced by valves made of metal or plastics.

XERODERMA PIGMENTOSUM

A rare inherited disorder in which the skin is extremely sensitive to the effects of sunlight. In those affected, even young children, the skin takes on the appearance of the elderly, sun-damaged type of skin seen in white races in the tropics. This is caused by an enzyme deficiency that seems to prevent the normal repair of sun-exposed skin. The main danger of the condition is the development of sun-induced skin cancers at an early age.

Treatment is entirely dependent upon reducing exposure to sunshine and genetic counselling where appropriate in the hope of preventing the birth of further affected children.

X-RAY

Electromagnetic radiation of very short wavelength generated by a high-velocity stream of electrons striking a metal target (often tungsten). A spectrum of X-rays of different wavelengths is produced.

Imaging of parts of the body by means of X-ray is possible because water-containing soft tissue, fat, gas, and bone calcium obstruct X-ray transmission to different degrees, some appearing on the X-ray as translucent and others opaque. Thus a contrast is produced between adjacent tissues of different composition. X-ray images transmitted through the body are recorded by one of the following methods:
- X-ray film
- a phosphor screen linked to an image intensifier and TV camera
- a selenium screen from which data is read and stored in digital form

- arrays of xenon-containing ionization chambers in computed tomography (CT) scanners

It is usual to screen other parts of the body, particularly the ovaries in women and the testes in men, in order to confine the radiation to the area being examined and avoid the risk of mutation in germ cells. X-rays should be avoided in early pregnancy, unless absolutely essential, because of the risk of teratogenesis (qv).

SEE ALSO *Arteriography, Barium enema/meal, Cholecystography, Magnetic resonance imaging, Phlebography, Radiotherapy, Tomography, Urography*

YAWS

A disease caused by the organism *Treponema pertenue*, which is similar to the one responsible for syphilis. Yaws, though, is not sexually transmitted. Common in Central America, Africa and the West Indies, it is a mild disease when it occurs in otherwise healthy people. Yaws begins as a scaly eruption about the legs and trunk in which small nodules grow, sometimes to several centimetres in diameter A yellow crust forms over the surface of the nodules, which in unhealthy people may develop into deep ulcers. Treatment is with penicillin.

Yaws is of particular concern to obstetricians because pregnant women who have had the disease give a positive result when their blood is tested for syphilis. Syphilis is a serious infection, especially in pregnancy, because it can harm the fetus (yaws will not). However, there is no test that can conclusively differentiate between yaws and syphilis. For this reason, all pregnant women who have a positive blood test for syphilis are treated with penicillin even if it is more likely that the positive test is due to a yaws infection.

YELLOW FEVER

An epidemic tropical viral haemorrhagic (bleeding) disease, occurring mainly in West Africa and South America. The virus is transmitted to humans by mosquito. The incubation period is 3—6 days. The illness begins with the sudden onset of fever, rigors, headache and backache; prostration, nausea and vomiting develop; and bleeding into the skin and from the gums and intestines occurs. When the infection is severe, death usually occurs within one week. Jaundice may occur but is more usual in patients who are convalescing. There is no treatment. Vaccination with an attenuated strain of the virus provides immunity.

ZOLLINGER-ELLISON SYNDROME

A rare disorder in which an excess of the hormone gastrin is produced by a tumour of the pancreas (occasionally the tumour is in the bowel wall). The tumour may be benign or malignant. The high concentrations of gastrin stimulate the stomach to over-produce acid, which results in severe peptic ulceration. The over-production of gastric acid can be controlled with drugs (particularly omeprazole), and all the symptoms can be relieved. Where possible, the tumour is removed surgically. Very rarely the syndrome may be associated with the over-production of other hormones by other glands.

ZOONOSIS

Zoonoses are infections which are transmitted from animals to humans. Examples of zoonoses include infection with salmonella (qv), anthrax (qv) and Q fever (qv).

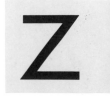